Industrial Environmental Health

THE WORKER AND THE COMMUNITY

Second Edition

ENVIRONMENTAL SCIENCES

An Interdisciplinary Monograph Series

Editors: Douglas H. K. Lee, E. Wendell Hewson, and Daniel Okun

A complete list of titles in this series appears at the end of this volume.

Industrial Environmental Health

THE WORKER AND THE COMMUNITY

Second Edition

Sponsored by Industrial Health Foundation, Inc.
Pittsburgh, Pennsylvania

EDITED BY

LESTER V. CRALLEY AND PATRICK R. ATKINS

Department of Health and Environment
Aluminum Company of America
Pittsburgh, Pennsylvania

ASSOCIATE EDITORS

Lewis J. Cralley
Formerly
Department of Health, Education and Welfare
Public Health Service
Health Services and Mental Health Administration
National Institute of Occupational Safety and Health
Cincinnati, Ohio

George D. Clayton
George D. Clayton and Associates
Southfield, Michigan

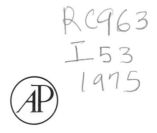

ACADEMIC PRESS   *New York   San Francisco   London   1975*
A Subsidiary of Harcourt Brace Jovanovich, Publishers

ACADEMIC PRESS, INC.
111 Fifth Avenue, New York, New York 10003

United Kingdom Edition published by
ACADEMIC PRESS, INC. (LONDON) LTD.
24/28 Oval Road, London NW1

Library of Congress Cataloging in Publication Data
Main entry under title:

Industrial environmental health.

    (Environmental sciences series)
    "Sponsored by Industrial Health Foundation, inc."
    Includes bibliographical references and index.
    1.   Industrial hygiene.   I.   Cralley, Lester Vincent,
(date)   ed.   II.   Atkins, Patrick R., ed.   III.   Industrial Health Foundation.   IV.   Series: Environmental sciences.   [DNLM: 1.   Environmental health.
2.   Industrial medicine.   WA400 I41]
RC963.I53 1975   613.6'2   75-1228
ISBN 0−12−195802−7

Contents

Epidemiologic Studies of Occupational Diseases

Howard E. Ayer

Toxicology

Emil A. Pfitzer

Noise

Paul L. Michael

Nonionizing Radiation

David H. Sliney and David L. Conover

Ionizing Radiation

McDonald E. Wrenn and Harry F. Schulte

Work in Hot Environments: Threshold Limit Values and Proposed Standards

Bruce A. Hertig

Evaluation of Chemical Hazards in the Environment

Robert G. Keenan and Richard R. Keenan

Hazard Evaluation and Control

Robert D. Soule

Personal Protective Devices

William A. Burgess and Bruce J. Held

The Off-Job Environmental Health Stress
as Related to the Workplace

Lester V. Cralley and Lewis J. Cralley

Impact of Governmental Environmental Regulations
upon Industrial Activities

Patrick R. Atkins

List of Contributors

Numbers in parentheses indicate the pages on which the authors' contributions begin.

PATRICK R. ATKINS, Environmental Health Services, Aluminum Company of America, Pittsburgh, Pennsylvania (330)

HOWARD E. AYER, Department of Environmental Health, Kettering Laboratory, University of Cincinnati, Cincinnati, Ohio (1)

WILLIAM A. BURGESS, Department of Environmental Health Sciences, Harvard School of Public Health, Boston, Massachusetts (293)

DAVID L. CONOVER, NIOSH, Physical Agents Branch, Cincinnati, Ohio (157)

LESTER V. CRALLEY, Environmental Health Services, Aluminum Company of America, Pittsburgh, Pennsylvania (311)

LEWIS J. CRALLEY, Formerly, Department of Health, Education and Welfare, Public Health Service, Health Services and Mental Health Administration, National Institute of Occupational Safety and Health, Cincinnati, Ohio (311)

BRUCE J. HELD, Los Alamos Scientific Laboratory, University of California, Los Alamos, New Mexico (293)

BRUCE A. HERTIG, Laboratory for Ergonomics Research, University of Illinois at Urbana-Champaign, Urbana, Illinois (219)

RICHARD R. KEENAN, Laboratory Services, George D. Clayton and Associates, Southfield, Michigan (233)

ROBERT G. KEENAN, Laboratory Services, George D. Clayton and Associates, Southfield, Michigan (233)

PAUL L. MICHAEL, Environmental Acoustics Laboratory, The Pennsylvania State University, University Park, Pennsylvania (129)

EMIL A. PFITZER, Department of Experimental Pathology and Toxicology, Hoffmann-La Roche, Inc., Nutley, New Jersey (67)

HARRY F. SCHULTE, Industrial Hygiene Group, Los Alamos Scientific Laboratory, University of California, Los Alamos, New Mexico (179)

DAVID H. SLINEY, Laser-Microwave Division, U.S. Army Environmental Hygiene Agency, Department of the Army, Edgewood Arsenal, Maryland (157)

ROBERT D. SOULE, Laboratory Services, George D. Clayton and Associates, Southfield, Michigan (259)

McDONALD E. WRENN, Department of Environmental Medicine, New York University Medical Center, New York, New York (179)

Foreword

The first edition of "Industrial Environmental Health: The Worker and the Community" could scarcely have been more timely. Since its publication there has been a dramatic increase in emphasis in this entire field. New regulatory agencies have been established, numerous standards have issued from them, and previously existing authorities and both the public and private sectors have shown a keenly increased awareness of the subject.

It is fitting, then, that the editors have accepted the task of updating the material in the first edition, taking into account the changes and the progress from 1971–1973. A further indication of their determination to make this volume completely current is the addition of chapters on the Impact of Governmental Environmental Regulations upon Industrial Activities and on The Off-Job Environmental Health Stress as Related to the Workplace.

The original volume presented the best available information from experts in government, industry, and universities, with the objective of leading to a safer and more healthful environment for all. This edition continues this worthy goal.

Dr. Cralley and Dr. Atkins and their associate editors and contributors are to be congratulated for their willingness to devote so much time to the production of this much needed compilation.

Daniel C. Braun
President
Industrial Health Foundation
Pittsburgh, Pennsylvania

Preface

The main objective of this second edition of "Industrial Environmental Health: The Worker and The Community" is to present new information on the environmental health hazards of the workplace in a thoughtful and meaningful manner for all those actively working in this area. It covers the period 1971–1973, and is a continuation of the information presented in the first edition and in "Industrial Hygiene Highlights." It is important that there be no unnecessary delay in highlighting the newer developments that are so vital in planning research or in the evaluation and control of environmental stress situations. However, in a field so broad as this, it is only possible to condense individual research or surveys into a meaningful summary. The comprehensive coverage provides a basis for those needing a greater in-depth understanding.

We live in an era where environmental regulations are mandated by Congress. It is disturbing that in many instances the scientific community cannot agree on either the adequacy or interpretation of the data which must serve as a basis for establishing regulations. This, combined with a safety factor having a magnitude which is also controversial, must inevitably lead to regulations that are both under- or overprotective. It is therefore imperative that limiting values not be frozen if we are to meet the major needs of society in a priority rating system commensurate with our available resources. Industrial participation in the regulatory process is imperative.

A second objective of this new edition is to broaden the scope of environmental health hazards in the workplace to include the off-job stresses that may either be additive or present a response incompatible with the known hazards of the job. It is not surprising to find increasing scientific concern about the potential environmental health stress in the home and the community. Much of this concern is based upon limited knowledge of the effect of long-term, low-level exposures and inadequate information on the actual exposure patterns. Even though there is not sufficient data to assess the importance of this area, those concerned with the in-plant environmental health stresses must remain alerted to its potential.

Lester V. Cralley
Patrick R. Atkins

Epidemiologic Studies of
Occupational Diseases

HOWARD E. AYER

Epidemiologic studies of disease in working populations are necessary to establish levels at which contaminants in the occupational environment are not causing injury. Studies in other animal species, although valuable, cannot completely assure safety in humans. Epidemiologic studies of working populations are especially important because the majority of toxic materials produce effects that are not unique to the occupational contaminant. For example, there are any number of particulate and gaseous air contaminants which can produce adverse effects on the respiratory tract similar to those produced by cigarette smoke. For such materials, the effect of the contaminant can only be determined by comparisons among populations standardized for age and degree of cigarette smoking.

In a previous edition of this treatise, which covered principally the years from 1968 to 1970, it was suggested that there might be a considerable increase in the number of epidemiologic studies, with more sponsorship by both government and industry. Such an increase was not noted from 1971 to 1973, although it still appears possible that the number of such studies will be considerably increased in the near future. However, no firm prediction can be made at this time.

A wide range of studies is represented in this chapter. Each was selected because it covered a sample of a working population and examined the effects of the material to which the workers were exposed. In reviewing the studies, it is evident that there is still a useful place for the small team examining tens or scores of workers, as well as for the industrywide studies of many hundreds, or even thousands, of workers. Likewise, although some problems are best handled by a long-term prospective study, many studies are able to draw valid conclusions from retrospective data.

The scope of this chapter has been restricted to chemical contaminants; ionizing radiation and other physical hazards are discussed elsewhere in the volume. It has also been restricted to those papers available in English. Where a number of successive or related papers on a study have been published, sometimes only one may be cited. It is inevitable that some valuable studies have been missed because the particular journal was not available when the subject was covered.

It is to be hoped that more occupational medical and environmental staffs will be able to add to data gathered in the course of their operations to produce valid epidemiologic studies, and that they will then be permitted to publish their data. Some of the most valuable studies available have been conducted in single companies or even single facilities. Gathering the data needed to make sure that all potential chemical contaminants are being handled in such a way as not to create health problems will continue to require the cooperation of labor, industry, and government.

ACRYLAMIDE

Takahashi *et al.*[1] report a study of 15 workers exposed to acrylamide in a factory manufacturing paper-coating materials. Exposure durations were from 2 months to 8 years and, based on the author's description of operations, opportunities existed for both inhalation and skin absorption. Three of the five workers who had handled acrylamide for 6 or more years complained of dizziness and ataxic gait, and displayed abnormalities in their EEG examinations. Electromyography revealed slight changes in 7 of the 15 workers. Slight abnormalities of motor nerve function were found in 9 of 15 workers. Nerve conduction studies showed a number of abnormalities. In the electrophysiologic examinations, abnormalities were noted in each of the 15 workers, with the number of abnormalities per worker varying from one to six and length of exposure having little apparent effect.

Controls used at the beginning of the study were apparently only "dust masks" and rubber gloves, and these had not always been worn. After the neurologic examinations, enclosure and ventilation were provided at the melting pot, the filtration was automated, bathing after work and frequent clean work clothes were provided, and worker exposure time was shortened. The report stated that these countermeasures, along with medication, resulted in improvement of worker health. Unfortunately, because no measurements were made of environmental conditions, the authors were not able to ascertain whether the effects occurred at concentrations above or below 0.3 mg/m^3, which is the OSHA exposure limit[2] and the ACGIH TLV.*[3] Thus the findings cannot be used to judge whether the limit is adequate for worker health protection.

* American Conference of Governmental Industrial Hygienists, Threshold Limit Value.

ACRYLONITRILE

A work force of 576 acrylonitrile workers from five artificial fiber plants was studied by Sakurai and Kusumoto.[4] Each worker had been examined an average of 7.7 times in 10 years. The workers were grouped into two exposure categories; group I was less than 5 ppm acrylonitrile, group II less than 20 ppm. The groups were further subdivided by age and length of service.

The incidence of subjective complaints and abnormal values of some objective findings increased with length of service, but not with age. The incidences were also higher in group II than group I. From the results, the authors concluded that a mild injury of the liver seemed to be caused by acrylonitrile at the levels found. The ill effects were believed to be of a cumulative nature.

The authors express doubt as to the adequacy of the 1973 Threshold Limit Value of 5 ppm which was adopted by the American Conference of Governmental Industrial Hygienists (ACGIH).

ALDRIN

Bonderman *et al.*[5] studied 20 formulators with occupational exposure to Aldrin, 2,4-D and 2,4,5-T. The formulators were matched with paired controls, and grouped according to type of compound formulated. The adaptive response of some esterase enzymes were tested and compared statistically. In the red blood cells, the "adaptive" enzyme tributyrinase was elevated for Aldrin formulators and for the total exposed group (seven Aldrin formulators, six herbicide formulators, and seven warehousemen and maintenance workers exposed to lower levels of both types of material) as compared with their matched controls. There was no effect found on blood plasma tributyrinase activity. An effect of exposure length was not found, but the minimum acclimatization time was not established. The group differences in enzyme levels were in the Aldrin formulators rather than the other groups. The level of insecticide (Aldrin) residue in the blood was correlated with cholinesterase levels. Unlike the study reported in a previous volume,[6] no symptoms were noted in the workers, and, in fact, the authors state: "In spite of the potential high exposures, the plant has experienced few job-related health incidences during its history" (over 20 years).

ARSENIC

Tarrant and Allard[7] reported on a study of three six-man U.S. Forest Service tree-thinning crews in north-central Washington. The men used cacodylic acid (dimethylarsenic acid) or monosodium methanearsonate with injection hatchets, a hack-squirt method, or an injector tool. The study was carried out over 9 weeks, and it compared exposures to workers who applied the two arsenical silvicides by two primary methods (injection hatchet and hack-squirt). Urine samples of Monday morning and Friday afternoon were analyzed for arsenic to determine absorption. Higher urine arsenic values for exposed workers were invariably found on Friday, and 14 of 15 workers exceeded the manufacturer's recommended limit of 0.3 ppm. The urine arsenics were low again on Monday, although there appeared to be an upward trend of Monday concentrations. There was substantially more arsenic absorption of both chemicals by workers using the injection hatchet, but differences neither between chemicals nor between application methods were statistically significant at the 5% probability level.

Wagner and Weswig[8] also monitored a crew of five forest workers applying cacodylic acid by the "hack and squirt" method. Careful crew supervision, education, and use of protective equipment were believed responsible for the fact that no worker exceeded the 0.3 ppm tentative limit of arsenic in urine. However, the excretion of arsenic in urine rose from an initial average of 38 μg/24 hr to an average of 149 μg/24 hr for weeks 3–8 of the study, returning to an average of 68 μg/24 hr after exposure ceased. Although no acute illness nor untoward health effects were observed, the authors caution that little is known of the behavior of organic arsenicals, and recommend strict environmental and medical supervision for workers. They also note an observation of a garlic odor in recently treated forests and suggest that monitoring for arsine be performed.

ASBESTOS

As in the first volume of this treatise, asbestos was the subject of many epidemiologic reports, and it leads the list of chemical substances reported on. The investigations run the gamut of the possible types of epidemiology, and, in addition to reinforcing the findings of previous studies, have given a considerable amount of new information on the relative hazard of lung cancer in asbestos workers. Unfortunately, the long-term nature of the hazard makes quantitative exposure data difficult to obtain or to interpret.

Further associations have been made between asbestos and mesothelioma by examination of the occupational and residential history of persons dying of mesotheliomas. Stumphius reports[9] on 25 cases of mesothelioma on Walcheren Island, The Netherlands. Excluding asbestos insulation workers, the shipyard workers were divided into five occupational groups, four of which had some exposure to asbestos dust and one group who did what was classified as "clean work." Considering both present occupation and occupation 5–10 years previously, a significant difference was found in the proportion of workers with asbestos bodies in their sputum (25.8% positive in "clean work" versus 85.2% in other groups combined). The mesotheliomas on Walcheren appeared to be associated with shipyard work. For Holland as a whole, the attack rate was 0.63/100,000 men per year. The attack rate for all shipyard workers was about 100/100,000 men/year. However, the attack rate for the occupational groups with some exposure to asbestos dust was 280 as compared to approximately 50 for "clean work." McEwan et al.[10] report on an investigation of 80 mesothelioma cases in Scotland, and two sets of controls: coronary artery disease deaths and cancer deaths, respectively. For each case, information was obtained from relatives or, in a few cases, from neighbors. Occupational history, residential history, and the possibility of domestic or family exposures were obtained from the interviews. Smoking histories were also obtained. Definite occupational exposure was found in 20 mesothelioma cases versus only two for the two control groups combined. There were significantly more cases of residential exposure in mesothelioma cases, but most of these cases also had occupational exposures. There was no statistical difference between the three groups with regard to either household or spare-time exposure to asbestos. Rubino et al.[11] looked at the epidemiology of mesothelioma in the Piedmont of northwestern Italy. They found 16% of 50 mesothelioma cases with definite occupational or familial exposure versus only 2% of the control group. Although significant, the degree of association between asbestos and mesothelioma is less striking than in many similar series.[12]

The studies of the research group at McGill University on asbestos mine and mill workers were mentioned in the previous volume of this study.[6] Published reports have now appeared to further document the preliminary findings already reported. Gibbs and LaChance[13] report on the dust exposure in the chrysotile asbestos mines and mills of Quebec. Systematic midget impinger sampling had been conducted since 1948. The results of over 4000 dust counts by the same individual were available. The chrysotile mines and mills covered by this investigation produce some 40% of the world's asbestos. Indices of exposure calculated for the workers in the industry included years of exposure, accumulated dust exposure or "dust index," accumulated dust exposure weighted for physical effort, accumulated dust exposure weighted for physical application, and time-weighted dust exposure. The indices were calculated for nearly 30,000 workers, each with an average of nearly 10 jobs. Conversion to fiber counts was considered, but variability of the impinger dust/membrane filter fiber count ratio and lack of sufficient membrane filter fiber count data made it impracticable. A later study of dust–fiber relationships[14] showed average fiber/cm^3 to mppcf* ratios to vary from 1.7 to 21.9 in five mines. Averages by operation varied from 1.7 to 14.2. The overall mean ratio was 9.3 fibers/cm^3 to

* Million particles per cubic foot.

1.0 mppcf, but they believed it best to continue to base standards in the mining industry on dust counts by impinger.

The quantitative assessment of dust exposure for each worker was used by McDonald et al.[15] to classify mortality, by Jodoin et al.[16] and Becklake et al.[17] to classify lung functions, by McDonald et al.[18] to classify symptoms, and by Rossiter et al.[19] to classify radiographic changes. The total effect on health was summarized by McDonald et al.[20] They found mortality from lung cancer to be three to five times as high in the most heavily exposed dust group, with about 2% of the total mortality representing excess deaths from cancer and lung disease. Forced vital capacity decreased with increasing dust exposure to a loss of 18% in the highest dust exposure group. The prevalence of breathlessness on exercise grew with increasing dust exposure as did persistent cough and phlegm production. The cough and phlegm production also increased, by about an equal amount, among smokers. The relationship of smoking to excess lung cancer was also investigated, and a higher proportion of nonsmokers was found among mine and mill workers, thus ruling out smoking as the primary cause of the lung cancer excess in the workers. The prevalence of irregular small opacities, particularly grade 2/1 or more, rose with increasing dust exposure, particularly for the highest dust group (>800 mppcf-years). If the criterion of a 1% risk of acquiring clinically significant disease in a working lifetime, as proposed by the British Occupational Hygiene Society, is accepted, this point is reached at the 100–200 mppcf-year level. McDonald et al.[20] thus suggest that a limit of 2–4 mppcf, as measured by the midget impinger, would be appropriate for Quebec mines and mills. They point out that little effect except at highest dust levels in mining and milling has also been observed in the Soviet Union[21] and in Italy.[22]

Considerable progress has been made in the study of workers in asbestos-product manufacturing plants. Wegmen et al.[23] demonstrated that it was possible to show the presence of excessive disease in a wallboard manufacturing plant by a voluntary worker study without company cooperation. El-Sewefy and Hassan[24] showed electrophoretic pattern changes in the sera of asbestos cement pipe manufacturing workers. Pleural hyalinosis was found more frequently in asbestos workers by Navratil and Dobias.[25]

Other types of asbestos have also been investigated. For example, the studies of Noro[26] on anthophyllite workers and community exposures in Finland have been followed up by studies of mortality among anthophyllite mining and milling workers.

Enterline and Henderson[27] and Enterline et al.[28,29] have reported on a study of retired asbestos factory workers. Past impinger sampling made it possible to estimate dust exposure by job and time period. Maintenance-service workers had a higher excess of lung cancers than production workers, but much lower death rates from asbestosis. For both groups combined, the ratio of observed to expected lung cancer deaths increased from 1.7 for the lowest dust exposure group to 5.6 for the highest. One possible reason was that 70% of maintenance-service workers had used amosite and/or crocidolite as opposed to only 21% of production workers. The effect on mortality seemed to become important at about 100–200 mppcf-years, and the relative effects of time and concentration appeared to be about the same. Separating for chrysotile only versus chrysotile and crocidolite, those who worked with only chrysotile had a lung cancer excess of 2.6 times, whereas those who worked with both types had a respiratory cancer risk 6.1 times expected.

Newhouse *et al.*[30] extended a previous study of male asbestos worker mortality[31] to females at the same factory. Of 928 women who had worked at the factory between 1936 and 1942, 77% were traced. Compared with overall British death rates, there was excess mortality in the group with low to moderate exposure, partly accounted for by deaths from cancer. In the "severe exposure" group that had worked less than 2 years there was an excess of cancer of the lung and pleura. The most marked increased exposure was in the group that had worked more than 2 years with severe exposure; among these workers there were excess deaths from cancer of the lung and pleura, from other cancers, and from respiratory diseases. Although information obtained on some of the deceased workers indicated a larger proportion of smokers than nationally, the greater mortality with increased asbestos exposure suggested the primary role of asbestos in the excess. Eleven mesothelioma deaths were found in the cohort. The proportionate mortality from lung cancer was much higher than in the male workers, but the absolute excess was similar. The authors therefore suggest that asbestos produces a similar effect in men and women, but that the effect is more easily detected in a cohort of women because of the lower lung cancer rates in the general population.

The mortality experience of insulation workers continued to show larger excesses of lung cancer, pleural and peritoneal mesothelioma, and cancer of the gastrointestinal tract than most other exposed groups. In an update of his continuing study of New York insulation workers, Selikoff[32] noted that of 425 deaths 20% were from lung cancer (versus 2.6% expected), 6.4% were from pleural or peritoneal mesothelioma, 9.6% were from cancer of the stomach, colon, and rectum (versus 2.9% expected), and 7.5% were from asbestosis. However, he does find similar excesses among a group of former amosite insulation factory workers; of 105 deaths, 25.7% were from lung cancer, 4.8% from pleural or peritoneal mesothelioma, 4.6% from cancer of the stomach, colon, or rectum, and 13.8% from asbestosis.[33] Selikoff observed more than an 11-fold excess of lung cancer in the amosite workers, and a 7.7 times excess in insulation workers; Enterline found a 6.1 times excess in factory workers with mixed asbestos exposure, while Elmes and Simpson[34] observed a 6-fold excess in Belfast insulation workers. These contrast with excesses of 2.6 times in chrysotile factory workers, 1.9–3.1 times in Soviet chrysotile mine and mill workers, and an overall excess of 1.0 to 1.5 among Quebec chrysotile asbestos mine and mill workers.[15] The excess of lung cancer among Finnish anthophyllite mine and mill workers occupied an intermediate place between the chrysotile workers and the amosite-crocidolite workers. As reported by Nurminen[35] in a cohort study of 1030 workers, the lung cancer was 2–3.5 times expected, but Kiviluoto and Meurman[36] found that when only workers with over 10 years' experience were considered, the lung cancer was 3–5 times expected.

The extensive former use of asbestos in shipbuilding and ship repair resulted in a number of studies of present and former ship workers. The mesothelioma experience of the Welcheren Island shipyards has already been noted. Ferris *et al.*[37] studied 63 pipe coverers in a repair yard, matching each with a welder and a pipe fitter. More lung x-ray changes and slightly lower pulmonary function were noted in pipe coverers as compared with the other two groups. Past impinger counts had shown many counts above the old 5 mppcf Threshold Limit Value, but the counts were reportedly made by a dark-field method that could be expected to yield higher counts than the standard method. Fiber counts taken in 1969 averaged 2.9 fibers/cm^3. Murphy *et al.*[38] reported on two studies of pipe coverers and controls in a shipyard, conducted 1 year apart. In the first survey, 11 of 101 pipe coverers were diagnosed with asbestosis by clinical criteria; by the second survey three of the 11 had died, but four more were diagnosed as asbestosis by the clinical criteria. Another followup, $3\frac{1}{2}$ years after the second study found eight surviving workers with asbestosis, and two additional cases. Pipe coverers as a group had significantly reduced forced vital capacities as well as single breath and exercise steady-state diffusing capacity. The overall average of dust counts taken in the shipyard was 5.2 mppcf. Harries *et al.*[39] examined a 10% sample (4072 men) in four British naval dockyards. An overall prevalence of 3.16% radiographic asbestos abnormalities was found. Considering only workers with more than 25 years' experience, the prevalence varied from 24% with asbestos abnormalities among asbestos laggers and related occupations to 5% in the "all other occupation" group. No environmental values were obtained. Lawton *et al.*[40] described the asbestos exposures in U.S. Navy shipyards, noting the increase in use of asbestos, primarily amosite, until about 1958, and the subsequent gradual substitution of nonasbestos insulating materials. One 1970 study was noted in which 21% of pipe coverers and insulation workers had pulmonary abnormalities, compared with 3.5% in boilermakers and less than 1% in clerks. Dust concentrations were generally maintained below 5 mppcf. Nicholson *et al.*[41] compared New York and New Jersey insulation worker asbestos dust samples with some engine room samples. They noted that when an asbestos worker producing an average exposure to himself of 11.5 fibers/cm^3, men in other trades nearby were exposed to an average of 2.5 fibers/cm^3. They also demonstrated that reductions by a factor of 10 in exposure were readily achievable by good practice. The mortality study of

Elmes and Simpson[34] was accompanied by a study of morbidity of insulation workers still on the job in Belfast shipyards by Langlands et al.[42] In 252 men examined, the frequency of chest x-ray abnormalities increased from 13% in men with less than 10 years' work to 85% in men who had been in the industry for 30 or more years. The men with lung field abnormalities tended to have other signs of asbestosis as well. No environmental data were presented in either study.

Other foreign studies included insulation workers in Finland as reported by Ahlman and Siltanen.[43] Although the prevalence of asbestosis was not available, 56 cases had been diagnosed between 1936 and 1968. Dust measurements indicated a large number of workers regularly exposed to concentrations over 10 fibers/cm^3, with some exposures over 100 fibers/cm^3. In contrast, asbestos fiber counts of only 1.3 fibers/cm^3 were found by Murphy et al.,[44] in a simulated asbestos tile floor sanding experiment undertaken in an attempt to explain asbestosis in two asbestos floor tile installers. A Singapore study of 114 employees exposed to asbestos demonstrated rales in nine workers, and "mild respiratory abnormality," but few workers had extensive length of service.

In summary, these reports and other reports of the same and similar studies, some as yet unpublished, have confirmed the carcinogenic potential of asbestos. The potential for production of lung cancer is strongly related to length of exposure, and appears to be stronger in cigarette smokers, with cigarette smoke perhaps acting as a cocarcinogen. The type of asbestos and the stage in which it is used appear to be almost as important as relative dust concentration for production of lung cancer. Mining and milling produces much less of an excess of lung cancer than asbestos textile manufacture, which in turn is less hazardous than insulation work. The amphiboles produce more lung cancer than chrysotile. Whether these differences in effect are related to the stage in subdivision and disagglomeration of the asbestos dust, to its morphology, or to chemical composition has not been determined. The amphiboles may also tend to be relatively dustier than chrysotile, but this has not been established. The production of mesothelioma, on the other hand, does not appear to bear any relationship to cigarette smoking, and is less strongly dose related than the production of lung cancer. Physiologic alterations are strongly dose related. A simple fiber-year concept appears to be predictive of changes in lung function, although the changes are not necessarily independent of dose rates. Roentgenographic changes are observed to be related to length of service as well as dose. Although studies of asbestos workers are reported to be continuing in the United States[45] and in the United Kingdom,[46] the emphasis in the past few years has been shifting toward control, with environmental and medical monitoring to assure that control is adequate.[47] The reservoir of asbestos-affected lungs will, however, make it difficult to assess the effectiveness of the controls for some years to come.

BENZENE

Studies related to benzene exposure are reported from England, Italy, Poland, and Turkey.

Parkinson[48] presents the most generally applicable study—on the hazard of benzene in gasoline in and around filling stations and in motor transport. Air sampling was done primarily by personal samples collected on silica gel for subsequent analysis. Filling stations, road car bulk loading of normal blends, rail car bulk loading of normal blends, and road car loading of gasoline containing added motor benzole (33% benzene) were studied. Urine samples were collected from most operators, drivers, and observers at the beginning and end of each working period for phenol content. Conclusions were that only trivial exposure to airborne benzene vapor occurred when gasoline of normal benzene content (up to 5% by volume) was dispensed at typical filling stations. The highest average air concentration was 2.4 ppm, and the peak was 3.2 ppm. Urine phenol values did not show significant absorption. All bulk-dispensing operations for normal blends produced average exposures below the TLV of 10 ppm, and peaks below the ceiling value of 25 ppm. Neither urine phenols nor expired air benzene demonstrated any significant absorption. The trials of bulk loading of 10 to 33% benzene in benzole-enriched gasoline produced no air samples above 10 ppm, and although urinary phenols were increased, the highest was increased by only 41 mg/liter and the average increase was only 10 mg/liter. Thus, neither air sampling nor urine sampling demonstrated dangerous exposure to benzene.

Forni et al.[49] studied 34 workers of a rotogravure plant and 34 controls. Ten of the workers had been exposed to benzene before 1953 and subsequently to toluene; the other 24 workers had been exposed only to toluene. The proportions of stable and unstable chromosome aberrations were significantly higher in the benzene group than in the toluene or the control group. No significant differences were found between the toluene and control groups. The exposures to benzene in 1953, at the time of an epidemic of chronic benzene poisoning, had ranged from 125 to 432 ppm, and may have been higher the preceding winter. Blood samples had been examined quarterly since the discontinuance of benzene in 1953; the chromosomal aberrations reported here were observed in 1968 and 1969.

Lange et al.[50] studied serum immunoglobulin levels of 35 workers occupationally exposed to benzene, toluene, and xylene. Benzene levels averaged 40 ppm in 1971 and 5 ppm in 1972; toluene levels, 60 ppm in 1971 and 40 ppm in 1972; and xylene levels, 60 ppm in 1971 and 75 ppm in 1972. A statistically significant decrease in the IgG and IgA levels, with an increase in IgM levels, was observed. Lange et al.[51] observed 76 workers including the 35 above. The other 41 workers had been isolated from solvent exposure in the period preceding the exposure. In this nonexposed group only one person showed the presence of leukocyte agglutins versus 10 of 35 persons in the exposed group. Smolik et al.[52] showed that in 62 of 79 workers in this same group, the serum complement level was lower than the mean value of a control group. The authors state that these data are consistent and suggest the involvement of immunologic factors in the mechanism of chronic exposure to benzene and its homologs.

Aksoy et al.[53] report a study of 217 workers manufacturing shoes in small shops under unhygienic conditions. The concentration of benzene in the workplaces ranged from 30 to 219 ppm, and the duration of exposure was 3 months to 17 years. Hematologic abnormalities were found in 23.5% of the workers. The authors discuss the nature of the abnormalities in some detail. There was no mention of substitution of other solvents for the benzene, or of other possible control measures.

A study of 220 benzene workers was conducted by Chung and Chang.[54] Abnormal hematologic findings were present in 23.5% of workers examined. Such changes occurred in workers exposed to as low as 20 ppm benzene in air. "Theoretically, it was derived that the threshold limit value for benzene exposure was 10.1 ppm."

A mortality study of pressmen, some with former exposures to benzene, is underway in the National Institute for Occupational Safety and Health.[45]

BENZIDINE

Zavon et al.[55] reported on 25 workers exposed to benzidine in its manufacture. Of the 25 workers, 13 developed bladder tumors. Those who developed tumors had an average exposure to benzidine of more than 13 years, with no tumors yet developing in any man with less than 6 years' exposure. For workers shoveling benzidine into drums, the airborne benzidine concentration was 17.6 mg/m^3. Concentrations at other locations were from <0.007 mg/m^3 to 0.415 mg/m^3. Manufacture was discontinued in 1958, when the first bladder tumors were observed; tumors have continued to occur for 12 years. Benzidine has been on the ACGIH TLV Committee's list of carcinogens since the original list in 1962, and was included in the Occupational Safety and Health Administration standard for carcinogens promulgated in 1974.

BERYLLIUM

Kanarek et al.[56] report a study of a beryllium extraction and processing plant that had been in operation for 14 years. High levels of beryllium which greatly exceeded the recommended peak limit of 25 $\mu g/m^3$ were noted in the plant. Of 245 full-time employees, 124 were studied. Thirty-one workers had chest radiographic abnormalities compatible with interstitial disease, and 11 of these had significant hypoxemia. Lung biopsies were performed in two subjects. One showed diffuse granulomas and increased lung tissue beryllium content, and the other had a markedly elevated lung tissue beryllium content with normal histology.

> It was concluded that in the presence of excessive air levels of beryllium, the combination of hypoxemia and radiographic evidence of a pulmonary interstitial process is suggestive of berylliosis. The evidence of beryllium disease in this population indicates the importance of rigorous implementation of industrial hygiene measures and the necessity for correlating the industrial exposure data with the status of the workers.

It was noteworthy that in this plant it was impossible to determine the actual exposure of workers because of an excessive reliance upon simple, half-mask filter type respirators. The authors thus determined ranges of concentration by high volume sampling. Several operations were noted where no samples were below the 8-hour mandatory limit of 2 $\mu g/m^3$, and four operations had peak concentration above 100 $\mu g/m^3$.

The National Institute for Occupational Safety and Health reports continuation of a long-term study of beryllium production workers to determine whether there is any excess of lung cancer.[45] They have not reported any such association.

BUDGERIGARS

Warren[57] reports an epidemic of hypersensitivity pneumonitis due to keeping budgerigars (zebra parakeets) in the home. Nine patients were treated in Toronto, the first report of this illness on the North American continent. Occupationally, there is the possibility of such illness in pet shops or among others who handle these birds.

CARBON DISULFIDE

Hanninen[58] administered a battery of psychological tests to 50 viscose rayon workers with carbon disulfide poisoning, 50 workers exposed to CS_2 without known poisoning, and 50 unexposed workers. There were large and statistically significant differences between the group means of the poisoned and the unexposed group in most performances involving speed, vigilance, manual dexterity, and intelligence. The exposed group also showed impairment, but the changes were less severe. The poisoned group could be reliably distinguished from the unexposed group by discriminant analysis (91% correct). It was suggested that the syndromes of latent and manifest poisoning differed not only in intensity, but also in quality. Latent poisoning was characterized by traits indicative of depressive mood, slight motor disturbances, and intellectual impairment, whereas clinically manifested poisoning resulted in lowered vigilance, diminished intellectual activity, diminished rational control, retarded speed, and motor disturbances. Exposures in the plant had averaged from 20 to 40 ppm during the years 1950–1959 and from 10 to 30 ppm from 1960 on.

Plasma and erythrocyte changes in zinc and magnesium levels such as those found in animals were investigated in Finnish and Norwegian workers exposed to carbon disulfide by Hernberg et al.[59] The magnesium levels were significantly reduced in erythrocytes of exposed Finnish workers, and zinc concentrations were lowered slightly. No such difference was found in Norwegian men. Plasma magnesium was higher for the exposed Finns, but not for the Norwegians; plasma zinc differences were not seen in either group. The geometric mean CS_2 concentrations were 4–15 ppm in the Finnish rayon factory, and 18 ppm in the Norwegian factory.

Mancuso and Locke,[60] in a mortality study using social security records, found an excess of suicides in workers first employed at one viscose factory between the years 1938 and 1948. In addition to an excess of recorded suicides, there were a number of deaths recorded as other causes which strongly resembled suicide. Certain departments of the plant were primarily responsible for the excess. Unfortunately, carbon disulfide concentrations were not available for the plant as a whole or for the departments with high suicide rates.

Hernberg et al.[61] examined blood lipids, glucose tolerance, and plasma creatinine in 343 viscose rayon workers who had been exposed to an average of 20–40 ppm CS_2 in the 1950's and 10–30 ppm in the 1960's. The study was part of a larger one of coronary risk factors and coronary disease. The only differences found between the workers and matched controls were in fasting glucose, where the difference correlated with the exposure time and exposure index, and in mean plasma creatinine, which was higher in the exposed group. When the mortality from coronary heart disease was examined prospectively,[62] it was found that in a 5.5-year period, 16 exposed men had died from coronary heart disease as compared with three controls. The difference was statistically significant, and the risk of death rose with increasing exposure. "The results agreed with earlier mortality studies, and strongly support the hypothesis of a causal relation between CS_2 exposure and coronary heart disease."

Sakurai[63] studied more than 10 years of blood pressure records in a Japanese viscose rayon plant. Blood pressures were reduced when workers were removed from a CS_2 environment and when the environment was improved from a level of 20–50 ppm to a level of 10–25 ppm.

Goto *et al.*[64] selected 214 carbon disulfide workers from 11 Japanese viscose rayon plants and 45 controls. They found a trend toward higher blood sugar levels with advancing age in carbon disulfide exposed workers, while hardly any such trend was seen in controls under age 50. A corticosteroid priming glucose tolerance test indicated a subclinical defect of carbohydrate metabolism in some apparently healthy CS_2 exposed workers, suggesting a mild diabetogenic action. The prevalence of retinal microaneurisms grew with increasing duration of exposure to CS_2, and the grade of the microaneurisms also increased. There was a trend toward higher blood sugar levels with increasing grade of micro- aneurisms. Unfortunately, no information as to intensity of carbon disulfide exposure is presented.

El-Gazzar *et al.*[65] examined 82 workers in the Egyptian viscose rayon industry and 33 controls. Carbon disulfide caused depletion of serum zinc by an increase in the rate of zinc excretion, and an increase in all serum protein fractions. The effects were temporary and improved on cessation of exposure.

CARBON MONOXIDE

Cohen *et al.*[66] examined inspectors at a United States–Mexico border station by collecting expired air carbon monoxide samples. Those inspectors who were smokers abstained during the working shift. During the day shift, with a mean CO concentration of 14 ppm, expired CO decreased in smokers and remained the same in nonsmokers. During the evening shift, with a mean CO level of 66 ppm, expired CO increased both in smokers and nonsmokers. During the night shift, with a mean CO concentration of 114 ppm, expired CO also increased both in smokers and nonsmokers. The authors concluded that the carboxyhemoglobin increases were comparable to those from cigarette smoking, and thus constitute a serious health problem for these workers. Revision of procedures could considerably reduce exposures to inspectors.

Burgess *et al.*[67] found that carbon monoxide exposures to traffic policemen in Boston were not well represented by conventional air pollution sampling programs. Carbon monoxide levels were found to be closely coupled to traffic activity. A personal sampling kit was proposed to better characterize officer exposure. A personal sampler for carbon monoxide exposure to firemen was subsequently developed.[68]

Ayres *et al.*[69] examined occupational exposures to carbon monoxide and other automotive emissions in 550 bridge and tunnel workers. A group of 619 workers examined in Union Square, New York City was used as a control. Over the 30-day period, CO concentrations averaged 63 ppm at the tunnel; bridge concentrations were lower, but were not presented. Respirable lead concen- trations at the tunnel averaged 11 $\mu g/m^3$; respirable particulate averaged

64 $\mu g/m^3$; NO_x averaged 1.4 ppm of which 0.07 ppm was NO_2. The authors show carboxyhemoglobin concentrations in bridge workers to be equivalent to that in Union Square people, but to be elevated by about 1% saturation in both smoking and nonsmoking tunnel workers. Mean carboxyhemoglobin (COHb) levels were about 5% for smoking tunnel workers, 4% for other smokers, 3% for nonsmoking tunnel workers, and 2% for others. Nonsmoking tunnel workers had lighter prevalence of respiratory symptoms than nonsmoking bridge workers; there was no difference between smoking groups. Expiratory flow rates at one-half and one-fourth of vital capacity were reduced in bridge and tunnel workers as compared with "normal subjects." Closing volumes were elevated in almost three-fourths of bridge and tunnel workers, as compared to a group of hospital maintenance workers. The authors attribute the respiratory abnormalities to automotive pollutants associated with carbon monoxide; it is unclear why bridge workers are not distinguished from tunnel workers in the closing volume studies Blood lead levels measured were higher than in other studies cited and did not correlate with aerometric data. Potential risks to tollbooth workers have been considerably reduced by installing ventilation systems with elevated air intakes, thus reducing CO concentration by a factor of four. The authors emphasize that the occupational contribution of CO, particulates, lead, and oxides of nitrogen are additive to those received off the job.

CHROMIUM OXIDE

Graham Jones and Warner[70] report a study of steel workers exposed to varying proportions of chromium oxide and nickel oxide in a predominantly iron oxide fume. They consider that effects on the workers are probably due to the admixture of the chromium and nickel oxide fumes with the iron oxide.

Their study was of ingot deseaming workers employed at this job for periods of up to 16 years. The nitrogen dioxide concentrations during deseaming of large stainless steel ingots averaged 2.1 ppm; that for small special steel ingots averaged 1.0 ppm or less. The respirable fume generated during the stainless steel operation (as collected by Hexhlet) consisted of 61.0% Fe_2O_3, 12.5% Cr_2O_3, and 10.4% NiO. During the special steel operation the respirable fume was 96.9% Fe_2O_3 and 1.3% Cr_2O_3. Deseaming and cutting of the stainless steel ingots and slabs was performed in a large bay with some natural ventilation. Concentrations of fume varied widely at this operation, but all were high. Deseaming the end resulted in an average of 77 mg/m^3, deseaming the top horizontal face resulted in only 13 mg/m^3, while deseaming the vertical end of the ingot gave 198 mg/m^3; cutting ends of ingots produced 70–124 mg/m^3. Cutting stainless slabs gave concentrations averaging from 32 to 28 mg/m^3 depending upon conditions. Deseaming small special steel ingots was conducted at an exhaust hood, and concentrations averaged only 9.1 mg/m³. The relevant airborne limits were 10 mg/m³ for iron oxide fume and 1 mg/m³ for nickel oxide and chromium oxide fume. All limits were exceeded by a great margin.

Seven of eighteen men showed definite signs of pneumoconiosis by x ray. Ventilatory function tests of all but one of the 14 workers were within the normal range. Four workers with category 2 or higher pneumoconiosis had more detailed pulmonary function tests performed, and it was concluded that two of the four showed evidence of pulmonary defects.

The authors point out that the operation continued for 16 years until 1963, with little or no complaint, because, the workers suffered no irritation and believed the fumes to be harmless. The authors feel that the pneumoconiosis should be classed as a mixed dust pneumoconiosis rather than siderosis because of the presence of chromium and nickel oxide with the iron oxide. No lung cancer had occurred in any of these workers over the 16 years of exposure and the subsequent 8 years. However, no conclusion as to the potential carcinogenicity of nickel oxide or chromium oxide fume can be drawn from this small negative sample.

PORTLAND CEMENT

The prevalence of nonspecific lung disease was studied in four groups of cement workers and in controls by Kalačic.[71] The British Medical Research Council's respiratory symptom questionnaire, chest x ray, electrocardiogram, blood pressure, and spirometric examinations were performed. The prevalence of respiratory symptoms and syndromes were significantly higher than in the controls. Major symptoms such as cough, expectoration, exertional dyspnea, and wheezing as well as chronic bronchitis syndromes were all more frequent in cement workers. Wives of both cement workers and controls were also examined. The two groups of wives demonstrated differences only in exertional dyspnea and occasional wheezing, which was more prevalent in cement workers' wives. The authors point out that a nonoccupational factor might be operating, but note also that these two conditions may have a psychologic component. Smoking was more pronounced in exposed groups, but a significantly higher prevalence was still found in cement workers when nonsmokers were compared with control nonsmokers. Dust concentrations were measured in two or three of the four plants. The concentration of 0.05 μm–5.0 μm particles ranged from 511/cm³ to 106,600/cm³. The permissible Yugoslav concentration is 450/cm³. These concentrations cannot be readily translated into count or mass concentration units in use in other nations. The authors suggests that occupational factors have played a role in the development of chronic nonspecific lung disease, but that the nature of this association requires further clarification.

The ventilatory lung function of these cement workers, the controls, and their wives was also compared.[72] The forced vital capacity (FVC) as a percent of that predicted was lower in all four groups of exposed workers. The FVC also decreased as length of service increased. The ratio of forced expiratory volume in 1 sec ($FEV_{1.0}$) to FVC also was lower in the cement workers. The $FEV_{1.0}/FVC$ decreased with increasing length of service. These studies may cause a reexamination of cement dust as an "inert" dust, although conclusions are difficult to draw until dust measurements are available in a more readily interpretable form.

CHLORINATED NAPHTHALENE

Kleinfeld *et al.*[73] described an exposure of 92 workers to a wax containing tetra- and pentachloronaphthalenes. Of 59 employees examined, 56 had skin lesions attributable to the exposure. Systemic effects noted included headache, fatigue, vertigo, and anorexia. Liver function tests on the most severely affected workers demonstrated no abnormalities. Excessive exposures were due mainly to an inadequate and poorly maintained ventilation system, indifference toward the use of preventive hygiene measures and protective clothing, and an inadequate medical program. Improvement of the environmental controls and the inplant medical program has effectively controlled the health hazard from exposure to chlorinated naphthalenes at this plant.

CHLOROMETHYL METHYL ETHER AND BISCHLOROMETHYL ETHER

Figuero *et al.*[74] observed 14 cases of lung cancer in a chemical plant manufacturing chloromethyl ether over a 5-year period. From this, they estimated an 8-fold risk of lung cancer. Further epidemiologic studies of bischloromethyl ether were being carried out by the New York University Institute for Environmental Medicine under the direction of R. E. Albert.[75] It is on the carcinogen list of the Threshold Limit Value Committee of the American Conference of Governmental Industrial Hygienists and included in the carcinogen standard of the Occupational Safety and Health Administration.

CHROMIC ACID

The frequency of skin ulceration, nasal ulceration, and perforation of the nasal septum is examined in Brazilian electroplaters by Gomes.[76] He examined 303 workers and took workplace air samples for chromic acid. Only 25% of the hard chrome workplaces had concentrations less than $0.1 \, mg/m^3$ of chromic acid, and all workers examined had either cutaneous lesions, mucous lesions, or both. In brilliant chrome workplaces, 52% of the measurements were less than $0.1 \, mg/m^3$ of chromic acid, but 83% of the workers had cutaneous lesions, mucous lesions, or both. However, 41.5% of the brilliant chrome workers were without nasal lesions, as compared with 11.4% of the hard chrome workers. In all, 86.8% of the workers showed some lesions due to chromic acid. In addition, the majority of those working with heated chromic acid suffered from coughing and expectoration, nasal irritation, sneezing when exposed to contaminants, and rhinorrhea, and over 30% had nosebleeds.

The authors note poor practices in personal protection, with inadequate or damaged gloves common. Exhaust systems, where installed, were frequently not used. The data as presented suggest that the recommended reduction in the occupational standard for chromic acid[77] may be required, but environmental data are scanty.

COAL

Epidemiologic studies of coal miners are by far the largest occupational studies underway. The groups of workers involved are in the hundreds of thousands in the United States, the United Kingdom, and other major coal-producing areas. The studies are national in scope. In the United States, the Coal Mine Health and Safety Act of 1969 established strict new requirements for dust control to prevent coal workers' pneumoconiosis (CWP) and gave statutory authority to the Department of Health, Education, and Welfare to conduct research into the prevalence, etiology, and prevention of CWP. In the United Kingdom, two decades had already gone into research on the problem, and new dust standards for the National Coal Board went into effect in 1970. Other coal-producing countries have also conducted epidemiologic studies.

It is fortunate that the Congress of the United States adopted by statute the horizontal elutriator sampler of the British National Coal Board as a standard, so that respirable dust concentrations in these two nations may be compared directly. In other coal-producing countries a variety of dust-measuring instruments are in use, but increasingly the British instrument concentrations are given for reference.

The classification of chest roentgenograms had also been aided by the international use of the UICC/Cincinnati classification.[78] Thus there are now standards for international comparison of dust exposures to workers and also for interpretation of miner chest x rays.

Overall mortality of British coal miners in 1961 was examined by Liddell.[79]

He examined deaths among coal miners age 20–64, including all those who had last worked at a coal mine. Detailed examination revealed overstatement of coal mining, and particularly face work, as an occupation. Collating data from the National Coal Board and the Registrar General, he classified men into their actual last occupation for determination of accurate death rate by occupation. A total of 5362 men age 20–64 who had last worked for the Coal Board died in 1961. Among working miners, death rates were lowest at the face and highest for surface workers; considering the rate for all occupied mineworkers as 100, the standardized mortality ratios (SMR's) were 77 and 127, respectively. Differences by geographic area were smaller, with ratios from 90 to 115 in the eight districts. Comparing working miners with all occupied and retired males as 100, the SMR for face workers was 60, for other underground workers 76, and for surface workers 108. Major advantages were noted for the face worker in all causes of death but pneumoconiosis and accidents. The proportion of various causes of death for current and former miners age 55–64 was similar to that of other males in most causes of death, but was significantly lower for lung cancer and significantly higher for bronchitis and pneumoconiosis.

Conflicting studies of coal miner mortality appeared in the United States. Enterline[80] examined U.S. Public Health Service data for 1950 and a 1967 actuarial study of insurance company policyholders. He found that in 1950 the overall death rate for coal miners was 14.8/1000 compared with 8.1 for all male workers. In 1967 the deaths of coal miners were 1.72 times those expected from deaths of other males. Excesses of deaths could not be explained by respiratory disease and accidents, known to be major causes of death among coal miners, but remained 1.4–1.7 times that expected when these causes of death were eliminated. The previous studies were confirmed by a prospective study of 553 miners for $28\frac{1}{2}$ years, which gave mortality excesses quite similar to those in the other studies. He concluded that death rates for coal miners were among the highest of any large, well-defined occupational group in the United States.

Ortmeyer et al.[81] compared death rates among coal miners compensated for disability in Pennsylvania with overall death rates for white males in Pennsylvania. The majority of the disabled miners were from the anthracite area. The number of deaths observed was 1.3 times the number expected, but when weighted for partial sampling, the standardized mortality ratio (SMR) was 1.19 for all compensated coal miners. Among anthracite miners 1.38 times the expected deaths were observed, with a SMR of 1.27. Among former bituminous miners the observed deaths were 1.10 times the expected, and the SMR was 1.00. SMR's calculated for those disabled former miners with simple pneumoconiosis were near 1.0; the SMR for category C complicated pneumoconiosis was 1.92 for the disabled former anthracite miners and 1.45 for the disabled former bituminous coal miners. Although the discrepancy between the overall mortality experience of this group and Enterline's is not explained, it appears that simple pneumoconiosis in disabled former coal miners does not result in higher death rates, while progressive massive fibrosis results in substantial excesses in mortality.

Overall morbidity among British coal miners was examined by Liddell.[82] Miners were found to suffer much more incapacity for work than men in other employment, even in those nonmining tasks considered to be very arduous. The lowest paid miners had the highest rates of incapacity. Miners living in rural areas had less incapacity than those in large towns. Men in deep mines tended to have more incapacity than those in shallow mines, particularly for psychoses, psychoneuroses, and acute bronchitis.

The relationship of prevalence of pneumoconiosis to coal dust exposure is still based largely on data gathered in the 20-year study of the British National Coal Board's Pneumoconiosis Field Research Unit.[83] The coal dust exposure standards of the United States and the United Kingdom, although different, are both based upon these data, which show 0.0 probability of a coal miner developing category 2/1 or higher pneumoconiosis after working 35 years at a concentration of 2 mg/m^3 of respirable dust.

The relationship of chronic bronchitis and dust exposure has been examined in a number of studies. Rogan et al.[84] report on a study of 3581 coal face workers in 20 British mines. A progressive reduction in forced expiratory volume 1.0 ($FEV_{1.0}$) with increasing coal dust exposure was demonstrated. Simple pneumoconiosis caused no reduction in $FEV_{1.0}$ not already accounted for by dust exposure, smoking habit, age, and physique. Increasing severity of bronchitic symptoms was accompanied by reductions in $FEV_{1.0}$ greater than that expected from effects of measured dust exposure, smoking, age, and physique. The bronchitic symptoms appear possibly related to dust exposure only during the early years of employment. These findings of problems of Bronchitis and coal mining in Britain confirm those of Lowe and Khosla[85] who studied ex-coal miners working in the steel industry and found substantially more chronic bronchitis and a poorer ventilatory capacity than nonminers irrespective of age and smoking habits. However, smoking was a more important factor than coal mining in production of chronic bronchitis. Ulmer and Reichel[86] point out that in West Germany chronic bronchitis and chronic obstructive bronchitis are very common diseases in the population not exposed to dust. They find simple pneumoconiosis to have no influence on chronic bronchitis, but category B and C complicated pneumoconiosis produces chronic obstructive bronchitis about twice as often as in nonexposed miners. However, category B and C can only be produced by producing simple coal workers' pneumoconiosis (CWP) so the solution to the excess rests in dust control. Higgins[87] also reviews chronic respiratory disease as a community and a coal mining problem. Studies of chronic respiratory disease were carried out in mining communities in England, Wales, and West Virginia. Miners, ex-miners, and nonminers were compared, using standard methods. A higher prevalence of symptoms and a lower average forced expiratory volume were consistently found in miners compared with nonminers. A greater prevalence of symptoms and decreasing lung function with increasing work underground was found in some studies, but not in others.

The continuing study of 31 large coal mines in the United States by the National Institute for Occupational Safety and Health in cooperation with the Bureau of Mines and the Mining Enforcement and Safety Administration has produced additional data on prevalence of CWP and on respiratory function of active coal miners. Morgan et al.[88] provide data on prevalence of CWP by type of coal and geographic area. In Pennsylvania, 45% of the anthracite miners had simple pneumoconiosis, and a further 14% had progressive massive fibrosis (PMF). In Appalachia, 29.3% of the miners had simple CWP, and 2.1% had PMF. In the Midwest mines the prevalence of simple CWP was 23.5%, and 0.9% of the miners had PMF. In Utah and Colorado, the prevalence of simple CWP was 10.5%, essentially all of it category 1, and the PMF was only 0.6%. These differences are not explained by dust measurements made by the Bureau of Mines in the mines studied. Sorenson et al.[89] have pointed out differences in trace metal composition of micronized samples from a high-prevalence Appalachian mine and a low-prevalence Utah mine, but the differences cannot be readily related to the miner exposure. Corn et al.[90] have described a dust sampling system used in two Appalachian mines capable of characterizing respirable dust by size and composition, but data for the interagency study are not available. Naeye et al.[91] have conducted a pathologic study of Appalachian miners classified by rank of coal and have found a greater degree of chronic cor pulmonale in miners of high-rank coal. They also found more pulmonary dust macules and nodules with more silica crystals and collagen than low-rank coal. The major differences were between bituminous coal and anthracite.

Major differences in prevalence by geographic area have also been noted in the United Kingdom[92] and in Poland.[93]

Morgan et al.[94] examined lung volumes and ventilatory capacity of coal miners in the U.S. interagency study. They found no relationship between ventilatory capacity and degree of simple CWP. However, complicated pneumoconiosis led to definite ventilatory impairment. Residual volume increased slightly with degree of simple CWP. There were significant geographic variations in ventilatory capacity and lung volumes, with pulmonary function being significantly better in miners in the western states than in Appalachian bituminous coal-miners, who were in turn of better health than the estern Pennsylvania anthracite miners.

Progression of pneumoconiosis in some United States coal miners also was found to vary by geographic area.[95] West Virginia had the highest rate of progression, followed by Pennsylvania, with the Midwest and West lower.

Lapp *et al.*[96] studied acute effects of mining on ventilatory function over a work shift. He found decreases in ventilatory capacity over a work shift in miners, compared with increases for nonminers. Although he believed dust exposure to be the likely cause, no dust measurements were available to determine degree of dust exposure.

Although mortality studies have tended to find a lower proportion of lung cancer in coal miners,[79] Scarano *et al.*[97] found 7% carcinoma of the lung in anthracosilicotics compared with 1.08% in nonanthracosilicotics.

New and improved instruments for personal sampling of respirable dust, as described in later sections, should materially aid the progress of epidemiologic studies of coal miners, if taken advantage of by the agencies conducting and sponsoring research in the mines.[98]

In summary, much more has been learned about the prevalence of pneumoconiosis, but many factors remain unevaluated. The reduction in dustiness following passage of the Coal Mine Health and Safety Act of 1969 should considerably reduce and, we hope, eventually eliminate coal workers' pneumoconiosis.

COKE MANUFACTURE

Further papers in the series on the long-term mortality study of a group of steel workers in the United States have appeared.[99,100]

They showed that the lung cancer excess in coke oven workers was associated primarily with employment in the full-time topside occupations. The lung cancer experience of coke oven workers never employed at full-time topside jobs was comparable to that of other steelworkers. The death rate from lung cancer for full-time topside workers was seven times expectation (19 versus 2.6). The previously observed differences in lung cancer by race were found to be merely a reflection of the fact that almost all of the topside workers were blacks; there were no excesses of lung cancer among blacks elsewhere in the coke plant. Excesses of lung cancer were also noted in men employed at the side of the oven for more than 5 years, but the differences were not statistically significant. An excess of nonrespiratory system cancers was also noted among coke oven workers, with the excess primarily in workers with 5 years at the coke plant, but less than 5 years topside on the coke oven. The lung cancer is believed to be due to inhalation of "coal tar," which is responsible for cancer in other industries as well. The study by Redmond *et al.*[100] is expanded from Allegheny County, Pennsylvania, to other areas. The findings of the Allegheny County study are confirmed. Overall, a relative risk for lung cancer of 6.9 is found for men employed 5 or more years full topside coke oven, 3.2 for men with 5 or more years of mixed topside and side oven experience, 2.1 for men with 5 or more years of side oven experience only, and 1.7 for all men with less than 5 years' experience at start of follow-up. A further finding in the expanded study was a $7\frac{1}{2}$-fold risk of dying from kidney cancers among coke oven workers. It also pointed out that measurements of coke oven effluents and the relationships between environmental measures, mortality, and illnesses should be studied in detail so that meaningful maximum allowable concentrations can be established for coke ovens.

Smith[101] describes the research on coke oven emissions. Polynuclear aromatic compounds (PNA's) constituted between 2 and 3% of the collected particulate matter above the coke oven, or between 4 and 6% of the benzene-soluble fraction of the collected volatiles emitted during the charging operation. A survey of three German coke plants determined that fume control equipment on larry cars, when operable, reduced employee exposure significantly, although leaving it still much in excess of the TLV of 0.2 mg/m^3 of benzene-soluble coal tar pitch volatiles. A powered air-purifying respirator was tested for coke oven use, and suggested as an interim measure for operator protection.

Walker et al.[102] examined the prevalence of bronchitis among men employed in National Coal Board coking plants. A strong association was found between bronchitis prevalence and cigarette smoking. In addition, the coke oven workers had more bronchitis than other coke plant workers. Both the presence of bronchitis and work at the coke ovens had significant and independent effects on ventilatory capacity. The combination of cigarette smoking and previous employment in a dusty industry also had a significant effect on ventilatory capacity.

COTTON (ALSO FLAX, HEMP, JUTE, AND SISAL)

The problems of byssinosis appear similar in many respects for a number of vegetable fibers, and they are thus considered together here, as in many of the epidemiologic studies.

Mortality in the cotton textile industry was reviewed by Henderson and Enterline.[103] They examined observed and expected deaths by cause among 5822 white males who worked sometime during 1938–1941 and 6316 white males who worked sometime during 1948–1951. They note an unusually low mortality from respiratory cancer, particularly in the latter cohort, where the SMR was only 20.5. Deaths from respiratory diseases were also considerably fewer than expected, with an SMR of 36.4 in the latter cohort. They cannot, however, separate out those textile workers with the major exposures to cotton dust. A retrospective cohort study is reported to be underway among a group of 10,000 cotton textile workers.[45]

Changes in the ventilatory capacity of Lancashire cotton mill workers were investigated by Berry et al.[104] A prospective study was carried out over a 3-year period in 14 cotton textile mills and two synthetic mills. A mean annual decline in forced expiratory volume in the first second ($FEV_{1.0}$) of 51 cm^3/yr was noted, which was comparable to some studies of noncotton workers, but greater than some others. The annual decline was not found to be related to symptoms of byssinosis or bronchitis, nor to present dust levels, bioactivity of the dust, or air pollution. The mean fall in $FEV_{1.0}$ over a Monday work shift was higher in cotton mills than in synthetic fiber mills among those without symptoms of byssinosis and was correlated with present dust levels. For those with symptoms of byssinosis an increased Monday fall was found only in those processing coarse cotton.

Fox et al.[105] performed two surveys of cotton blow- and cardroom workers between 1966 and 1970. There were 2316 workers in the first study and 2556 in the second, including 886 in both studies. Symptoms and ventilatory changes of byssinosis were found in workers in all mills except the two fine cotton mills. Some workers with less than 10 years' exposure were classified as byssinotic in both surveys. The 886 workers in both studies had a greater fall in $FEV_{1.0}$ between the two surveys than a local control population. Even symptom-free workers showed a 10% excess in the rate of decrease of $FEV_{1.0}$ with age. But neither the ventilatory tests nor the symptoms were of value in predicting the rate of deterioration between the two studies.

Also Fox et al.[105] examined the effect of dust levels and smoking on byssinotic symptoms. They found that dust levels were 1.15 to 4.8 mg/m^3, excluding fly. There was an increase in symptoms and a greater reduction in ventilatory capacity in those exposed to the higher dust levels. Smokers showed more frequent symptoms and a greater loss in ventilatory function at all dust levels. The correlation between dust levels and frequency of byssinotic symptoms and loss of ventilatory function was increased by including a time factor. By expressing dust levels as mg-yr/m^3, it could be predicted that about 10% of workers exposed to 0.5 mg/m^3 of dust for 40 years would have symptoms of byssinosis.

Imbus and Suh[107] reported on a study of 10,133 American textile workers. They found an overall byssinosis prevalence (all grades) of 5.7% in males and 3.0% in females. The highest prevalence was found in preparation areas, with a much lower prevalence in other areas. Chronic bronchitis was found to be associated with byssinosis, and smokers had a higher prevalence of bronchitis with or without byssinosis. The $FEV_{1.0}$ as a percent of predicted in nonsmoking byssinotic males began to drop off sharply after about 18 years of employment. Nonbyssinotic smokers had lower $FEV_{1.0}$'s, which gradually decreased; the

$FEV_{1.0}$'s for smoking byssinotics were lower than those for nonsmoking byssinotics for the first 20 years, and then the difference narrowed. A drop in $FEV_{1.0}$ during the working shift, although associated with, was often present without, byssinosis symptoms. The authors emphasized that a combined program of dust control and medical surveillance is required to protect cotton textile workers.

A survey of cotton and synthetic textile mills in Israel[108] found no byssinosis.

Two studies present suggestions as to possible causes of some of the effects of cotton dust. Certain similarities in the effects of proteolytic enzymes and cotton dust, and the association of enzymes and signs and symptoms are presented by Tuma *et al.*[109] They believe that control of enzymes will be necessary to prevent byssinosis. Taylor *et al.*[110] extracted a condensed polyphenol based on leucocyanidin from the cotton plant which reacted differently in byssinotics and controls. The mean titers of the two groups differed significantly. Inhaling an aerosol of this solution by nonbyssinotic workers produced neither symptoms nor changes in $FEV_{1.0}$. Inhalation by byssinotic cardroom workers produced symptoms identicial to those of the Monday morning cardroom without a fall in the $FEV_{1.0}$.

The effects of a number of vegetable dusts upon workers have been studied in Zagreb, Yugoslavia. Valic and Zuskin[111] compared the effects of cotton and jute dusts in female textile workers. Cotton workers were found to have a significantly higher prevalence of byssinosis, persistent cough, and dyspnea than jute workers. Byssinosis prevalence in cotton workers was 28.3% compared with none in jute workers. Cotton and, to a lesser degree, jute caused reduction of $FEV_{1.0}$ over a work shift. Among cotton workers, 28% had a reduction of 0.2 liters or more in $FEV_{1.0}$, while 13% of jute workers experienced such a reduction. Dust concentrations and other parameters were similar for the two groups. The effects of hemp were examined in a group of 102 female, nonsmoking workers.[112] Symptoms of byssinosis were found in 39% of the workers. A higher prevalence of chronic bronchitis was found in the byssinotics. $FEV_{1.0}$ decreased during the work shift in both byssinotics and nonbyssinotics. A chronic effect of hemp dust on ventilatory function was indicated by comparison with a control group. Dust concentrations were 6.2–26.9 mg/m^3 respirable (as sampled by a horizontal elutriator meeting the Johannesburg criteria).

Another study ranked biologic acitivity of cotton, flax, hemp, jute, and sisal by comparing five groups of nonsmoking female workers exposed to similar dust concentrations.[113] The total dust concentrations varied from 16 mg/m^3 in the hemp mill to 1.9 mg/m^3 in the sisal mill; respirable dust concentrations, from 1.8 mg/m^3 in the hemp mill to 0.6 mg/m^3 in the cotton mill. Byssinosis symptoms were found in 39% of the hemp workers, 40% of the flax workers, 11% of the cotton workers, and none of the sisal or jute workers. The hemp, flax, and cotton workers also had more chronic respiratory symptoms than controls. Monday reductions in $FEV_{1.0}$ were 19% in hemp workers, 11% in flax, 8% in cotton, 7% in sisal, and 5% in jute. A mixed exposure to hemp and flax dust in high concentrations (14–16 mg/m^3) resulted in 80% byssinosis in the mill with 2/3 flax, and 47% in the mill with 2/3 hemp.[114] Almost half the byssinotic workers had grade 2 or 3 symptoms. The two mixtures were compared with hemp only[112] and flax only[115] and the mixtures were found to have about the same acute effect as flax, while the effect of "hemp only" appeared somewhat greater.

Braun et al.[116] studied a stratified random sample of United States cotton textile mills belonging to the American Textile Manufacturers Institute. The study was structured to represent four grades of cottons and three card speeds, each with and without card ventilation. Air samples were collected by high volume samples at a number of locations in each plant. Dust that passed through a screen ahead of the filter was designated as "fines"; that collected on the screen was "fly." A very weak correlation was observed between chest tightness or decrease in $FEV_{1.0}$ on the one hand, and card speed or cotton grade on the other hand, even though both the latter were related to dust concentration. Exhausting of the card machines reduced prevalence of symptoms only from 25% to 19% and of signs from 26% to 17%. If tightness in the chest on any Monday, a drop of more than 10% in the $FEV_{1.0}$, and an $FEV_{1.0}$ less than 80% of predicted were considered as abnormalities; then 49% of the carders were "normal," 34% had one abnormality, 12% had two abnormalities, and 5% had all three abnormalities. Length of service was directly related to a decline in $FEV_{1.0}$ on Mondays as well as to an $FEV_{1.0}$ less than 80% of predicted. Smoking had little effect on either prevalence or degree of positive findings. The reliability of the questionnaire in determining chest tightness was considered somewhat less than 50%. The authors concluded that two to three times as many carders as noncarders were affected by the occupational respiratory condition studied.

An historical note is provided by Bouhuys et al.[117] They examined a restored flax mill at Philipsburg Manor, North Tarrytown, New York, where flax is processed in a barn as in colonial times. Exposure to the dust for about 5 hr caused minor symptoms of chest tightness in five healthy persons accompanied by decreases in maximum expiratory flow rates. Total dust concentrations were 2.1 mg/m^3, considerably less than those reported in the Yugoslav mills, but they probably were higher in colonial times when operations were performed in winter in closed barns.

A group of female nonsmoking sisal workers was examined for byssinosis.[118] Higher frequencies of persistent cough and phlegm, chronic bronchitis, and nasal catarrh were found in sisal workers than in controls, but no byssinosis was observed. Ventilatory function parameters decreased significantly over the work shift in sisal workers, but not in controls. Extracts of the sisal dust released histamine from pig and human but not from rat tissue,[115] suggesting that histamine release might be the cause of acute ventilatory capacity changes in sisal dust exposure.

The effect of cotton dust has been investigated in cotton gins and in a mattress factory,[45] but reports are not yet published.

DDT [2,2-BIS(p-CHLOROPHENYL)-1,1,1-TRICHLOROETHANE]

Agriculture provides one of the principal interfaces of the worker and the community. Exposure to persistent pesticides, such as DDT among production workers and insecticide applicators, may give some indication of the effect of much lower levels on the general population. A study of 31 production workers exposed to 3.6–18 mg DDT daily for an average of 21 years was done by Laws et al.[119] The same workers had been studied in 1966, but were restudied for liver function because of animal studies demonstrating DDT-induced effects on the liver. A series of liver function tests and detailed history failed to show any evidence of DDT-induced hepatotoxicity, hepatic enlargement, or liver dysfunction. DDT workers have shown increased activity of hepatic microsomal enzymes, but "there is no evidence that this effect is detrimental to health, nor is it qualitatively different from the enzyme stimulations produced by drugs, other pesticides, foods, or food additives."

A group of persons occupationally exposed to DDT and Lindane was examined by Kolmodin-Hedman et al.[120] The DDT exposures were to nurserymen who received dermal exposure from planting trees dipped in a 1% DDT solution and three groups of fishermen exposed to DDT in the flesh of fish from the Baltic sea. The plasma p,p-DDT was 10 ng/ml, compared with 654 ng/ml in the production workers of Laws et al.[119] Plasma p,p-DDE was 15 ng/ml compared with 598 ng/ml in the production workers. In the fishermen, plasma p,p-DDE averaged 31 ng/ml, and the p,p-DDT in plasma averaged 14 ng/ml. No health effects were found in either the nurserymen or the fishermen.

DICHLORVOS (DDVP)

A study was made of 13 workers exposed to DDVP vapors while processing a DDVP releasing product.[121] The employees were exposed to an average concentration of 0.7 mg/m^3 for a period of 8 months, with the highest value recorded being 3 mg/m^3. During the period of production, the cholinesterase activity in plasma (ChE) was inhibited by approximately 60%, while the erythrocyte acetylcholinesterase (AChE) was reduced by an average of 35%. Age and sex had no influence on the cholinesterase-inhibiting effect of DDVP and there were no differences between the mean DDVP concentrations in the two buildings, nor did the long working hours in the processing building (up to 216 hours per month) have any effect. The authors believe the 1 mg/m^3 limit in force in the United States and elsewhere is adequate, and that cholinesterase monitoring should be performed to protect workers. The cholinesterases of these workers returned to initial levels within 1 month after cessation of exposure. All other hematologic, biochemical, and urinalysis measurements during the exposure "were considered to be within physiological limits." One wonders whether routine reduction of cholinesterases by a factor of two would be considered universally acceptable for long periods of time.

DIPHENYL

Hakkinen *et al.*[122] report a study of 31 workers in a plant producing diphenyl-impregnated paper for wrapping citrus fruit. When the investigation was instigated by the death of a worker, concentrations in the paper machine room varied from 4.4 to 128 mg/m^3, and were 74.5 mg/m^3 while the "oilman" was adding diphenyl to the paraffin oil. Twenty-two men were examined neurophysiologically and nine were hospitalized. Of the twenty-two men examined, only three were without pathologic findings and of the nine hospitalized, five had liver damage.

The authors point out that the diphenyl producer was somewhat responsible, having stated in his technical bulletin that "Laboratory and practical investigations have shown that diphenyl is completely harmless in quantities several times greater than that to which workers are exposed in the manufacture or use of diphenyl impregnated paper." Although this statement was proven false, the authors cannot attest to the safety of the TLV of 1 mg/m^3, considering that concentrations were so far above it. The prognosis of the poisoning at the time of the paper was still unknown, as some patients were still deteriorating.

It is hoped that a study will be conducted on workers exposed to levels at or below the TLV to attest to its safety. Monitoring air concentrations at any operation where diphenyl is impregnated on paper should be considered mandatory.

FARMER'S LUNG

Farmer's lung is an occupational disease caused by inhalation of moldy hay or other moldy matter. Like many other agricultural problems, it is diffuse, difficult to study and to prevent. Morgan *et al.*[123] report a community survey in Devon, England among 91 farmers and their families. A questionnaire and a blood sample were used. Precipitin reactions to the fungus *Micropolyspora faeni* occurred in the serums of 35 of 124 persons. Nonsmokers had more positive serologic results than smokers. Of the men, 35% of those with breathlessness had positive serology compared with 28% of the positives who did not report such attacks. Some also had attacks of shivering with breathlessness. Of 22 men with a past serious illness, 10 had positive precipitins. Six persons were known to their practitioners to have had farmer's lung. Five reported attacks of breathlessness associated with fever and shivering, and four reported shortness of breath when hurrying on the level. All six were farming actively and wore some kind of mask at times during their work. The authors believe that some persons with negative serology probably had had farmer's lung, based on their symptoms.

The study presents an interesting problem—one which would be formidable for a manufacturing operation—but no suggestions for prevention.

FERROSILICON

Pneumoconiosis in ferrosilicon workers has been reported previously, and Swensson *et al.*[124] present a follow-up of 10 workers diagnosed as having silicosis by Bruce in a small melting plant in 1937. Follow-up examination in 1943–1944 is now reported. They found that silicosis as a diagnosis could be supported in only one case. The disease regressed in those who had roentgenograms 7–8 years later; of the seven who have died, only one (of two autopsies) had silicosis by autopsy. Although the authors exclude silicosis, no conclusion can be drawn as to other hazards of amorphous silica fume at this time.

FIBROUS GLASS

The analogy between the mineral fibers of asbestos and the skin irritation experienced from handling fibrous glass is probably a major cause of the recurring interest in possible long-term effects of this material. For example, Gross *et al.*[125] report on a study of the lungs of 20 deceased fibrous glass workers with exposures ranging from 16 to 32 years. Average dust content of lungs of the fibrous glass workers was 2.0%, close to the average for Pittsburgh residents of 2.1%. The average fiber content of dry lung was 95,000/gm of dry dust, compared with 105,000/gm of dry lung in Pittsburgh residents. Average diameters of fibers were 2.0 and 2.0 μm in glass workers and Pittsburghers, respectively, and lengths were 27 and 23 μm for the two groups. There was one case of lung cancer among the 20 glass workers and none in the 26 controls. No relationship between duration or severity of exposure and lung fiber concentration could be established. No consistent difference in any respect could be established between the glass workers' lungs and those of the Pittsburgh residents.

Nasr et al.[126] examined 2028 workers employed in a glass factory, more than half of them employed for more than 10 years. Approximately 16% were found to have radiographic abnormalities; increased lung markings, abnormal aorta, emphysema, and abnormal heart were the most frequent. The prevalence of abnormalities was about equally associated with increasing age and duration of employment. No difference in prevalence of abnormalities could be found between office workers and production workers.

Another group of 70 production workers was compared with a control group by Hill et al.[127] The workers had an average exposure of 19.85 years and were matched with the controls for age, sex, height, weight, and location of residence. Radiography, the British Medical Research Council's respiratory symptom questionnaire, and pulmonary function measurements were compared. Statistical analysis showed the control group to be at a slight disadvantage with respect to complaints of phlegm and forced vital capacity. There is no evidence of any respiratory hazard from glass fiber.

As in previous volumes of this treatise, all studies on fibrous glass have produced negative findings. It is reassuring to have relatively continuous surveillance of this type; one can only hope that materials which are known hazards will be examined as frequently.

FLUORIDES

The production of aluminum, by electrolysis of alumina (Al_2O_3) in cryolite (Na_3AlF_6), has always had fluoride exposures in the pot rooms where electrolysis takes place. A health study of pot room workers at two facilities is reported by Kaltreider et al.[128] The Niagara Falls Works was one of the early aluminum reduction plants, and a survey of pot room workers was done in 1945–1946 prior to termination of the unit. Estimated average 8-hr exposures to airborne fluoride varied from 2.4 to 6.0 mg/m^3, with one-third to one-half gaseous. The average urine concentration was 8.7–9.8 ppm fluorine. Medical examination of pot room workers revealed no great differences from the control group of laborers, tradesmen, and others, except for slight to moderate limitation of motion of the dorsolumbar spine in 22 of 107 workers. By roentgenogram, however, only 7 employees had no hypertrophic arthritis of the spine, 21 were slight, 2 moderate, and 49 marked. The degree of increase in bone density was normal in 3.8%, slight in 58.3%, moderate in 5.1%, and marked in 33.0%. Ten of 79 workers had calcification of pelvic ligaments and 17 had marked increase in density of ribs. The workers with marked fluorosis of the spine showed rather restricted movements of the spine. There was no restriction of the other joints except for the elbow, which was considered to have traumatic damage because of the continuous handling of heavy tools. The cases of skeletal fluorosis were, in summary, asymptomatic, free of physical impairment and disability.

The Massena facility used the prebake process with one row of pots in each building, but the pots were hooded and exposures were a fraction of those at Niagara Falls. Because of the local nature of the contamination, and the mobility of the workers, the exposure was monitored regularly by urinary fluoride analysis. Fluoride concentrations in the urine were 2.7–4.0 ppm at the first survey in 1960, and 2.1–4.6 in 1970. Concentrations were higher in 1966 and 1967; otherwise they were the same over the 11-year period. A detailed breakdown of occupations and distribution of concentrations reveals nothing startling. After 72 hr away from work, concentrations in 1970 averaged 1.5 ppm. No skeletal fluorosis has yet occurred, and the health status of the pot room workers (as detailed in the report) is equivalent to that of the controls in other respects. The two studies demonstrated that in a modern plant with adequate ventilation and modest fluoride concentrations there is no discernable fluorosis over exposure periods of up to 40 years. No nonskeletal phase of fluorosis could be detected at either plant.

A study of aluminum reduction workers, which will include some exposure to fluorides, is reported to be underway by the National Institute for Occupational Safety and Health.[45]

FOUNDRY MEN

Just as safety standards may either apply to one industry grouping, such as pulp, paper, and paperboard mills, or cut across general industry lines, so some health effects are difficult to classify in terms of a single contaminant. In foundries, for example, with heat, organic smoke, and iron fume as well as dust, it would not seem reasonable to attribute all respiratory disease to silica dust.

A study of British foundries, begun in 1964 and completed in 1965, was reported to the Industrial Health Advisory Committee in 1968 and published in 1971.[129] The survey used the standard British Medical Research Council Questionnaire on Respiratory Symptoms and standard ventilatory function tests. A sample of 1 in 40 of the 130,000 foundry workers was drawn from four size ranges of four types of foundries—iron, steel, nonferrous, and mixed. Some 1780 foundry workers, age 35 to 64, and 1730 factory workers as controls were examined.

A condition called sputum-chest illness was defined, consisting of bronchitis with sputum for 3 months of the year, loss of work and one or more chest illnesses. This condition was found more frequently in foundry workers than in controls, and, in smokers than in nonsmokers.

Only simple pneumoconiosis was seen, and this was found in 14.1% of the foundry floor men, and 34.6% of those in the cleaning room. It was estimated that between 2500 and 7800 men were potentially eligible for industrial injury benefit for pneumoconiosis category 2 or 3.

No dust measurements are mentioned in the excellent short review by McCallum,[130] but the report itself is well worth obtaining for those interested in foundries.

An additional hazard noted for foundries by Mintz and Fraga[131] is severe osteoarthritis of the elbow in workers who use tongs for lifting and twisting metal rods. There was an average loss of 45° for extension and 60° for flexion in these workers.

A mortality study of 5000 foundry workers is reported to be underway in the National Institute for Occupational Safety and Health.[45]

GAS WORKERS

With the decreasing supply of natural gas, and the gradual moves toward coal gasification in the United States, it is instructive to have a long-term study completed in England. A 12-year study was conducted in four area gas boards, and 8 years' mortality experience are available from an additional four. Doll *et al.*[132] reported on 2444 coal-carbonizing process workers and 579 process and maintenance workers in chemical and by-products plants in the four original gas works, and 4687 men in the four additional works. An excess of lung, bladder, and scrotal cancer was observed in the carbonizing workers. It appeared to make little difference whether the retorts were vertical, horizontal, or mixed. In the four additional gas boards, the lung cancer death rate was as high or higher in those intermittently exposed as in those exposed full time. The data are consistent with those of Lloyd[99] relating to coke oven workers and, with similar data from Japanese gas works, amply demonstrate that exposure to coal tar particulates will give rise to lung cancer. It is of interest that even in this high risk group of gas workers, 60% of the expected lung cancer deaths are the result of cigarette smoking.

Cancer of the bladder was $2\frac{1}{2}$ times the national rate. It is known that β-naphthylamine is present, but a measurement of airborne concentrations results in a calculated amount that might have been achieved by smoking one cigarette per day. However, the bladder cancer victims may have been more highly exposed, and may also have had skin absorption.

Scrotal cancer was present only in men who had worked in the gas houses prior to 1925, before any hygienic precautions were taken.

The excess of chronic bronchitis found in the first four gas works was not present in the additional works, and cannot be considered a proven hazard.

These studies point out the care with which coal gasification plants, shale oil plants, and other operations in which tars are involved will have to be designed and operated to prevent lung cancers in the next generation of workers.

GRAIN

Respiratory abnormalities from grain handling were investigated by Tse *et al.*[133] They surveyed 68 grain elevator agents within 110 km of Winnipeg, Manitoba. More than 75% of the agents had respiratory symptoms. Chronic cough, sputum production, and shortness of breath associated with grain dust were common. More than half the smokers and exsmokers and a quarter of the nonsmokers reported these symptoms. In 19 of the 68 (28%), flu-like symptoms of malaise, muscle aches, and headaches and even chills and fever developed some hours after exposure to grain dust; these symptoms have sometimes been called grain fever. The fever bore no relationship to the dyspnea which developed on exposure to grain dust. Skin irritation (32%), eye irritation (49%), and nasal catarrh (62%) were also commonly associated with exposure to grain dust.

Abnormal ventilatory function was found by spirometry in 41% of the smokers, 36% of the exsmokers, and 27% of the nonsmokers. Abnormalities in closing volume measurement were found in 42% of the elevator agents.

Only 8 of the 68 agents reacted positively to prick skin testing with grain mill dust extract, and there was no correlation between positive skin tests and either symptoms or abnormal lung function.

The seeds stored in the elevators included wheat, corn, barley, rye, buckwheat, flax, rape, and less commonly, pea, sunflower, and mustard. Rye, flax, and rape had been most common in recent years. The elevator agents themselves felt that old or moldy grain, oats, and barley were particularly liable to cause respiratory symptoms. Although most grain is mechanically loaded, it still creates much dust and final emptying is often done by hand. Masks were usually provided but seldom used, because they are uncomfortable during heavy exertion. Dust-collecting apparatus is not helpful while shoveling grain. This is another of the problems for which some combination of personal protection, education, and revision of procedures is going to be necessary to protect the health of the workers.

GRANITE

A survey of monument workers in Aberdeen, Scotland is reported by Lloyd Davies *et al.*[134] The medical study consisted of chest radiography; the environmental survey included high volume samples for general air, and personal size-selecting samplers for respirable dust. The investigators found 3% of "all occupations" or 4.6% of "dusty" workers to have category 1 or greater pneumoconiosis. Only 4.1% had category 2 silicosis, and none had category 3. The hazard among monument workers does not appear to have increased in recent years as sheds have been enclosed and local exhaust ventilation has been added. Respirable dust averaged less than $2 \, mg/m^3$. The quartz content of respirable dust was not measured, but assuming it to be one-third that of the total dust, the average TLV, using the formula of the American Conference of Governmental Industrial Hygienists, was equal to the average respirable dust concentration.

Pulmonary function among the granite shed workers in Vermont is reported by Theriault *et al.*[135] and related to roentgenographic changes[136] as well as to worker dust exposure in the sheds.[137] Current dust exposure was estimated by personal, respirable dust samples on 784 workers in 13 occupational groups in 49 sheds, and 483 of the samples were directly analyzed for quartz. A lifetime estimate of dust exposure was calculated for each worker from the dust concentration data and a complete occupational history. The "dust-year" was selected from among various indices tested as that most closely related to changes in forced vital capacity (FVC). Based on the large number of samples, they calculated a concentration for each occupational group in each shed, and used the previous studies of dustiness in these same sheds to estimate exposures of older workers. Because it seemed more direct and relevant, they favored a limit directly in $\mu g/m^3$ of quartz rather than in mg/m^3 of dust based on the percentage of quartz.

The ventilatory function in the Vermont granite workers was correlated with age, height, smoking, and dust. It was found that 1 dust year ($523 \, \mu g/m^3$ of granite dust for 1 year) produced a decrease of $2 \, cm^3$ in the FVC. Thus a carver or pneumatic-handtool operator could be expected to lose 2.8% of his forced vital capacity in a 45-year exposure. A dose-response curve between granite dust and quartz showed a 50% point to be at 32.5 dust years and 35 quartz years, suggesting that quartz in granite is not as harmful as total granite.

Roentgenographic findings were that 28% of the workers had profusion grade

1 or more, 7% had profusion grade 2 or more, and 0.3% had profusion grade 3. If rounded opacities of profusion grade 2 or more are considered silicosis, then silicosis could be said to have existed in 5.7% of these workers by x ray. The rounded opacities appeared related to dust, the irregular opacities were more coincidental with smoking. Drawing a dose-response curve, the 50% point was observed at 46 dust-years, or 13.5 years later than the similar point from the FVC curve.

The authors make no recommendations in these papers as to the desirable limit for granite dust or for quartz.

GRAPHITE

A survey of 344 workers in a graphite mine was carried out by Ranasinha and Uragoda.[138] The 308 men in the study worked underground (at a depth of 670 m) and the 36 women were on the surface in the curing shed where the graphite is separated from the rock. The prevalence of radiographic abnormalities by chest x ray was 22% in the men and 25% in the women. A control population had only 2% abnormalities. Of the workers with radiographic abnormalities, 19% had respiratory symptoms, the most common being dyspnea. Finger clubbing was noted in 22%. Only one man, with massive fibrosis, was disabled to the extent that it hindered his work. Chronic bronchitis is uncommon in Ceylon, so the authors believed that predisposing factors were not present. They consider the condition to be a graphite pneumoconiosis.

There are no dust measurements available, nor is even a qualitative description of dustiness given. Although synthetic graphite is listed by the Threshold Limit Values Committee as an inert dust, it is evident that this is not the case for natural graphite.

GUM ACACIA

An outbreak of rhinitis and asthma in the summer of 1970 in a small printing plant was investigated by Cuthbert.[139] Sixteen men were involved, and gum acacia was implicated as a possible cause. The substance was used in an offset lotion and its presence was determined in the environment by air sampling. Two men gave positive skin and nasal provocation responses to gum acacia. The authors believe that the extent to which gum acacia remains a hazard requires further investigation.

HAIR SPRAY LACQUER

The existence of pulmonary infiltration caused by hair spray lacquer (thesaurosis) is debatable. Gowdy and Wagstaff[140] surveyed beauty operators in the Washington, D.C. area. In a preliminary survey, 227 beauticians were examined; only 96 of these could be obtained on a resurvey 5 years later. A high prevalence of pulmonary abnormalities was noted (31%), but in only 11 (5%) was thesaurosis suspected. The authors review the problems in diagnosis of thesaurosis and conclude that it can only be made by exclusion. The results of their survey were not sufficient to draw any general conclusions.

A mortality study of 10,000 Connecticut workers and a prevalence study of 800 beauticians is reported to be underway in the National Institute for Occupational Safety and Health.[45]

IRON OXIDE

The pulmonary function of 14 workers in a plant manufacturing pure red iron oxide (rouge) was investigated by Tecelescu and Albu.[141] The workers were selected from a group with opacities on their chest x rays. The results of the pulmonary function tests were all considered negative by the authors. This was in spite of measured concentrations of iron oxide from 10 to 15 mg/m^3 in the reaction room, 45 to 700 mg/m^3 in the drying room, 306 to 770 mg/m^3 in the calcination room, and 330 to 500 mg/m^3 in the packing room.

Graham Jones and Warner, in their study,[70] considered a predominantly iron oxide exposure to be mixed fume because of the chromium oxide (see section on chromium oxide) and nickel oxide present in the fume. Thus it cannot be concluded from either of these studies that iron oxide is an occupational health hazard. Nevertheless, it would be prudent to keep concentrations below 10 mg/m^3 as recommended by the Threshold Limit Value Committee, and OSHA regulations require that concentrations in the United States average below 15 mg/m^3.

LEAD

The number of occupational lead poisonings reported and compensated in West Germany is tabulated by Neubert.[142] Although the nature of the data is such that rates cannot be calculated, the number of cases reported has dropped, and the lost-time per case, as represented by compensation, has dropped. From 1950 to 1960, the drop paralleled that in other occupational accidents and disease; from 1960 on, it dropped at a more rapid rate. In 1950, lead poisoning was 27.3% of all occupational diseases reported; in 1968, it was 20.4%.

All three storage battery factories in Finland and the five storage battery repair shops in Helsinki were surveyed by Tola et al.[143] Blood leads averaged 68 μg/dl and 60 μg/dl in the two factories, 52 μg/dl in the assembling shop, and 35 μg/dl in the repair shops. The most heavily exposed occupations were the lead oxide mill and paste mixing at 79 μg/dl. In the two factories some 44% of the workers had blood lead concentrations above the Finnish limit of 70 μg/dl. The authors conclude that storage battery work is a high risk occupation and should be kept under close medical and technical supervision.

The lead absorption in Finnish garages and service stations was investigated by Tola et al.[144] In 10 of 80 service stations and 13 of 118 garages, all workers were examined. Average blood lead concentrations in garages were 35 μg/dl, higher than the 21 μg/dl in the service stations. Two workers were found above the Finnish limit of 70 μg/dl, but their excessive lead was difficult to explain. The most exposed workers used molten lead to smooth surfaces of dented bodies. The authors believe the blood lead results to be low compared with other industrialized countries.

The δ-aminolevulinic acid dehydrase (ALA dehydrase) activity in 27 tetraethyllead manufacturing employees was found by Millar et al.[145] to be significantly lower than a control group (220 versus 677) while the blood lead was significantly higher in the production workers (42.5 μg/dl versus 15 μg/dl). All workers were within recommended blood lead limits of 80 μg/dl, and no clinical effects were manifested. "The results suggest that exposure to tetraethyllead can cause a decrease in erythrocyte ALA-dehydrase activity."

A group of 33 new workers just starting in two storage battery factories with poor hygiene in some departments (up to 2, 3, and 4 mg/m^3 Pb in air) was followed with a battery of tests by Tola et al.[146] It was found that blood lead rose and ALA-dehydrase fell with no demonstrable time lag, while the latency periods of urinary ALA, urinary lead, and urinary coproporphyrin concentrations were about 2 weeks each. All indices reached a steady state during follow-up. ALA-dehydrase showed the highest correlation to blood lead and proved to be the most sensitive indicator. Although both the urinary coproporphyrin and ALA were useful, coproporphyrins had a better explaining power. Mean hemoglobin values were lower at the end of the 100-day period, providing an indication that anemia begins to develop early.

A governmental committee was appointed under the chairmanship of Lord Windeyer[147] to inquire into circumstances that gave rise to lead poisoning at the RTZ smelter at Avonmouth. A summary of the report is given by Bonnell.[148] Lead concentrations in the smelter were well above the ACGIH TLV of 0.2 mg/m^3 used in England; in fact as many as 62% of the readings were more than 10 times the TLV, with some individual samples above 45 mg/m^3.

Considerable reliance was placed on respiratory protection. Recommendations were made for more frequent biologic monitoring, but mainly for improvements in the exposure situation at the smelter. There is considerable emphasis on the need to distinguish between lead poisoning and lead absorption.

Tsuchiya et al.[149] examined 58 workers in electric wire production exposed to an average of 12 $\mu g/m^3$ for 6 hr per day, 6 days per week. The examination included blood-specific gravity, hemoglobin, hematocrit, urinary copro-porphyrins, protein, δ-ALA, and blood lead. "All of the items, except for the red blood system, did not show any difference from those of control workers." The authors concluded that "the exposure to 12 $\mu g/ms^3$ of lead in the air 6 hr a day for 6 days a week would not produce any biological responses so far."

Nineteen printing shops in Helsinki, representing 10% of the total, were studied by Hernberg et al.[150] There were 105 workers in the exposed group, including all workers in the small shops and a sample in the large shops. Blood was analyzed for lead and ALA-D in subjects and 23 controls, and urine was analyzed for ALA in the exposed only. The mean blood lead concentration for smelters was 38 $\mu g/dl$, for typesetters 29 $\mu g/dl$, and for controls 10 $\mu g/dl$. These differences were statistically significant as were inhibitions of ALA-D among exposed workers. Urine ALA was not useful. It was concluded that risk of lead poisoning was minimal with the possible exception of smelters who should have annual examinations.

LINDANE

Samuels and Milby,[151] following up on a previous study, looked at 71 workers in two plants processing Lindane-containing products and eight persons (including seven children) in homes using Lindane-vaporizing devices for insect control. The workers had been exposed to Lindane for several months to several years. Comprehensive clinical and laboratory appraisals were conducted to detect, if possible, any clinical or laboratory evidence of disease attributable specifically to Lindane, particularly with reference to hematopoietic depression and renal or hepatic dysfunction. No clinical symptomatology nor physical evidence of disease clearly attributable to this exposure could be demonstrated. Elevation in mean monocyte counts and uric acid levels was shown, but could not be related to blood Lindane content or duration of Lindane exposure.

Milby and Samuels[152] compared the above exposed group to a control group of health department employees matched for sex, race, and age. Statistically significant differences were observed in blood Lindane content, blood creatinine level, reticulocyte count, white blood cell count, and polymorphonuclear leukocyte count. All levels except blood Lindane were in the normal range. None of the differences gave any indication of evidence of hypoplastic or aplastic anemia. Not seeing any differences relevant to this, they concluded that "within the limits of this study, Lindane does not appear to produce hematologic disorders on a basis of toxic suppression of hematopoiesis." Blood Lindane levels in the exposed group averaged 11.9 parts per billion compared with 0.1 ppb for the control group.

Spray men exposed to Lindane were examined by Kolmodin-Hedman et al.[120] The men did not always wear gloves and masks, so there was the possibility of both respiratory and dermal exposure. The spray men were routinely examined for health status, and laboratory examinations were also made. All were healthy except two suffering from a Lindane skin allergy. The median Lindane concentration in one group was 6.4 ng/ml, while the other two groups had means of 7.5 and 9.9 ng/ml. No hematologic changes or neurologic symptoms were noted. The men had blood levels of Lindane similar to those of the production workers of Milby and Samuels.

MANGANESE

Overexposures to manganese in dry battery manufacture, resulting in chronic manganese poisoning, are reported by Emara et al.[153] Thirty-six workers were exposed to dust containing 60–70% manganese oxide. Dust concentrations averaged 6.8 mg/m^3 in the compressing area and 33–42 mg/m^3 in the mixing area. Under these conditions, eight workers (22%) had neuropsychiatric manifestations; six (17%) of these had chronic manganese psychoses, one had left hemiparkinsonism, and one had left choreoathetosis. The manganese level in blood was almost within the normal range. Urine coproporphyrin was normal. The period of exposure of the affected workers was 1–16 years. The three affected workers with the longest exposures (10, 13, and 16 years) worked in the compression department where concentrations were only about one-seventh those in the mixing department and, in fact, may not have been much above the TLV. The longest exposure in the mixing room of an affected employee was 7 years.

Another group of workers with high exposure at a manganese alloy foundry is reported by Jonderko et al.[154] Manganese concentrations in air were up to "125 multiple MAC"* (no detailed environmental data are given). Blood manganese levels were greater than the 20 μg/% used as a working threshold for manganese retention in 46 of 119 workers. Differences in exposed workers were found in a number of biochemical tests. All exposed workers had at least one positive test,

* The "MAC," presumably a maximum allowable concentration, is not given by the authors.

and 37 of 46 had three or more positive tests, whereas no controls had as many as three positive tests. Upon removing the workers from exposure, the blood levels returned to normal rather rapidly, but the neurologic symptoms did not improve as quickly.

An excellent study, combining thorough environmental assessments and medical examinations, is reported by Smyth et al.[155] A ferromanganese facility had been in operation since 1923. Excessively dusty conditions formerly existed at crushing with concentrations up to over 1000 mg/m^3. After a mandatory respirator program, dust concentrations were reduced by enclosure and local exhaust ventilation of the operations to well within the TLV. However, at casting operations, high concentrations of fume to which certain employees were exposed regularly existed for 20–30 min during the cast. There was also exposure to fume at the pig casting machine which lasted for $1\frac{1}{2}$–2 hr per pouring operation (5 times per 24-hr period). Fifteen positions were sampled, nine at the production (fume) area, and six at the dust area. Sampling was by a combination of breathing zone and personal samples. All workers but the pig caster were under 5 mg/m^3 as a time-weighted average, but almost all of the men were over the ceiling limit a substantial number of times. In the crushing and screening plant, the TLV was exceeded at three of the six positions. The clinical study involved 71 men in 15 positions on three shifts and an equal number of matched controls from nonmanganese exposure areas of the plant. Examination of the 142 employees elicited five cases with signs and symptoms of central nervous impairment suggestive of manganism. All were from the exposed group, and all but one occurred in positions of highest manganese exposure. Large amounts of manganese were excreted in the urine after treatment with calcium EDTA. Two of the cases regained normal associated arm movements. The other three did not regain function, but have not progressed in the following six years with no further exposure to manganese. The authors stress the fact that blood and urine concentrations of manganese are poor indicators of exposure, and the value of periodic medical examinations for exposed workers. In particular, they note that one of the five employees with manganism apparently had a relatively low exposure.

MERCURY

A study of 25 workers exposed to mercury in a chlorine plant by Hernberg et al.[156] demonstrated that mercury exposure had no effect on erythrocyte δ-aminolevulinic acid dehydratase at the levels encountered. They suggest that general population mercury exposures would not interfere with ALA-D as a lead absorption index.

Danziger and Possick[157] studied 75 workers in 13 laboratory glassware manufacturing plants in New Jersey. Concentrations averaged 0.08 mg/m³ Hg overall, with four plants averaging 0.1 mg/m³ or more. Only one of 13 plants possessed an effective local exhaust ventilation system, only four of 13 had properly designed workbenches, and only 2 of 13 had properly constructed floors. Only one of the 75 workers showed a tremor; however, he also had a number of other mercury symptoms. Other than this worker, no other could be definitely diagnosed by signs and symptoms. It was noted that 59 of 75 workers were myopic as determined by the Snellen test. Six workers showed presence of proteinuria. Urine mercury concentrations varied from 0 to 2.2 mg per liter. The authors emphasize the preventable nature of the conditions they encountered, and the need for adequate environmental control.

Bell *et al.*[158] describe mercury exposure evaluations of four workers by personal sampling, using a monitoring train developed for the purpose. Substantial mercury exposure fluctuations were noted, and the possibility of mercury exposure from contaminated clothing is suggested. Personal sampling appears advisable in these circumstances.

Lovejoy *et al.*[159] examined the eyes of 68 men who worked in cell areas of two chlor-alkali plants. They found no cases of mercurialentis. They conclude that mercurialentis does not occur at urine levels of less than 1.0 mg/liter. Because the condition is considered permanent, they suggest that employees with potential high exposure to mercury should have regular ophthalmologic examinations.

A group of 40 technicians exposed to mercury vapor at an average level of 0.03 mg/m³ was examined by Lauwerys and Buchet.[160a] They detected the following changes: increased blood and urine mercury concentrations, increased plasma galactosidase and plasma catalase activities, and decreased red blood cell (RBC) cholinesterase activity. Weak but statistically significant correlations were found between air and urine mercury and, on a group basis, the RBC cholinesterase activity was related to intensity of exposure. They conclude that 0.05 mg/m³ Hg in air would correspond to about 50 μg/liter in urine. They therefore suggest that a group mean urine mercury concentration of 50 μg/liter should trigger corrective industrial hygiene action.

METHYL *n*-BUTYL KETONE

An extensive investigation by the Ohio State Department of Health and the National Institute for Occupational Safety and Health of a number of cases of peripheral neuropathy in a coated fabrics plant has identified exposures to methyl *n*-butyl ketone as the most likely cause. Detailed results of the investigation had not been published at the time this section was assembled, although a report has been presented.[160b]

METHYLENE CHLORIDE (DICHLOROMETHANE)

The safety of methylene chloride (dichloromethane) as a solvent is challenged by the evidence that it is converted to carbon monoxide in the body. Ratney *et al.*[161] investigated the effect of methylene chloride on four workers in a plastic film plant. The three investigators also were sampled. The workers had been exposed 8 hr per day, 6 days per week for several years to these concentrations.

Air samples were taken during a continuous 42-hr period while the plant was operating without interruption. Alveolar air samples were taken from the workers at regular intervals during a 24-hr period beginning 18 hr after air sampling had started. All alveolar air samples were analyzed for CO, and some were analyzed for methylene chloride.

Workroom air concentrations averaged 286 ppm on the day before alveolar air sampling and 183 ppm on the day of sampling. Alveolar carbon monoxide in the four nonsmoking workers averaged 29 and 33 ppm at the start of the 2 days. After 5 hr of exposure the average alveolar CO was 48 ppm, and it reached a plateau of 52 ppm at 7 hr. After cessation of exposure, the concentration dropped exponentially, but the rate was slower than in subjects exposed experimentally to methylene chloride.

The authors calculate that the 180 ppm CH_2Cl_2 exposure resulted in a 24-hr average carboxyhemoglobin concentration about double that produced by an 8 hr exposure to 50 ppm CO. Thus, the methylene chloride concentration should be kept below 75–100 ppm to make it equivalent to the CO limit.

The 1973 TLV (intended change since 1972) was 250 ppm. The OSHA Standard, taken from the American National Standards Institute, was 500 ppm average, 1000 ppm ceiling, and 2000 ppm peak (5 min each 2 hr).

NEWSPAPER WORKERS

A mortality study of 3485 newspaper workers in London and Manchester who died in the period 1952–1966 was analyzed for occupation and cause of death.[162,163] The printing trade workers had a moderate but statistically significant excess of cancer of the lung and bronchus in both cities. White collar workers showed no excess in London and an excess that was not statistically significant in Manchester. There appeared to be a concentration of lung cancer deaths (about 100% excess) in the machine room men in Manchester, but not in

London. The origin of the excess could not be determined. The possibility of excess smoking being responsible is discounted by the fact the bronchitis deaths are rather less than expected, whereas they ordinarily occur in greater frequency among smokers.

Greenberg,[164] in investigating a rumored bladder cancer excess in a London newspaper plant, studied death certificates for the years 1954–1966. Using proportionate mortality, he too came to the conclusion that there was an excess of carcinoma of the bronchus. Only death by suicide was in excess among causes of death other than cancer. He concluded that a prospective study would be required if occupation were to be implicated as a hazard.

NITROGEN OXIDES

Kennedy[165] presented a summary of experience with 100 miners who had exposure to nitrous fumes from shotblasting in coal mines. He believed that low exposures to these fumes over a period of years was associated with development of an emphysemalike condition. Many miners who developed acute pulmonary edema or severe acute chest illness also had prolonged exposure to fumes and subsequently developed emphysema. No control population was used.

A group of 70 male workers exposed to nitrogen oxides in a chemical factory at levels of 0.4–2.7 ppm were studied by Kosmider and Misiewicz.[166] The control group was 80 healthy nonexposed people. Total, free, and esterified cholesterol, lipids and lipidogram were investigated. The exposed group had increased levels of serum total lipids, β- and γ-lipoproteins as well as a fall in α-lipoproteins. The authors concluded that chronic exposure to nitrogen oxides causes impaired lipid metabolism in humans and animals. The problem of a possible effect of nitrogen oxides on arteriosclerotic processes needs further investigation.

OIL MIST

Pasternack and Ehrlich[167] present results of a 12-year mortality study of pressmen and compositors. For unexplained reasons, pressmen who were first employed at 40 or more years of age and worked 20 or more years had significantly higher death rates than compositors. No such significant difference was found for pressmen employed before the age of 40. Although the pressmen were exposed to more than 5 mg/m^3 of oil mist, the respirable fraction was less than 5 mg/m^3.

Speculation concerning the reason for increased scrotal cancer in the

Birmingham, England area was expressed by Waterhouse.[168,169] He noted the presence of oil mist in a number of light engineering shops. Men with scrotal cancer also had a higher frequency of other cancers. A detailed study of oil mist and scrotal cancer in the light engineering factories was underway.

Lee et al.[170] also considered scrotal cancer, but in northwest England. Of 103 cases of scrotal cancer between 1962 and 1968, occupational histories were obtained on 89. Fifty-one had been mule spinners. Another 19 had worked in other industries with a recognized scrotal cancer hazard; among these, the authors included machine shop occupations with oil or oil mist, as well as tar, exposures. They particularly noted automatic lathe operating, road making, dye making, and chain making.

The changes in composition of American oils suggest that surveillance should be maintained on workers who may have heavy exposures to oil mist.

PARATHION

The absorption of Parathion by spraymen in Wenatchee Valley apple orchards was studied by Durham et al.[171] Significant amounts of urinary metabolite, p-nitrophenol, were detected in the urine of spraymen as long as 10 days after the last exposure to Parathion. About 2 days after exposure, excretion was insignificant during late night and early morning hours, but reached higher levels during midday. The height of immediate postexposure excretory peaks and the delayed rises in midday exposure seemed to vary directly with the temperature. Bathing after exposure was accompanied by a rapid decrease in p-nitrophenol excretion. Under the conditions of this study, the dermal route of absorption appeared to be responsible for the greater absorption. However, the authors conclude that, with equivalent absorbed dosages, the respiratory route is the more hazardous.

Guthrie et al.[172] monitored 44 tobacco harvesting workers in Florida through the season. There was Parathion absorption as measured by p-nitrophenol excretion in urine, and up to 5 ppm of toxicant on leaves, but no member of the harvesting teams examined showed significant depression of red blood cell cholinesterase. One worker had slight inhibition of plasma cholinesterase. The authors caution that reentry times and other instructions must be observed to assure prevention of Parathion poisoning.

PARAQUAT

A survey of 296 spray operators on a sugar plantation in Trinidad exposed to diluted Paraquat was carried out by Hearn and Keir.[173] Nail damage was found in

55 of the workers. The most common damage was transverse white bands of discoloration, but loss of nail surface, transverse ridging, gross deformity of the nail plate, and loss of nails also occurred. The index, middle, and ring fingers were most often affected, and this could be ascribed to leakage from the knapsack sprayer. Although diluted Paraquat can cause nail damage, simple hygienic precautions and maintenance of sprayers can prevent its occurrence. Periodic medical examinations are recommended. The nail damage is the result of a local action. Following cessation of exposure, subsequent nail growth is normal.

PESTICIDES

Although animal studies are usually run on single pesticides, and some agricultural workers are only exposed to one or two pesticides, many workers are exposed to a large variety of pesticides. Even when effects are found, it may be difficult to attribute them to a particular pesticide; the situation is common enough to warrant investigation.

A 4-year investigation of pesticide exposures in South Carolina was conducted by Sandifer et al.[174] Exposures of the 120 workers averaged 12 years. The control group was taken from a roofing shingle plant, a phosphoric acid plant, a detergent producer, truck drivers, and firemen. The exposed were divided into five subgroups with diminishing exposure. The blood pressure was elevated in the most intensively exposed formulators and pest control as was plasma DDT and DDE. No significant differences in illnesses, work absences, or death were noted. Several biochemical indices were significantly different in the exposed workers.

A study of Utah workers occupationally exposed to pesticides was reported by Warnick and Carter.[175] The exposed group included 70 men, and the control group had 30 workers. About 50 tests were given every participant each quarter for 4 years. No significant differences in illness or death rate could be found. There were differences in various biochemical tests, but they were not consistent from season to season. No conclusion as to long-term effects could be made.

Neuromuscular function in agricultural workers using pesticides was investigated by Drenth et al.[176] Electromyographic (EMG) examinations were given to 102 men. Abnormal EMG patterns were observed in 40% of the workers. Upon reexamination of 53 workers, about half changed from normal to abnormal or vice versa. All blood cholinesterase activities were within normal limits and were unrelated to EMG status. No special causal agents were identified, and no dose response relationship was established.

The adrenocortical function of a group of Arizona workers was investigated by Morgan and Roan.[177] Occupational exposure of workers averaged 11 years; there were 133 in a group tested for urinary steroids, and 257 tested for serum cortisol. There were no significant effects such as might have been seen if there had been a significant exposure to op' DDD.

The health of workers exposed to a "cocktail of pesticides" was investigated by Ensberg et al.[178] The workers, intensively exposed for more than 4 years, experienced "diminished well-being" (more subjective symptoms). There were no statistically significant differences between workers and controls in physical examination. Small biochemical differences were observed, but these could not be interpreted in terms of health. The authors conclude that in the highly exposed group there very probably existed a *"toxic overload of biological systems* which should be regarded as *unacceptable* from the viewpoint of *occupational* health" (authors' emphasis). The data, however, strengthened the view "that 'normal' everyday exposure has no direct health effect in the general population."

POLYVINYL CHLORIDE

Dinman et al.[179] present the results of an epidemiologic study covering 5011 employees engaged in various phases of vinyl chloride (VC) and polyvinyl chloride (PVC) manufacturing in 32 plants in the United States and Canada. A total of 25 definite and 16 suspicious cases of acroosteolysis was found. The condition was clearly associated with the hand cleaning of polymerizers. Workers engaged in other phases of VC and PVC manufacture were not affected. The importance of Raynaud's phenomenon as a concomitant of acroosteolysis is emphasized. Although neither the etiologic agent nor the portal of entry is known, acroosteolysis appeared to be a systemic rather than a local disease.

Meatwrapper's asthma was first described by Sokol et al.[180] It was reported to be associated with the cutting of polyvinyl chloride film with a hot wire. The wrappers developed respiratory symptoms when exposed and demonstrated reversible airway obstruction on pulmonary function testing. Environmental measurements had not yet been reported.

Angiosarcomas were reported from vinyl chloride production facilities, and an emergency standard for vinyl chloride was adopted by the Occupational Safety and Health Administration in the spring of 1974.[181] Epidemiologic studies were underway,[182] but it would be some time before they were available. In the meantime, extreme caution was being urged on PVC fabricators as well as producers.

POTASH

The mortality of potash miners and millers was investigated by Waxweiler et al.[183] Some 2743 surface workers and 1143 underground workers were included in the analysis. No excesses from lung cancer were noted. There was an unexplainable deficit of other than lung cancer among surface workers. There was an excess of on-the-job fatal accidents among underground miners with less than 15 years' experience. No excess mortality was attributable to the presence of diesel engines in the mines. There was an excess of "other" respiratory disease, which includes silicosis, among underground miners, several of whom had other underground mining experience. There were no excesses of mortality which could be attributed to potash exposure.

PROTEOLYTIC ENZYMES

Mitchell and Gandevia[184] surveyed 98 workers exposed periodically to high concentrations of proteolytic enzymes. They found that symptoms suggestive of asthma developed in 50% of the workers on exposure either within $\frac{1}{2}$ hr, after 4 or 5 hr, or at night. The symptomatic reactors were not well predicted by skin tests. Familial histories of allergies were not particularly helpful, with the exception of a history of food or drug allergy. Smoking or current bronchitis also did not influence the development of symptoms. Tests of ventilatory diffusion capacity showed no evidence of permanent damage in sensitized or unsensitized workers, whether symptomatic or not. Concentrations of enzyme after the first 18 months averaged about 5 glycine units/m^3, with values up to 150 glycine units/m^3 when a major spill occurred.

Weill et al.[185] studied two detergent plants in the United States where enzymes derived from *Bacillus subtilis* were in use. Plant A was a new plant with current dust supression measures, and Plant B was an older plant, where higher concentrations of enzyme, particularly peaks, occurred. "Low" concentrations of enzyme were $<1 \mu g/m^3$ (μg of 3% crystalline subtilisin Carlsberg), "moderate" concentrations were $1-5 \mu g/m^3$ average with peaks to $20 \mu g/m^3$, and "high" concentrations averaged $3-18 \mu g/m^3$ in plant A with peaks to $60 \mu g/m^3$, and $3-30 \mu g/m^3$ and peaks to $1000 \mu g/m^3$ in plant B. Close to half the workers in the moderate and high exposure groups in both factories had positive prick tests. Thirteen of 60 workers in plant B had symptoms indicating lower respiratory tract disease. Eleven had a typical symptom complex including wheezing, tightness in chest, shortness of breath, and cough occurring at night, often several hours after leaving work. Pulmonary function tests in plant A were essentially normal. Seven of the 13 plant B workers with symptoms and 24 of 47 workers without symptoms displayed some evidence of obstructive ventilatory impairment. No statistically significant differences for any of the functional measurements were found between the different exposure groups in plant B, and the only significant difference between plant A and plant B was in the forced expiratory flow in the middle 50% of vital capacity (FEF 25–75). Since the study, control measures at plant B have been markedly improved and both averages and peak levels have been reduced. It was thought that average levels could be reduced to 1 $\mu g/m^3$ or less, which the authors believed would be adequate to prevent respiratory problems.

Another study of enzymes was conducted in two plants in Sweden.[186] Plant A handled enzymes largely without control for almost 3 years. Plant B started with incomplete enclosure of the enzyme mixer, but was increasingly enclosed over the years. In plant A the concentrations were 1.3–10.6 glycine units per cubic meter (GU/m^3). In plant B the concentrations were 45 GU/m^3 in the enzyme room and under 1.2 GU/m^3 in the rest of the plant. An airline respirator and a protective rubber gown were worn by the worker in the enzyme room in plant B. Based on symptoms and sensitivity developed in plant A and some problems before controls were completed in plant B, the authors recommended a time-weighted average limit of 1 GU/m^3 which the authors estimate to be about one-half the 1973 intended change TLV of 0.06 $\mu g/m^3$ pure enzyme. There was no OSHA limit for proteolytic enzyme concentrations in early 1974.

The proteolytic enzymes are of some interest as an industrial sensitizer. It was understood that some, but not all detergent manufacturers had discontinued the addition of enzymes to household detergents. One of the theories[109] about the action of cotton dust suggests that it is proteolytic enzymes that are responsible for at least part of the problem. Since detergent manufacturers can apparently keep concentrations at lower levels, it would seem advisable to reduce the limit to one that does not produce effects.

SILICA

A survey of silicosis in Finland over 30 years was presented by Ahlman.[187] He analyzed 878 cases during the period 1935–1964. Silicosis decreased among miners and in steel foundries, but increased among stone and iron foundry workers. Progression was most rapid in those workers who had the shortest exposure before diagnosis. Progression occurred in about half the miners who stopped mining upon diagnosis. Lung function tests showed reduction of forced vital capacity and the forced expiratory volume with progression to stages II and III. Although the current incidence of silicosis among Finnish workers was not known, it was still considered a problem from the standpoint of occupational health.

Pneumoconioses in Bulgaria from 1950 to 1968 were discussed by Zolov and Dobreva.[188] They reported that dust concentrations have been reduced on average from 10 mg/m^3 to between 2 and 3 mg/m^3 in the last 10 years. Between 1950 and 1968 the number of silicosis cases reported per year decreased by a factor of 15.

Woitowitz et al.[189] proposed that a dust-ranking system rather than absolute dust concentrations be used for epidemiologic studies. They stated that this would give more satisfactory results when complete data were not available.

Phibbs et al.[190] reported a study of silicosis in Wyoming bentonite workers. Dust counts were 2–10 times the ACGIH impinger count TLV. A review of chest x rays of 32 bentonite mill workers revealed 14 cases of silicosis. The confirmed cases of silicosis made it necessary to add Wyoming bentonite to the list of silicosis-producing minerals, because of its free crystalline silica content.

Brinkman et al.[191] reported a study of bronchitis, silica exposure, and ventilatory function. Initially, 1142 men were selected from a group undergoing study in 1959. They were restudied in 1964 and 1970. A total of 301 men completed all three examinations. They were classified into three groups; industrial exposure but no silica dust, at least 20 years' silica dust exposure but normal x ray, and at least 20 years' silica dust exposure with x ray evidence of silicosis. Those who in 1959 were classified as bronchitics having daily cough for at least 6 months with at least a teaspoon of sputum per day remained in that category throughout the study. Both forced expiratory volume in the first second ($FEV_{1.0}$) and maximum midexpiratory flow rate (MMEF) showed a consistent difference between bronchitics and normals. The difference was maintained in 1964 and 1970 with no accelerated decline for bronchitis. The degree of cigarette smoking was classified in 1959 and this classification was maintained throughout the study. There was an inverse relationship between the extent of cigarette smoking and $FEV_{1.0}$ and MMEF, but no accelarated decline for moderate or heavy smokers. The men in group 1 were auto assembly workers; groups 2 and 3 were foundry workers. There was a consistent difference in $FEV_{1.0}$ and MMEF by occupational group, with the assembly line workers highest and the men with silicosis lowest. There was no accelarated decline of ventilatory function in the silicotics. Both $FEV_{1.0}$ and MMEF showed the expected decline with age. Analysis of covariance was used to adjust the samples for age makeup. The adjusted groups showed a more linear decline in MMEF with smoking; adjustment produced a more clearcut difference in MMEF between occupational groups, but it was not statistically significant. The difference between bronchitics and normal lessened with correction for age, but deterioration in MMEF was similar in bronchitics and normals. Thus, neither the presence of bronchitis nor foundry work had apparent effect on the deterioration of MMEF with age. Likewise, degree of smoking produced a difference that was maintained over the 11-year period, with changes due mainly to age.

Brinkman and Block[192] also examined frequency of early retirement and death rates in the above population. They found that bronchitis did not significantly affect either early retirement or death rate. Occupation was more important; both groups of foundry workers had significantly increased death rates, but early retirement was not influenced by occupation. Cigarette smoking resulted in increased morbidity and mortality. Those men who entered the study with an $FEV_{1.0}$ below 2.0 liters or an MMEF below 1.5 liters/sec had an increased incidence of early retirement and an increased death rate over the 11-year study period.

Clarke[193] presented a report of his examinations of 1058 men retired from a large iron foundry. In the group examined, there were more blacks than whites, the blacks were younger and had proportionately less silicosis. The majority of those with silicosis were nonsmokers. There was proportionately less heart disease among silicotics. Only nine of 76 men classified by Clarke as disabled were disabled by silicosis. This constituted 0.9% of his sample and 12% of those in the sample with roentgenographic silicosis. These findings supported his view that "compensation be granted only when demonstrable disability solely from silicosis has developed, or (has) been proved conclusively to have aggravated existing disease."

Vekeny[194] presented a method of evaluating dust hazard in terms of a "moment," that is, the proportion of new silicotics times the number of years worked. He illustrated his concept with an example from Hungarian coal mines, examining its suitability over three periods.

Viswanathan et al. [195] surveyed 1977 employees in dust areas of an Indian ordnance factory. The factory areas were classified as "dusty" and "less dusty"; no dust measurements are reported. Overall, there was radiographic evidence of pneumoconiosis in 3.5% of the workers and 4.2% tuberculosis, about half again as high in the "dusty" areas. Prevalence of pneumoconioses was 5.9% in the heavy steel foundry, 4.7% in the iron foundry, 4.1% in the light steel factory, 2.8% in the hand grenade section, and 1.5% in the rest of the factory. The ventilatory capacity of the group with pneumoconosis was similar to a group without silicosis, but both were significantly less than a group of "normal males" from outside the factory.

It should be pointed out that the most quantitative epidemiologic study on the effect of silica dust is that conducted in the Vermont granite sheds, which is discussed under "Granite."

STYRENE

Gotell et al. [196] present the results of a study of 17 workers in four shops making fibrous-glass-reinforced, styrene-modified polyester plastic products. The workers were often exposed to several times the Swedish limit of 50 ppm or the American TLV of 100 ppm. It was found possible to monitor the environment by charcoal tubes, impingers, indicating tubes, or combustible gas indicator. Symptoms were not remarkable. They included gastritis, tiredness, sleep disturbances, and memory disturbances, but were difficult to relate to the environment. A simple reaction time was measured, and was found to be longer in the subgroup exposed to more than 150 ppm than in the controls. The subgroup exposed to less than 150 ppm did not have an average reaction time different from that of the controls.

The metabolites mandelic acid and phenylglyoxylic acid were positively correlated with styrene exposures for the low exposure groups, but negatively correlated for the high exposure group. The author cautioned against using these metabolites as exposure indices because of these inconsistencies.

The authors concluded that an average exposure of 150 ppm is probably too high. If a safety factor of 3 is desired, the TLV should be 50 ppm. The ACGIH TLV for 1973 was 100 ppm; there was no OSHA standard as of mid 1974.

SOLVENTS—MIXED

A major problem in industrial hygiene is the evaluation of mixed exposures to solvents of various types. This is an even greater problem in epidemiology, where the type of solvent exposure is often determined by occupational history— sometimes secondhand.

Beirne and Brennan[197] reported a retrospective case study of autoimmune glomerulonephritis in 13 patients. Eight patients were available for history, and six of the eight had a history of intensive exposure to various industrial solvents. Petroleum products included paint removers, degreasing solvents, hair sprays, and paint solvents. No specific component could be implicated. The authors proposed that the first stage in this disease might be chemical injury to lung or kidney. The antibodies to glomerular basement membrane, according to this theory, would be considered a secondary response to chemical injury to lung or kidney basement membranes. This theory, if true, would appear to be of more assistance to the clinician in diagnosis of this rare disease than to the industrial hygienist.

SULFURIC ACID

Thirty-three workers in two storage battery factories were examined by El-Sadik et al.[198] Concentrations of sulfuric acid were 26–35 mg/m^3 in one plant and 13–14 mg/m^3 in the other. At these high concentrations, a reduction in vital capacity, as compared with a control group, was not noted. The mean forced expiratory volume in 1 sec was reduced slightly in the exposed group. The sulfuric acid exposures did not appear to result in significantly increased chronic bronchitis or chronic asthmatic bronchitis. Tooth erosion or other dental lesions among the exposed workers were noted in 20 of 26 workers with more than 1 year of exposure.

The threshold limit value for sulfuric acid and the OSHA standard were 1 mg/m^3 in 1974.

TALC

A clinical and environmental study was made of a group of 39 workers exposed to commercial talc dust by Kleinfeld et al.[199] All workers studied were exposed more than 10 years, with an average exposure of 16.2 years. The major fibrous components were tremolite and anthophyllite. Concentrations of dust averaged 6 mppcf* by impinger in mine drilling, 13–20 mppcf in most other operations, and 68 mppcf in railroad car loading. Fiber counts in fibers longer than 5 μm/cm^3 were 8 fibers/cm^3 in drilling, 13–30 fibers/cm^3 in most other operations, and 260 fibers/cm^3 in crushing. Only one of the talc workers showed a chest roentgenogram consistent with a diagnosis of pneumoconiosis. There was a dyspnea prevalence of 23% in the exposed group compared with 7% in the control group; this was the only significant difference between the talc workers and their controls. The duration of exposure was too short (22 years maximum) to determine whether lung cancer would occur in these workers.

The talc workers in this study were compared with another group studied previously that had similar lengths of exposure to concentrations from 1.1 to 30 times those in the study reported in 1973, with half the reported operation in the 5–7 times range. The group with the higher exposures had significantly greater prevalences of dyspnea, lung crepitations, clubbing, and radiographic findings compatible with pneumoconiosis.

The talc miner and miller experience was considerably less severe than some manufacturing and other workers using chrysotile or amosite at apparently similar levels of fiber. The experience seemed more similar to the experience of the Quebec chrysotile mine and mill workers (see section on asbestos).

TRICHLOROETHYLENE

Lowry et al.[200] report a survey of 19 workers exposed to trichloroethylene with nine nonexposed controls. Estimated average exposures to trichloroethylene based on charcoal tube sampling and gas chromatographic analysis ranged from 170 to 420 ppm. Subjective symptoms were reported by more than

* Million particles per cubic foot.

half the exposed workers. Urine specimens collected before and after the workshift were analyzed for the metabolites trichloroacetic acid and trichloroethanol. Their data were consistent with the observations that trichloroacetic acid was excreted slowly over several days, and trichloroethanol was excreted rapidly within a few hours following exposure. They concluded that the former can indicate cumulative exposure during the work week and the latter can indicate exposure during the workday on which samples were collected.

Pfaffli and Backman[201] looked at 31 workers occupationally exposed to trichloroethylene at seven different workplaces. Of these workers 17 were exposed only to trichloroethylene and 14 to mixtures of trichloroethylene with 1,1,1-trichloroethane or tetrachloroethylene. Expired air and blood samples were taken before, during, and after exposure. Ambient air samples were collected in plastic bags throughout the workshift. All samples were analyzed by gas chromatography, the blood samples after extraction with hexane. A curvilinear relationship between concentrations of trichloroethylene in ambient and expired air was shown for pure exposure, but concomitant exposure to 1,1,1-trichloroethane resulted in lower concentrations in expired air. Trichloroethylene could also be measured in expired air before exposure; concentrations were 0.3–4.9 ppm, with a slight day-to-day increase for workers exposed at 70–115 ppm. Blood samples also exhibited a curvilinear relationships to ambient air exposure, and trichloroethylene was detectable in the blood 15 hr after the exposure. As with the expired air, 1,1,1-trichloroethane was observed to delay excretion, resulting in higher before-work concentrations of trichloroethylene. The authors concluded that either expired air or blood analysis for trichloroethylene could be used for estimation of occupational exposure, but that expired air was simpler. They believed that examination before the beginning of the following work shift was important, and that special attention should be paid to workers exposed to other halogenated hydrocarbons with trichloroethylene.

TRICHLOROTRIFLUOROETHANE (REFRIGERANT 113)

A group of 50 workers exposed to refrigerant 113 and an equal number of controls were investigated by Imbus and Adkins.[202] Exposure ranged from 46 to 4700 ppm with an average of 70 ppm over a mean exposure period of 2.77 years. The maximum period of exposure was $4\frac{1}{2}$ years. Although there were more respiratory symptoms among those exposed, all had antedated exposure and did not appear to be work related. Only one exposed worker had an abnormal timed vital capacity. Blood cholesterol levels were slightly lower for the exposed workers, and protein levels were slightly higher. There appeared to be no great differences between the exposed and control groups in the blood chemistry studies. One worker had an abnormal alkaline phosphatase and was diagnosed as possible hepatic cirrhosis, but he had a history of excessive ethanol ingestion.

2,4,5-T (2,4,5-TRICHLOROPHENOXYACETIC ACID)

Seventy-three workers in a factory manufacturing 2,4,5-T and 2,4-D were studied by Poland et al.[203] Acne was found in 48 of the 73 workers; 36 of these had scarring. Mucous membrane irritation was noted in 42% of the workers. Eye irritation was noted in 19%, and acne in 29%. A number of gastrointestinal symptoms were noted, but no comparison standard was available for judging prevalence. Various neurologic findings were noted, but conclusions were not drawn. The Minnesota Multiphasic Personality Inventory (MMPI) was administered. Although the group was significantly different from the "normal" scores, the group was not considered comparable to the small group on which "normals" was determined. A significant correlation was found between the score on severity of acne and the hypomanic scale on the MMPI.

The esterase enzyme activity in 2,4,5-T and 2,4-D workers was compared with Aldrin formulators and controls.[5] Only the Aldrin workers showed significant differences.

VIBRATION

Although physical hazards are covered in another section, the extensive epidemiology in the past 3 years should be noted.

Banister and Smith[204] noted significant losses in manipulative skill associated with the use of power-driven saws.

Chain-saw operators in forests were studied by Taylor et al.[205] who found increased prevalence of vibration-induced white fingers (Raynaud's phenomenon); Hellstrom and Andersen[206] and Kakosky and Szepesi,[207] who also found such an excess; and Seppalainen,[208] who found Raynaud's phenomenon and damage to the peripheral nerves.

WELDING FUMES

Welders are exposed to a wide variety of air contaminants. A group of 61 shipyard welders was studied by Peters et al.[209] The exposure of these men, as measured by samples from inside their welding helmets, averaged 4.3 mg/m³ iron oxide while performing conventional welding and 1.9 mg/m³ iron oxide during inert gas-shielded arc welding. Zinc oxide averaged 2.0 and 0.3 mg/m³ respectively. Copper, chromium, manganese, and nickel averaged 0.1 mg/m³ or less, and cadmium oxide averaged 0.01 mg/m³. Ozone averaged 0.10 ppm and oxides of nitrogen, 0.04 ppm.

The welders, when compared with a group of pipefitters, showed no significant differences by questionnaire, partial physical examination, pulmonary function tests, or chest x ray. However, both groups had depressed pulmonary function as compared with policemen. Compared with pipe coverers exposed to asbestos, the welders appeared to have more obstructive lung disease, while the pipe coverers tended to have restrictive lung disease. However, nonsmoking welders appeared to have normal pulmonary function.

WOOD

The excess of adenocarcinomas in the furniture workers of Buckinghamshire and Oxfordshire was previously reported. Cancer registries in other areas of England were queried by Acheson et al.[210] to determine whether this excess of adenocarcinoma was general. A total of 107 patients with adenocarcinoma (80 men and 27 women) were accepted for analysis, along with 110 matched controls. Thirty-four of the adenocarcinoma patients, but only nine of the control patients had at one time or another worked with wood, mostly in the furniture industry. The control group of nasal cancers other than adeno-carcinoma also had a higher proportion in the furniture industry than expected, and there may also be a slight excess risk of nasal cancers in the furniture industry.

Occupational asthma from western red cedar (*Thuja plicata*) is the subject of a report from Ishizaki et al.[211] A population of 1797 workers was investigated. Occupational, medical, and personal histories were obtained by a questionnaire, a medical history was taken, and a clinical examination performed. The total prevalence of patients with allergic symptoms including asthma (3.4%), rhinitis (9.4%), uticaria (3.6%), dermatitis (4.5%), and conjunctivitis (9.5%) was 24.5%. Epidemiologic analysis of these data showed that sawmill workers had more conjunctivitis, and carpenters had more asthma and rhinitis. The wood, most of which came from Washington, was distributed throughout Japan, causing problems in all parts of the country.

Twenty-two British Columbia woodworkers with respiratory symptoms after exposure to western red cedar were studied by Chan-Yeung et al.[212] The workers developed characteristic nocturnal attacks of cough and asthma. Most recovered within 6 weeks after cessation of exposure. Inhalation provocation was the only method of confirming the diagnosis. Plicatic acid, a major fraction of red cedar extract, produced bronchial symptoms similar to those produced by whole extract, and is probably the active agent.

Chan-Yeung[213] also studied 11 patients before and during broncho-constriction caused by plicatic acid. Decreases in maximum midexpiratory flow, forced vital capacity, forced vital capacity in the first second, and vital capacity were noted.

XYLENE

The use of xylene- and toluene-containing paints by ships' painters was investigated by Mikulski et al.[214] Toluene and xylene were determined from gas syringe samples by gas chromatography. The toluene comprised only about 10% of the solvents, and a joint determination of hippuric acid and methyl hippuric acid in the urine was used as an index of exposure. There was a good correlation between the urine excretions and the environmental exposure. There was an inhibition of uric acid excretion by the xylene–toluene concentrations, which ranged up to 540 ppm xylene and 88 ppm toluene. The authors concluded that determination of the hippuric acid in urine was a reasonable way to monitor mixed exposures to xylene and toluene.

Mixed exposures to benzene, toluene, and xylene were investigated by Lange et al.,[50,51] and by Smolik et al.[52] In their group of workers they report differences between the solvent workers and controls in serum immunoglobulin levels, serum complement levels, and leukocyte agglutinins. Although xylene concentrations were higher than benzene or toluene, it is not possible to say which of the compounds or combinations was responsible for these effects.

REFERENCES

1. Takahaski, M., Ohara, T., and Hashimoto, K., Electrophysiological study of nerve injuries in workers handling acrylamide. *Int. Arch. Arbeitsmed. 28,* 1–11 (1971).
2. Occupational Safety and Health Administration, Occupational safety and health standards. *Fed. Regist. 37,* 22102 (1972).
3. TLV Airborne Contaminants Committee, "TLVs, Threshold Limit Values for Chemical Substances and Physical Agents in the Workroom Environment with Intended Changes for 1973." Amer. Conf. Govt. Ind. Hyg., Cincinnati, Ohio, 1973.
4. Sakurai, H., and Kusumoto, M., Epidemiological study of health impairment among acrylonitrile workers. *Rodo Kagaku 48,* 273 (1972).
5. Bonderman, D. P., Mick, D. L., and Long, K. R., Occupational exposure to aldrin, 2,4-D and 2,4,5-T and its relationship to esterases. *Ind. Med. Surg. 40,* 23 (1971).

6. Cralley, L. J., Epidemiological studies of occupational diseases. *In* "Industrial Environmental Health: The Worker and the Community" (L. V. Cralley, ed.), p. 1. Academic Press, New York, 1972.

7. Tarrant, R. F., and Allard, J., Arsenic levels in urine of forest workers applying silvicides. *Arch. Environ. Health 24,* 277 (1972).

8. Wagner, S. L., and Weswig, P., Arsenic in blood and urine of forest workers. *Arch. Environ. Health 28,* 77 (1974).

9. Stumphius, J., Epidemiology of mesothelioma on Walcheren Island. *Brit. J. Ind. Med. 28,* 59 (1971).

10. McEwen, J., Finlayson, A., Mair, A., and Gibson, A. A. M., Asbestos and mesothelioma in Scotland. *Int. Arch. Arbeitsmed. 28,* 301 (1971).

11. Rubino, G. F., Scansetti, G., Donna, A., and Palestro, G., Epidemiology of pleural mesothelioma in North-western Italy (Piedmont). *Brit. J. Ind. Med. 29,* 436 (1972).

12. Wagner, J. C., Gilson, J. C., Berry, G., and Timbrell, V., Epidemiology of asbestos cancers. *Brit. Med. Bull. 27,* 71 (1971).

13. Gibbs, G. W., and LaChance, M., Dust exposure in the chrysotile asbestos mines and mills of Quebec. *Arch. Environ. Health 24,* 189 (1972).

14. Gibbs, G. W., and LaChance, M., Dust-fiber relationships in the Quebec chrysotile industry. *Arch. Environ. Health 28,* 69 (1974).

15. McDonald, J. C., McDonald, A. D., Gibbs, G. W., Siemiatycki, J., and Rossiter, C. E., Mortality in the chrysotile mines and mills of Quebec. *Arch. Environ. Health 22,* 677 (1971).

16. Jodoin, G., Gibbs, G. W., Macklem, P. T., McDonald, J. C., and Becklake, M. R., Early effects of asbestos exposure on lung function. *Amer. Rev. Resp. Dis. 104,* 525 (1971).

17. Becklake, M. R., Fournier-Massey, G., Rossiter, C. E., and McDonald, J. C., Lung function in chrysotile asbestos mine and mill workers of Quebec. *Arch. Environ. Health 24,* 401 (1972).

18. McDonald, J. D., Becklake, M. V., Fournier-Massey, G., and Rossiter, C. E., Respiratory symptoms in chrysotile asbestos mine and mill workers of Quebec. *Arch. Environ. Health 24,* 358 (1972).

19. Rossiter, C. E., Bristol, L. J., Cartier, P. H., Gilson, J. G., Grainger, T. R., Sluis-Cremer, G. K., and McDonald, J. C., Radiographic changes in chrysotile asbestos mine and mill workers of Quebec. *Arch. Environ. Health 24,* 388 (1972).

20. McDonald, J. C., Becklake, M. R., Gibbs, G. W., McDonald, A. D., and Rossiter, C. E., The health of chrysotile asbestos mine and mill workers of Quebec. *Arch. Environ. Health 28,* 61 (1974).

21. Kogan, F. M., Guselnikova, N. A., and Gulevskaya, M. R., The cancer mortality rate among workers in the asbestos industry of the Urals. *Gig. Sanit. 37,* 29 (1972).

22. Vigliani, E. C., Asbestos exposure and its results in Italy. *In* "Pneumoconiosis" (H. A. Shapiro, ed.), p. 192. Oxford Univ. Press, London and New York, 1970.

23. Wegan, D. H., Theriault, G. P., and Peters, J. M., Worker-sponsered survey for asbestosis. *Arch. Environ. Health 27,* 105 (1973).

24. El-Sewefy, A. Z., and Hassan, F., Immunoelectrophoretic pattern changes in asbestosis. *Ann. Occup. Hyg. 14,* 25 (1971).

25. Navratil, M., and Dobias, J., Development of pleural hyalinosis in long term studies of persons exposed to asbestos dust. *Environ. Res. 6,* 455 (1973).

26. Noro, L., Occupational and non-occupational asbestos in Finland. *Amer. Ind. Hyg. Ass., J. 29,* 195 (1968).

27. Enterline, P. E., and Henderson, V., Type of asbestos and respiratory cancer in the asbestos industry. *Arch. Environ. Health 27,* 312 (1973).

28. Enterline, P., DeCoufle, P., and Henderson, V., Mortality in relation to occupational exposure in the asbestos industry. *J. Occup. Med. 14,* 897 (1972).

29. Enterline, P., DeCoufle, P., and Henderson, V., Respiratory cancer in relation to occupational exposures among retired asbestos workers. *Brit. J. Ind. Med. 30,* 162 (1973).

30. Newhouse, M. L., Berry, G., Wagner, J. C., and Turok, M. E., A study of the mortality of female asbestos workers. *Brit. J. Ind. Med. 29,* 134 (1972).

31. Newhouse, M. L., A study of the mortality of workers in an asbestos factory. *Brit. J. Ind. Med. 26,* 294 (1969).

32. Selikoff, I. J., Disease prevention in asbestos insulation work. *In* "Safety and Health in Shipbuilding and Ship Repairing," p. 13. ILO Occupational Safety and Health Series, No. 27, International Labour Office, Geneva, 1972.

33. Selikoff, I. J., Hammond, E. C., and Churg, J., Carcinogenicity of amosite asbestos. *Arch. Environ. Health 25,* 187 (1972).

34. Elmes, P. C., and Simpson, M. J. C., Insulation workers in Belfast. 3. Mortality 1940–66. *Brit. J. Ind. Med. 28,* 226 (1971).

35. Nurminen, M., A study of the mortality of workers in an anthophyllite asbestos factory in Finland. *Work-Environ.-Health 9,* 112 (1972).

36. Kiviluoto, R., and Meurman, L., Results of asbestos exposure in Finland. *In* "Pneumoconiosis" (H. A. Shapiro, ed.), p. 107. Oxford Univ. Press, London and New York, 1970.

37. Ferris, B. G., Ranadive, M. V., Peters, J. M., Murphy, R. L. H., Burgess, W. A., and Pendergrass, H. P., Prevalence of chronic respiratory disease. *Arch. Environ. Health 23,* 220 (1971).

38. Murphy, R. L. H., Gaensler, E. A., Redding, R. A., Belleau, R., Keelan, P. J., Smith, A. A., Goff, A. M., and Ferris, B. G., Jr., Low exposure to asbestos. *Arch. Environ. Health 25,* 253 (1972).

39. Harries, P. G., MacKenzie, F. A. F., Sheers, G., Kemp, J. H., Oliver, T. P., and Wright, D. S., Radiological survey of men exposed to asbestos in naval dockyards. *Brit. J. Ind. Med. 29,* 274 (1972).

40. Lawton, G. M., Barboo, S. H., and Sullivan, E. J., Significance and description of exposures in the fabrication, installation and removal of asbestos material in the U.S. Navy shipyards. *In* "Safety and Health in Shipbuilding and Ship Repairing," p. 77. International Labour Office, Geneva, 1972.

41. Nicholson, W. J., Holaday, D. A., and Heimann, H., Direct and indirect occupational exposure to insulation dusts in U.S. shipyards. *In* "Safety and Health in Shipbuilding and Ship Repairing," p. 37. International Labour Office, Geneva, 1972.

42. Langlands, J. H. M., Wallace, W. F. M., and Simpson, M. J. C., Insulation workers in Belfast. 2. Morbidity in men still at work. *Brit. J. Ind. Med. 28,* 217 (1971).

43. Ahlman, K., and Siltanen, E., Exposure of insulation workers to asbestos dust. *Work-Environ.-Health 8,* 1 (1971).

44. Murphy, R. L., Levine, B. W., Al Bazzaz, F. J., Lynch, J. L., and Burgess, W. A., Floor tile installation as a source of asbestos exposure. *Amer. Rev. Resp. Dis. 104,* 576 (1971).

45. U.S. Department of Health, Education and Welfare, Report on occupational safety and health. *In* "The President's Report on Occupational Safety and Health." US Govt. Printing Office, Washington, D.C., 1973.

46. Lloyd Davies, T. A., Study of asbestos workers. *Abstr., Int. Congr. Occup. Health, 17th, 1972,* p. 94 (1972).

47. Key, M. M., "Criteria for a Recommended Standard . . . Occupational Exposure to

Asbestos." National Institute for Occupational Safety and Health, Rockville, Maryland, 1972.

48. Parkinson, G. S., Benzene in motor gasoline—an investigation into possible health hazards in and around filling stations and in normal transport operations. *Ann. Occup. Hyg. 14,* 145 (1971).

49. Forni, A., Pacifico, E., and Limonta, A., Chromosome studies of workers exposed to benzene or toluene or both. *Arch. Environ. Health 22,* 373 (1971).

50. Lange, A., Smolek, R., Zatonski, W., and Szymanska, J., Serumimmunoglobulin levels in workers exposed to benzene, toluene and xylene. *Int. Arch. Arbeitsmed. 31,* 37 (1973).

51. Lange, A., Smolik, R., Zatonski, W., and Glazman, H., Leukocyte agglutins in workers exposed to benzene, toluene and xylene. *Int. Arch. Arbeitsmed. 31,* 45 (1973).

52. Smolik, R., Grzybek-Hryncewicz, K., Lange, A., and Zatonski, W., Serum complement level in workers exposed to benzene, toluene and xylene. *Int. Arch. Arbeitsmed. 31,* 243 (1973).

53. Aksoy, M., Dincol, K., Akgun, T., Erdem, S., and Dincol, G., Haematological effects of chronic benzene poisoning in 217 workers. *Brit. J. Ind. Med. 28,* 296 (1971).

54. Chung, K. C., and Chang, I. W., A study on benzene poisoning. *Abstr., Int. Congr. Occup. Health, 17th, 1972* p. 22 (1972).

55. Zavon, M. R., Hoegg, V., and Bingham, E., Benzidine exposure as a cause of bladder tumors. *Arch. Environ. Health 27,* 1 (1973).

56. Kanarek, D. J., Wainer, R. A., Chamberlin, R. I., Weber, A. L., and Kazemi, H., Respiratory illness in a population exposed to beryllium. *Amer. Rev. Resp. Dis. 108,* 1295 (1973).

57. Warren, W. P., Hypersensitivity pneumonitis due to exposure to budgerigars. *Chest 62,* 170 (1972).

58. Hanninen, H., Psychological picture of manifest and latent carbon disulfide poisoning. *Brit. J. Ind. Med. 28,* 374 (1971).

59. Hernberg, S., Mowe, G., Virkola, P., Partanen, T., and Nordman, C., Magnesium and zinc values of erythrocytes and plasma for workers exposed to carbon disulfide. *Work-Environ.-Health 6,* 9 (1969).

60. Mancuso, T., and Locke, B. Z., Carbon disulfide as a cause of suicide. *J. Occup. Med. 14,* 595 (1972).

61. Hernberg, S., Nordman, C., Partanen, T., Christiansen, V., and Virkola, P., Blood lipids, glucose tolerance and plasma creatinine in workers exposed to carbon disulfide. *Work-Environ.-Health 8,* 11 (1971).

62. Hernberg, S., Nurminen, M., and Tolonen, M., Excess mortality from coronary heart disease in viscose rayon workers exposed to carbon disulfide. *Work-Environ.-Health 10,* 93 (1973).

63. Sakurai, H., Hypertension induced by the occupational exposure to carbon disulfide. *Abstr., Int. Congr. Occup. Health, 17th, 1972* p. 182 (1972).

64. Goto, S., Hotta, R., and Sugimoto, K., Studies on chronic carbon disulfide poisoning. *Int. Arch. Arbeitsmed. 28,* 115 (1971).

65. El-Gazzar, R., El-Sadik, Y. M., and Hussein, M., Changes in zinc and serum proteins due to carbon disulfide exposure. *Brit. J. Ind. Med. 30,* 284 (1973).

66. Cohen, S. J., Dorion, G., Goldsmith, J. R., and Perrnutt, S., Carbon Monoxide uptake by inspectors at a United States-Mexico border station. *Arch. Environ. Health 22,* 47 (1971).

67. Burgess, W., DiBerardinis, L. J., and Speizer, F. E., Exposure to automobile exhaust. *Arch. Environ. Health 26* (1973).

68. Sidor, R., Peterson, N. H., and Burgess, W. A., A carbon monoxide-oxygen sampler for evaluation of fire fighter exposure. *Amer. Ind. Hyg. Ass., J. 34,* 264 (1973).

69. Ayres, S. M., Evans, R., Licht, D., Griesbach, J., Reimold, F., Ferrand, E. F., and Criscitello, A., Health effects of exposure to high concentrations of automotive emissions. *Arch. Environ. Health 27,* 168 (1973).

70. Graham Jones, J., and Warner, C. G., Chronic exposure to iron oxide, chromium oxide, and nickel oxide fumes of metal dressers in 9 steelworks. *Brit. J. Ind. Med. 29,* 169 (1972).

71. Kalačic, I., Chronic nonspecific lung disease in cement workers. *Arch. Environ. Health 26,* 78 (1973).

72. Kalačic, I., Ventilatory lung function in cement workers. *Arch. Environ. Health 26,* 84 (1973).

73. Kleinfeld, M., Messite, J., and Swencicki, R., Clinical effects of chlorinated naphthalene exposure. *J. Occup. Med. 14,* 377 (1972).

74. Figuero, W. G., Raszkowski, R., and Weiss, W., Lung cancer in chloromethyl methyl ether workers. *N. Engl. J. Med. 288,* 1096 (1973).

75. National Institute for Occupational Safety and Health, "NIOSH Contracts and Research Agreements." U.S. Dept. of Health, Education and Welfare, Rockville, Maryland, 1973.

76. Gomes, E. R., Incidence of chromium induced lesions among electroplating workers in Brazil. *Ind. Med. Surg. 41,* 21 (1972).

77. National Institute for Occupational Safety and Health, "Criteria for a Recommended Standard: Occupational Exposure to Chromic Acid." U.S. Dept. of Health, Education and Welfare, Rockville, Maryland, 1973.

78. Jacobsen, G., and Gilson, J. C., Present status of the UICC/Cincinnati classification of radiographic appearances of the pneumoconioses. *Ann. N.Y. Acad. Sci. 200,* 552 (1972).

79. Liddell, F. D. K., Mortality of British coal miners in 1961. *Brit. J. Ind. Med. 30,* 15 (1973).

80. Enterline, P. E., A review of mortality data for American coal miners. *Ann. N.Y. Acad. Sci. 200,* 260 (1972).

81. Ortmeyer, C. E., Baier, E. J., and Crawford, G. M., Life expectancy of Pennsylvania coal miners compensated for disability. *Arch. Environ. Health 27,* 227 (1973).

82. Liddell, F. D. K., Morbidity of British coal miners in 1961–62. *Brit. J. Ind. Med. 30,* 1 (1973).

83. Rae, S., Pneumoconiosis and coal dust exposure. *Brit. Med. Bull. 27,* 53 (1971).

84. Rogan, J. M., Attfield, M. D., Jacobsen, M., Rae, S., Walker, D. D., and Walton, W. H., Role of dust in the working environment in development of chronic bronchitis in British coal miners. *Brit. J. Ind. Med. 30,* 217 (1973).

85. Lowe, C. R., and Khosla, T., Chronic bronchitis in ex-coal miners working in the steel industry. *Brit. J. Ind. Med. 29,* 45 (1972).

86. Ulmer, W. T., and Reichel, G., Epidemiological problems of coal workers bronchitis in comparison with the general population. *Ann. N.Y. Acad. Sci. 200,* 211 (1972).

87. Higgins, I. T. T., Chronic respiratory disease in mining communities. *Ann. N.Y. Acad. Sci. 200,* 197 (1972).

88. Morgan, W. K. C., Burgess, D. B., Jacobson, G., O'Brien, R. J., Pendergrass, E. P., Reger, R. B., and Shoub, E. P., The prevalence of coal workers' pneumoconosis in U.S. coal miners. *Arch. Environ. Health 27,* 221 (1973).

89. Sorenson, J. R. J., Kober, T. E., and Petering, H. G., The concentration of Cd, Cu, Fe, Ni, Pb, and Zn in bituminous coals from mines with differing incidences of coal workers' pneumoconiosis. *Amer. Ind. Hyg. Ass., J. 35,* 93 (1974).

90. Corn, M., Stein, F., Hammad, Y., Manekshaw, S., Freedman, R., and Hartstein, A. M., Physical and chemical properties of respirable coal dust from two United States mines. *Amer. Ind. Hyg. Ass., J. 34,* 279 (1973).
91. Naeye, R. L., Mahon, J. K., and Dellinger, W. S., Rank of coal and coal workers' pneumoconiosis. *Amer. Rev. Resp. Dis. 103,* 350 (1971).
92. McLintock, J. S., The changing prevalence of coal workers' pneumoconioses in Great Britain. *Ann. N.Y. Acad. Sci. 200,* 278 (1972).
93. Zahorski, W. W., Trends in coal workers' pneumoconiosis in Poland. *Ann. N.Y. Acad. Sci. 200,* 292 (1972).
94. Morgan, W. K. C., Handelsman, L., Kibelstis, J., Lapp, N. L., and Reger, R., Ventilatory capacity and lung volumes of U.S. coal miners. *Arch. Environ. Health 28,* 182 (1974).
95. Amandus, H. E., Reger, R. B., Pendergrass, E. P., Dennis, R. M., and Morgan, W. K. C., The pneumoconioses: Methods of measuring progression. *Chest 63,* 736 (1973).
96. Lapp, N. L., Hankinson, J. L., Burgess, D. B., and O'Brien, R., Changes in ventilatory function after a work shift. *Arch. Environ. Health 24,* 204 (1972).
97. Scarano, D., Fadali, A. M. A., and Lemole, G. M., Carcinoma of the lung and anthracosilicosis. *Chest 62,* 251 (1972).
98. National Institute for Occupational Safety and Health, "The Federal Coal Mine Health Program in 1972." U.S. Dept. of Health, Education and Welfare, Rockville, Maryland, 1973.
99. Lloyd, J. W., Long-term mortality study of steelworkers. *J. Occup. Med. 13,* 53 (1971).
100. Redmond, C. K., Ciocco, A., Lloyd, J. W., and Rush, H. W., Long-term mortality study of steelworkers. *J. Occup. Med. 14,* 621 (1972).
101. Smith, W. M., Evaluation of coke oven emissions. *J. Occup. Med. 13,* 69 (1971).
102. Walker, D. D., Archibald, R. M., and Attfield, M. D., Bronchitis in men employed in the coke industry. *Brit. J. Ind. Med. 28,* 358 (1971).
103. Henderson, V., and Enterline, P. E., An unusual mortality experience in cotton textile workers. *J. Occup. Med. 15,* 717 (1973).
104. Berry, G., McKerrow, C. B., Molyneux, M. K. B., Rossiter, C. E., and Tombleson, J. B. L., A study of the acute and chronic changes in ventilatory capacity of workers in Lancashire cotton mills. *Brit. J. Ind. Med. 30,* 25 (1973).
105. Fox, A. J., Tombleson, J. B. L., Watt, A., and Wilkie, A. G., A survey of respiratory disease in cotton operatives. Part I. *Brit. J. Ind. Med. 30,* 42 (1973).
106. Fox, A. J., Tombleson, J. B. L., Watt, A., and Wilkie, A. G., A survey of respiratory disease in cotton operatives. Part II. *Brit. J. Ind. Med. 30,* 48 (1973).
107. Imbus, H. R., and Suh, M. W., Byssinosis. *Arch. Environ. Health 26,* 183 (1973).
108. Israeli, R., Maldgolowkin, M., and Amar, R., Variation of lung function among textile workers in the southern district of Israel. *Ind. Med. 41,* 26 (1972).
109. Tuma, J., Parker, L., and Braun, D. C., The proteolytic enzymes and the prevalences of signs and symptoms in U.S. cotton textile mills. *J. Occup. Med. 15,* 409 (1973).
110. Taylor, G., Massoud, A. A. E., and Lucas, F., Studies on the aetiology of byssinosis. *Brit. J. Ind. Med. 28,* 143 (1971).
111. Valic, F., and Zuskin, E., A comparative study of respiratory function in female nonsmoking cotton and jute workers. *Brit. J. Ind. Med. 28,* 364 (1971).
112. Valic, F., and Zuskin, E., Effects of hemp dust exposure on nonsmoking female textile workers. *Arch. Environ. Health 23,* 359 (1971).
113. Valic, F., and Zuskin, E., Effects of different vegetable dust exposures. *Brit. J. Ind. Med. 29,* 293 (1972).
114. Zuskin, E., and Valic, F., Respiratory response in simultaneous exposure to flax and hemp dust. *Brit. J. Ind. Med. 30,* 375 (1973).

115. Nicholls, P. S., Evans, E., Valic, F., and Zuskin, E., Histamine releasing activity and bronchoconstricting effects of sisal. *Brit. J. Ind. Med. 30,* 142 (1973).
116. Braun, D. C., Jurgiel, J. A., Kaschak, M. C., and Babyak, M. A., Prevalence of respiratory signs and symptoms among U.S. cotton textile workers. *J. Occup. Med. 15,* 414 (1973).
117. Bouhuys, A., Mitchell, C. A., Schilling, R. S. F., and Zuskin, E., A physiological study of byssinosis in colonial America. *Trans. N.Y. Acad. Sci. [2] 35,* 537 (1973).
118. Zuskin, E., Valic, F., Nicholls, P. J., and Evans, E. L., Respiratory symptoms and ventilatory function in sisal dust exposure. *Int. Arch. Arbeitsmed. 30,* 105 (1972).
119. Laws, E. R., Jr., Maddrey, W. C., Curley, A., and Burse, V. W., Long-term occupational exposure to DDT. *Arch. Environ. Health 27,* 318 (1973).
120. Kolmodin-Hedman, B., Palmer, L., Gotell, P., and Skerfving, S., Plasma levels of Lindane, p,p-DDE and p,p-DDT in occupationally exposed persons in Sweden. *Work-Environ.-Health 10,* 100 (1973).
121. Menz, M., Luetkemeier, H., and Sachsse, K., Long-term exposure of factory workers to dichlorvos (DDVP) insecticide. *Arch. Environ. Health 28,* 72 (1974).
122. Hakkinen, I., Siltanen, E., Hernberg, S., Seppalainen, A. M., Karli, P., and Vikkula, E., Diphenyl poisoning in fruit paper production. *Arch. Environ. Health 26,* 70 (1973).
123. Morgan, D. C., Smyth, J. T., Lister, R. W., and Pethybridge, R. J., Chest symptoms and farmer's lung: A community survey. *Brit. J. Ind. Med. 30,* 259 (1973).
124. Swensson, A., Kvarnstrom, K., Bruce, T., Edling, N. P. G., and Glomme, J., Pneumoconiosis in ferrosilicon workers—a follow-up study. *J. Occup. Med. 13,* 427 (1971).
125. Gross, P., Tuma, J., and deTreville, R. T. P., Lungs of workers exposed to fiber glass. *Arch. Environ. Health 23,* 67 (1971).
126. Nasr, A. N. M., Ditchek, T., and Schlotens, P. A., The prevalence of radiographic abnormalities in the chests of fiber glass workers. *J. Occup. Med. 13,* 371 (1971).
127. Hill, J. W., Whitehead, W. S., Cameron, J. D., and Hedgecock, G. A., Glass fibres: Absence of pulmonary hazard in production workers. *Brit. J. Ind. Med. 30,* 174 (1973).
128. Kaltreider, N. L., Elder, M. J., Cralley, L. V., and Colwell, M. O., Health survey of aluminum workers with special reference to fluoride exposure. *J. Occup. Med. 14,* 531 (1972).
129. Lloyd Davies, T. A., "Respiratory Disease in Foundrymen, Report of a Survey." HM Stationery Office, London, 1971.
130. McCallum, R. I., Respiratory disease in foundrymen. *Brit. J. Ind. Med. 29,* 341 (1972).
131. Mintz, G., and Fraga, A., Severe osteoarthritis of the elbow in foundry workers. *Arch. Environ. Health 27,* 78 (1973).
132. Doll, R., Vessey, M. P., Beasley, R. W. R., Buckley, A. R., Fear, E. C., Fisher, R. E. W., Gammon, E. J., Gunn, W., Hughes, G. O., Lee, K., and Norman-Smith, B., Mortality of gasworkers—final report of a prospective study. *Brit. J. Ind. Med. 29,* 394 (1972).
133. Tse, K. S., Warren, P., Janusz, M., McCarthy, D. S., and Cherniack, R. M., Respiratory abnormalities in workers exposed to grain dust. *Arch. Environ. Health 27,* 74 (1973).
134. Lloyd Davies, T. A., Doig, A. T., Fox, A. J., and Greenberg, M., A radiographic survey of monumental masonry workers in Aberdeen. *Brit. J. Ind. Med. 30,* 227 (1973).
135. Theriault, G. P., Burgess, W. A., DiBerardinis, L. J., and Peters, J. M., Dust exposure in the Vermont granite sheds. *Arch. Environ. Health 28,* 12 (1974).
136. Theriault, G. P., Peters, J. M., and Fine, L. J., Pulmonary function in granite shed workers of Vermont. *Arch. Environ. Health 28,* 18 (1974).

137. Theriault, G. P., Peters, J. M., and Johnson, W. M., Pulmonary function and roentgenographic changes in granite dust exposure. *Arch. Environ. Health 28,* 23 (1974).

138. Ranasinha, K. W., and Uragoda, C. G., Graphite pneumoconiosis. *Brit. J. Ind. Med. 29,* 178 (1972).

139. Cuthbert, O. D., Investigation into an outbreak of rhinitis and asthma in a printing works. *Ann. Occup. Hyg. 16,* 203 (1973).

140. Gowdy, J. M., and Wagstaff, M. J., Pulmonary infiltration due to aerosol thesaurosis. *Arch Environ. Health 25,* 101 (1972).

141. Teculescu, D., and Albu, A., Pulmonary function in workers inhaling iron oxide dust. *Int. Arch. Arbeitsmed. 31,* 163 (1973).

142. Neubert, H., Lead poisoning in the industrial economy—a statistical survey. *Staub 30,* 7 (1970).

143. Tola, S., Hernberg, S., Nikkanen, J., and Valkonen, S., Occupational lead exposure in Finland. I. Electric storage battery manufacturing and repair. *Work-Environ.-Health 8,* 81 (1971).

144. Tola, S., Hernberg, S., and Nikkanen, J., Occupational lead exposure in Finland. II. Service stations and garages. *Work-Environ.-Health 9,* 102 (1972).

145. Millar, J. A., Thompson, G. G., Goldberg, A., Barry, P. S. I., and Lowe, E. H., δ-aminolevulinic acid dehydrase activity in the blood of men working with lead alkyls.1 *Brit. J. Ind. Med. 29,* 317 (1972).

146. Tola, S., Hernberg, S., Asp, S., and Nikkanen, J., Parameters indicative of absorption and biological effect in new lead exposure: A prospective study. *Brit. J. Ind. Med. 30,* 134 (1973).

147. Report of a Committee under the Chairmanship of Sir Brian Windeyer Appointed to inquire into Lead Poisonings at the RTZ Smelter at Avonmouth. HM Stationery Office, London, 1972.

148. Bonnel, J. A., Lead smelting at Avonmouth. *Brit. J. Ind. Med. 30,* 199 (1973).

149. Tsuchiya, K., Takahashi, K., Sugita, M., and Seki, Y., Biological response to low level exposure to lead. *Abstr., Int. Congr. Occup. Health, 17th, 1972,* p. 129 (1972).

150. Hernberg, S., Lilius, H., Mellin, G., and Nikkanen, J., Lead exposure of workers in printing shops. *Work-Environ.-Health 6,* 5 (1969).

151. Samuels, A. J., and Milby, T. H., Human exposure to Lindane. *J. Occup. Med. 13,* 147 (1971).

152. Milby, T. H., and Samuels, A. J., Human exposure to Lindane. *J. Occup. Med. 13,* 256 (1971).

153. Emara, A. M., El-Ghawabi, S. H., Madkour, O. I., and El-Samra, G. H., Chronic manganese poisoning in the dry battery industry. *Brit. J. Ind. Med. 28,* 78 (1971).

154. Jonderko, G., Kujawska, A., and Langauer-Lewowicka, H., Problems of chronic manganese poisoning on the basis of investigations of workers at a manganese alloy foundry. *Int. Arch. Arbeitsmed. 28,* 250 (1971).

155. Smyth, L. T., Ruhf, R. C., Whitman, N. E., and Dugan, T., Clinical manganism and exposure to manganese in the production and processing of ferromanganese alloy. *J. Occup. Med. 15,* 101 (1973).

156. Hernberg, S., Nikkanen, J., and Hosanen, E., Erythrocyte δ-aminolevulinic acid dehydratase in workers exposed to mercury vapor. *Work-Environ.-Health 8,* 42 (1971).

157. Danziger, S. J., and Possick, P. A., Metallic mercury exposure in scientific glassware manufacturing plants. *J. Occup. Med. 15,* 15 (1973).

158. Bell, Z. G., Jr., Wood, M. W., and Kuryla, L. A., Mercury exposure evaluations and their correlation with urine mercury excretions. 2. Time-weighted average (TWA) exposures. *J. Occup. Med. 15,* 420 (1973).

159. Lovejoy, H. B., Berry, J., and Bell, Z. G., Jr., Mercury exposure evaluations and their correlation with urine mercury excretions. 5. Occurrence of mercurialentis. *J. Occup. Med. 15,* 647 (1973).

160a. Lauwerys, R. R., and Buchet, J. P., Occupational exposure to mercury vapors and biological action. *Arch. Environ. Health 27,* 65 (1973).

160b. Billmaier, D. J., Peripheral neuropathy in a coated fabrics plant. *Proc. Industrial Med. Ass.,* Bal Harbour, Florida, May 1974. (To be published.)

161. Ratney, R. S., Wegman, D. H., and Elkins, H. B., *In vivo* conversion of methylene chloride to carbon monoxide. *Arch. Environ. Health 28,* 223 (1974).

162. Moss, E., Scott, T. S., and Atherly, G. R. C., Mortality of newspaper workers from lung cancer and bronchitis 1952–66. *Brit. J. Ind. Med. 29,* 1 (1972).

163. Moss, E., A mortality survey in the newspaper industry. *Ann. Occup. Hyg. 16,* 195 (1973).

164. Greenberg, M., A proportional mortality study of a group of newspaper workers. *Brit. J. Ind. Med. 29,* 15 (1972).

165. Kennedy, M. C. S., Nitrous fumes and coal-miners with emphysema. *Ann. Occup. Hyg. 15,* 285 (1972).

166. Kosmider, S., and Misiewiez, A., Experimental and epidemiological investigations on the effect of nitrogen oxides on lipid metabolism. *Int. Arch. Arbeitsmed. 31,* 249 (1973).

167. Pasternack, B., and Erlich, L., Occupational exposure to oil mist atmosphere. *Arch. Environ. Health 25,* 286 (1972).

168. Waterhouse, J. A. H., Cutting oils and cancer. *Ann. Occup. Hyg. 14,* 161 (1971).

169. Waterhouse, J. A. H., Lung cancer and gastro-intestinal cancer in mineral oil workers. *Ann. Occup. Hyg. 15,* 43 (1972).

170. Lee, W. R., Alderson, M. R., and Downes, J. E., Scrotal cancer in the north-west of England, 1962–68. *Brit. J. Ind. Med. 29,* 188 (1972).

171. Durham, W. F., Wolfe, H. R., and Elliott, J. W., Absorption and excretion of parathion by spraymen. *Arch. Environ. Health 24,* 381 (1972).

172. Guthrie, F. E., Tappan, W. B., Jackson, M. D., Smith, F. D., Krieger, H. C., and Chasson, A. L., Cholinesterase levels of cigar-wrapper tobacco workers exposed to parathion. *Arch. Environ. Health 25,* 32 (1972).

173. Hearn, C. E. D., and Keir, W., Nail damage in spray operators exposed to paraquat. *Brit. J. Ind. Med. 28,* 399 (1971).

174. Sandifer, S. H., Keil, J. E., Finklea, J. F., and Gadsden, R. H., Pesticide effects on occupationally exposed workers. *Ind. Med. Surg. 41,* 9 (1972).

175. Warnick, S. L., and Carter, J. E., Some findings in a study of workers occupationally exposed to pesticides. *Arch. Environ. Health 25,* 265 (1972).

176. Drenth, H. J., Ensberg, I. G. G., Roberts, D. V., and Wilson, A., Neuromuscular function in agricultural workers using pesticides. *Arch. Environ. Health 25,* 395 (1972).

177. Morgan, D. P., and Roan, C. C., Adreno cortical function in persons occupationally exposed to pesticides. *J. Occup. Med. 15,* 26 (1973).

178. Ensberg, I. F. G., deBruin, A., and Zielhus, R. L., Health of workers exposed to a cocktail of pesticides. *Int. Arch. Arbeitsmed. 32,* 191 (1974).

179. Dinman, B. D., Cook, W. A., Whitehouse, W. M., Magnuson, H. J., and Ditchek, T., Occupational acroosteolysis. *Arch. Environ. Health 22,* 61 (1971).

180. Sokol, W. N., Aelony, Y., and Beall, G. N., Meat-wrapper's asthma—a new syndrome? *J. Amer. Med. Ass. 226,* 639 (1973).

181. Occupational Safety and Health Administration. Emergency temporary standard for exposure to vinyl chloride. *Fed. Regist. 39,* 12342 (1974).

182. Question on effects of vinyl chloride exposure. *Amer. Ind. Hyg. Ass., J. 35,* 61 (1974).

183. Waxweiler, R. J., Wagoner, J. K., and Archer, V. E., Mortality of potash workers. *J. Occup. Med. 15,* 486 (1973).

184. Mitchell, C. A., and Gandevia, B., Respiratory symptoms and skin reactivity in workers exposed to proteolytic enzymes in the detergent industry. *Amer. Rev. Resp. Dis. 104,* 1 (1971).

185. Weill, H., Waddell, L. C., and Ziskind, M., A study of workers exposed to detergent enzymes. *J. Amer. Med. Ass. 217,* 425 (1971).

186. Gothe, C., Westlin, A., and Sundquist, S., Air-borne *b. subtilis* enzymes in the detergent industry. *Int. Arch. Arbeitsmed. 29,* 201 (1972).

187. Ahlman, K., Silicosis in Finland. *Work-Environ.-Health 4,* Suppl. 1 (1968).

188. Zolov, C., and Dobreva, M., Development of dust control and silicosis morbidity in Bulgaria. *Staub 30,* 9 (1970).

189. Woitowitz, H., Schacke, G., and Woitowitz, R., Ranking estimation of the dust exposure and industrial-medical epidemiology. *Staub 30,* 15 (1970).

190. Phibbs, B. P., Sundin, R. E., and Mitchell, R. S., Silicosis in Wyoming bentonite workers. *Amer. Rev. Resp. Dis. 103,* 1 (1971).

191. Brinkman, G. L., Block, D. L., and Cress, C., Effects of bronchitis and occupation on pulmonary ventilation over an 11-year period. *J. Occup. Med. 14,* 615 (1972).

192. Brinkman, G. L., and Block, D. L., Chronic bronchitis in a working population. *J. Occup. Med. 14,* 825 (1972).

193. Clarke, N. E., Silicosis and diseases of retired iron foundry workers. *Ind. Med. Surg. 41,* 22 (1972).

194. Vekeny, H., A dynamic index of the silicosis epidemiology. *Staub 32,* 27 (1972).

195. Viswanathan, R., Boparai, M. S., Jain, S. K., and Dash, M. S., Pneumoconiosis survey of workers in an ordnance factory in India. *Arch. Environ. Health 25,* 198 (1972).

196. Gotell, P., Axelson, O., and Lindelof, B., Field studies on human styrene exposure. *Work-Environ.-Health 9,* 76 (1972).

197. Beirne, G. J., and Brennan, J. T., Glomerulonephritis associated with hydrocarbon solvents. *Arch. Environ. Health 25,* 365 (1972).

198. El-Sadik, Y., Osman, H. A., and El-Gazzar, R. M., Exposure to sulfuric acid in manufacture of storage batteries. *J. Occup. Med. 14,* 224 (1972).

199. Kleinfeld, M., Messite, J., and Langer, A. M., A study of workers exposed to asbestiform minerals in commercial talc manufacture. *Environ. Res. 6,* 132 (1973).

200. Lowry, L. K., Vandervort, R., and Polakoff, P. L., Biological indicators of occupational exposure to trichloroethylene. *J. Occup. Med. 16,* 98 (1974).

201. Pfaffli, P., and Backman, A., Trichloroethylene concentrations in blood and expired air as indicators of occupational exposure. *Work-Environ.-Health 9,* 140 (1972).

202. Imbus, H. R., and Adkins, C., Physical examinations of workers exposed to trichlorotrifluoroethane. *Arch. Environ. Health 24,* 257 (1972).

203. Poland, A. P., Smith, D., Metter, G., and Possick, P., A health survey of workers in a 2,4-D and 2,4,5-T plant. *Arch. Environ. Health 22,* 316 (1971).

204. Banister, P. A., and Smith, F. V., Vibration-induced white fingers and manipulative dexterity. *Brit. J. Ind. Med. 29,* 264 (1972).

205. Taylor, W., Pearson, J., Kell, R. L., and Keighley, G. D., Vibration syndrome in Forestry Commission chain saw operators. *Brit. J. Ind. Med. 28,* 83 (1971).

206. Hellstrom, B., and Andersen, K. L., Vibration injuries in Norwegian forest workers. *Brit. J. Ind. Med. 29,* 255 (1972).

207. Kakosy, T., and Szepesi, L., Effects of vibration exposure on the localization of Raynaud's phenomenon in chain saw operators. *Work-Environ.-Health 10,* 134 (1973).

208. Seppalainen, A. M., Peripheral neuropathy in forest workers: A field study. *Work-Environ.-Health 9,* 106 (1972).
209. Peters, J. M., Murphy, R. L. M., Ferris, B. G., Burgess, W. A., Ranadive, M. V., and Pendergrass, H. P., Pulmonary function in shipyard workers. *Arch. Environ. Health 26,* 28 (1973).
210. Acheson, E. D., Cowdell, R. H., and Rang, E., Adenocarcinoma of the nasal cavity and sinuses in England and Wales. *Brit. J. Ind. Med. 29,* 21 (1972).
211. Ishizaki, T., Shida, T., Miyamoto, T., Matsumara, Y., Mizuno, K., and Tomaru, M., Occupational asthma from Western red cedar dust (*Thuja plicata*) in furniture factory workers. *J. Occup. Med. 15,* 581 (1973).
212. Chan-Yeung, M., Barton, G. M., MacLean, L., and Grzybowski, S., Occupational asthma and rhinitis due to Western red cedar (*Thuja plicata*). *Amer. Rev. Resp. Dis. 108,* 1094 (1973).
213. Chan-Yeung, M., Maximal expiratory flow and airway resistance during induced bronchoconstriction in patients with asthma due to Western red cedar. *Amer. Rev. Resp. Dis. 108,* 1103 (1973).
214. Mikulski, P. I., Wiglusz, R., Bublewska, A., and Uselis, J., Investigation of exposure of ships painters to organic solvents. *Brit. J. Ind. Med. 29,* 450 (1972).

Toxicology

EMIL A. PFITZER

CMT-GENICITY: THE TRIAD OF GENESES

Carcinogenesis (C), mutagenesis (M), and teratogenesis (T)—how does one test chemicals for these actions? Are current procedures satisfactory for decision making about safety? Are the results reproducible? Toxicologists have been struggling with these questions with increasing intensity. The research output providing new published knowledge about the potential for CMT-genicity of numerous chemicals has been phenomenal, including 2,4,5-T, PCBs, NTA, cyclamate, saccharin, methylmercury, lead, cadmium, and many pesticides. At the same time a major fraction of the effort of many toxicologists has been spent on developing guidelines for toxicologic testing procedures which will provide a basis for sound, but reasonable, decisions for the evaluation of safety. Much of this effort has not been published as yet.

A comprehensive review of testing chemicals for CMT-genicity has been published by the Departments of Health and Welfare of Canada.[1] This document considers methodology, general principles, and the problem areas both of documentation and interpretation of the tests. In the United States, the Food and Drug Administration Panel on Carcinogenesis published a report on cancer testing in the safety evaluation of food additives and pesticides.[2] Additional documents on CMT-genicity, as well as other toxicologic testing procedures, will be published; many of these documents will have a marked regulatory impact.

Much of the uncertainty surrounding testing the CMT-genicity lies in the fact that cancer, mutations, and terrata occur in the general population for both man and experimental animals. This makes cause-and-effect relationships extremely difficult to ascertain when the effect of treatment is barely different from observations in the nonexposed. C. S. Weil has discussed this dilemma and recommended the use of variable factors of safety established by properly informed, scientific judgment.[3]

Of course, the monumental dilemma is the definition by different scientists and laymen of what they mean by safety—"absolute safety" or "practical certainty." L. Golberg has dealt with the question, "Is practical certainty acceptable when the potential hazard, however remote, is one that may be shared unwittingly by vast numbers of people of various states of health?" He notes that "in many instances the most we can hope to do is to try to define as clearly as possible the likely hazard associated with particular conditions of exposure; in other words the price, in terms of potential harm, that the consumer may be expected to incur for a certain increment of contaminant level in his diet."[4] He suggests that the evaluation of safety is a continuing, in fact an unending, process and greater leadership must be displayed in devising continuing systems of review and developing improved testing procedures.[5]

The President's Science Advisory Committee, Panel on Chemicals and Health has presented these issues as key principles in an extremely clear and comprehensive way. Their recommendations in part call for the establishment of an Advisory Board of Review to assist with the decision-making procedures, the publication of the issues and rationale for decision making in a way understandable to the public, and the advancement of scientific knowledge of chemical impacts so that those who use, regulate, or produce chemicals may act more prudently.[6]

Guidelines for Safety in Man

C. S. Weil prepared a statement of guidelines believed to be valid and applicable to experiments where the results are used to predict the degree of safety of a chemical for man. His statement was slightly revised after receiving comments from 66 toxicologists or scientists from related fields, and is presented here verbatim.[7]

1. Use, wherever possible, species that biologically handle the material as similarly as possible to man.

2. Where practical, use several dose levels on the principle that all types of toxicologic and pharmacologic actions in man and animals are dose related.

3. Effects produced at higher dose levels are useful for delineating mechanisms of action, but for any material and adverse effect, some dose level exists for man or animal below which this adverse effect will not appear. This biologically insignificant level can and should be set by use of a proper safety factor and competent scientific judgment.

4. Statistical tests for significance are valid only on the experimental units (e.g., either litters or individuals) that have been mathematically randomized among the dosed and concurrent control groups.

5. Effects obtained by one route of administration to test animals are not *a*

priori applicable to effects by another route of administration to man. The routes chosen for administration to test animals should, therefore, be the same as those to be used in man. Thus, for example, food additives for man should be tested by admixture of the material in the diet of animals.

METHODOLOGY

Mutagenicity Testing

An ad hoc committee of the Environmental Mutagen Society and the Institute for Medical Research reported the following conclusions about chromosome methodologies in mutation testing.

> The committee concluded that a provisional recommendation for cytogenetic methodologies to be used as one of a group of tests for mutagenicity should include an *in vivo* and an *in vitro* mammalian system. The *in vivo* system should employ a metaphase system from the bone marrow of the rat or mouse. The *in vitro* system should employ an anaphase system from a diploid mammalian cell line with low background. Protocol, scoring, and terminology should be sufficiently standardized to permit comparisons of results from various laboratories. The committee emphasized that these suggestions are a starting point, that suggestions and criticism are welcomed, that a frequent reevaluation of methods used and methods available should be undertaken, and that further developments and research should be encouraged.[8]

Skin and Eye Irritation Tests

Twelve chemicals were tested for their ability to cause skin irritation in male white adult human volunteers and New Zealand white rabbits according to the standard Draize skin irritancy test. The Draize rabbit test accurately predicted the severe human skin irritants and the nonirritants; however, it failed to distinguish the mild and moderate skin irritants. The rabbit was more sensitive in these cases, indicating skin irritation for several chemicals that proved nonirritating to human skin.[9] A variety of methods for detecting primary skin irritants has been recently reviewed.[10]

An objective assessment of eye irritation has been proposed using a depth-measuring attachment to a slit lamp to determine corneal thickness. This procedure should be free of the individual observer bias inherent in the widely used Draize rabbit eye test.[11]

In order to minimize any confusion with staining of normal rabbit corneas, it was recommended that a fluorescein staining time of 15 sec be used.[12]

Twenty-five laboratories collaborated in a joint study to test skin and eye irritation for 12 materials. These studies emphasized the large differences that may occur between observers evaluating skin and eye reactions to irritants. Some laboratories tended to rate materials consistently more severely than others, and some consistently rated materials nonirritating. Some laboratories showed an inconsistency in that certain materials were either more or less severely rated when compared with other laboratories.[13]

Lung Models: Ventilation, Clearance, Residues

Respired air and flow rates of small animals can be measured without head and neck attachment, anesthesia, or trachea intubation. The volume-related surface area changes of the thorax and abdomen are detected by measuring changes in the frequency of an oscillating capacitor circuit.[14]

A technique has been developed to quantitate simultaneously several variables of mucociliary clearance in the lungs of the living cat. The procedure requires surgery that could be repeated several times for serial observations during exposure to hazardous inhalants. In young cats the mucous blanket depth was usually less than 10 μm, ciliary beat frequency averaged 876 ± 151 beats/min, transport rate was 10.5 ± 3.7 mm/min, average mucous viscosity was 248 ± 106 poises at a shear rate of 1/sec, and recoverable shear strain (elasticity) was 3.1 ± 1.1 units at 100 dynes/cm^2.[15]

An *in vivo* method for determination of the rate of mucociliary transport in the rat trachea utilized an aqueous suspension of barium sulfate deposited in the trachea followed by x ray photographs, taken over a period of several minutes at 30-sec intervals through a radiopaque measuring grid. Normally, the transport rate was 6–10 mm/min. The effects of injected substances as well as environmental contaminants may be determined by this method using the same animal repeatedly.[16]

The pulmonary defense mechanisms are sufficiently good that it has been difficult to study the interrelationships between infection and response to inhaled pollutants except with large and lethal exposures to infective organisms. It has, however, been possible to infect mice with nonlethal doses of influenza virus and to verify infection by positive hemagglutinin inhibition titers 2 weeks after inoculation. Infected mice showed a marked deficiency in pulmonary clearance as measured with $^{51}Cr_2O_3$ given by intratracheal injection. Although not all of the mice with positive titers showed a deficiency in pulmonary clearance, some of the deficiencies that did occur persisted for a considerable time after the infectious episode.[17,18]

The recovery of inhaled mineral dusts, from lung tissue, with minimal physical damage is important for studying deposition and clearance mechanisms. Clorox solution and Hydroxide of Hyamine were considered to be reagents of choice and to have the least effect on mineral dusts. However, Clorox solution was not suitable for extraction of coal dusts, owing to apparent oxidation.[19]

Inhalation Exposure Systems

An apparatus to allow an exposure limited to the nasal area of rodents has been described. The system provides for the generation and dispersion of radioactive aerosols and will allow simultaneous exposure of 88 mice, hamsters, or rats.[20]

A convenient exposure system for long-term inhalation studies has been described which will house approximately 100 rodents. The system has been used for aerosol exposures of cobalt oxide and nickel oxide using a Wright dust feed generator and for chrysotile asbestos using a specially designed generator.[21]

A fluidizing dust generator has been developed to provide consistent levels of respirable particles for inhalation toxicity studies. The system proved to be practical for redispersing bulk dust obtained from bag filters at a polyester–fiber glass manufacturing plant.[22]

Variables Influencing Mortality

Chemicals that are weak acids or weak bases with limited water solubility are toxic at lower doses when given in dilution rather than in concentrated solution. It was suggested that two mechanisms may be involved: (1) a more rapid stomach emptying with larger volumes, and (2) exposure to a larger absorptive surface in a relatively large fluid volume.[23]

Water is essential for the normal physiologic functions of experimental animals. One critical function is the defense mechanism for the lungs involving clearance of particulates and microorganisms by alveolar macrophages. It was shown that dehydration in rats resulted in a marked decrease in the number of macrophages which could be recovered from the lungs.[24] Deprivation of water for 48 hr increased mortality of rats and mice when injected with the water-soluble compounds of lead and antimony, but did not alter mortality following injections of the lipid-soluble compounds trichloroethylene, benzene, and Parathion.[25]

Predictive Toxicology

Toxicologists have attempted to develop data that would allow reasonable prediction of life-span toxicity from shorter periods such as one-tenth life span (about 90 days for the rat). The 90-dose ED_{50}, 90-dose LD_{50}, the chronicity factor (relation of 90-dose LD_{50} to single-dose LD_{50}), and the concentration index (relation of concentration in blood at steady state to that at the first dosage interval) have been discussed as available measurements, in combination with measurements already accepted as standard, for a more general understanding of the effects of long-term exposure.[26]

Percutaneous absorption was studied in rats and rabbits with either 4-hr or 24-hr contact with the skin. The 4-hr versus 24-hr LD_{50} values were well correlated for both rats and rabbits. The 4-hr rat values and the 24-hr rabbit values were best correlated on a logarithmic basis. A formula was derived to predict 24-hr LD_{50} values in rabbits from 4-hr LD_{50} values in rats. This procedure will be particularly valuable when the initial sample of a new chemical is too small to allow LD_{50} values for skin penetration in the rabbit.[27]

Organ Weight as a Criterion of Effect

Organ weights have been one of the more sensitive parameters of toxic effect due to treatment with chemicals. However, organ weights also vary as a function of body weight. Thus the toxicologist must judge whether or not changes in organ weights are related to reduced growth independent of the effect of the compound. In rats it was found that brain weight is mainly a function of actual age and that it alters little with changing body weights. It was suggested that organ weight/brain weight ratios may lead to erroneous conclusions in cases of animals in which growth has been retarded.[28]

MINERAL AND FIBROUS DUSTS

Asbestos

A major review of literature pertaining to worker exposure to asbestos dust was published. The standard recommended was based upon dose-response relationships that estimate the risk of contracting asbestosis by less than 1% of those exposed for a lifetime, and upon a factor for prudence in consideration of the carcinogenesis risk.[29] A monograph on the evaluation of carcinogenic risk of asbestos to man is available.[30]

A new theory has been proposed that the locus of pathogenicity of asbestos dusts resides in their polyfilamentous structure. Monofilamentous or fused polyfilamentous fibers appear to have less pathogenic potential in experimental studies to date.[31]

Lung Clearance Not Size Selective for Fiber Glass?

Rats exposed to fiber glass dust clouds for 2 months were examined for postexposure clearance of fibers. Both optical and electron microscopy gave results suggesting that clearance was independent of fiber diameter over the range of 0.28–1.10 μm. With regard to fiber length, electron microscopy data indicated that fibers with lengths up to 3 μm were all cleared at the same rate, while optical microscopy data indicated that fibers below 4 μm in length were cleared more rapidly than longer fibers. Papain-induced emphysema in the rats had no effect on clearance except that the optical microscopy data suggested a more rapid clearance of fibers less than 4 μm in the papain-treated rats.[32]

Cotton Bract Extract = Byssinosis?

The acute reversible bronchoconstriction that occurs as a part of the disease byssinosis has been considered to be related to the local release of histamine in the lung airways. Many attempts have been made to localize the responsible component of cotton dust and to develop animal models for such tests. An extract from cotton bracts, but not pericarps or fibers per se, released histamine from human lung autopsy specimens. The responsible component in the extract was not positively identified, but it has properties similar to methyl piperonylate, a steam-volatile naturally occurring compound. The action of the cotton bract extract and the methyl piperonylate was specific for human lung and was inactive with rat and guinea pig lungs.[33]

LEAD AND ITS COMPOUNDS

Clinical Significance of ALA-D

δ-Aminolevulinic acid dehydrase (ALA-D) is the enzyme that catalyzes the conversion of δ-aminolevulinic acid (ALA) to porphobilinogen in heme synthesis. Its measurement in circulating erythrocytes has been shown again and again to have a striking negative correlation with the measurement of lead in blood.[34] Nevertheless the clinical significance of the measurement remains obscure.

The lead-induced decrease in ALA-D in erythrocytes had no effect on the regenerating ability of the hematopoietic system of dogs. After being fed high concentrations of lead for 46 weeks, dogs had accumulated burdens of lead as demonstrated by increases in blood and urine lead concentrations, increased urinary ALA excretion, and decreased red blood cell ALA-D activity. Withdrawal of one-half the estimated blood volume from each dog resulted in a 30–40% reduction in hemoglobin concentration, red cell count, and hematocrit ratio; the recovery curves were not affected by the presence of the lead.[35]

Measurements of lead and ALA-D in blood were made for lead workers prior to exposure at their preemployment physical examination and then 2–3 times during the first week, once a week for 3 months, and twice during the fourth month of their work exposure. The rise in lead in blood and the decrease in ALA-D activity in the erythrocytes were virtual mirror images of each other, providing additional confirmation of the sensitivity of ALA-D activity for lead exposure and emphasizing the reliability of the test during the first few days of initial exposure.[36]

Hair and Urine Tests: Exposure Indications

Hair samples from individuals without known exposure to lead showed concentrations ranging from 3 to 26 μg/gm with an average value of 9.4 μg/gm. With workers exposed to lead, a correlation was found between levels of lead in hair and biochemical and clinical findings. Lead in hair at concentrations greater than 30 μg/gm were associated with signs of excessive lead exposure.[37]

The excretion of δ-aminolevulinic acid in the urine appears to correlate slightly better than urinary coproporphyrin with lead in urine and blood.[38]

Solubility and Macrophages

Exposures to aerosols of $PbCl_2$, Pb_2O_3, $NiCl_2$, or NiO produced variable changes in numbers and size of free alveolar macrophages. The two relatively soluble compounds, $NiCl_2$ and $PbCl_2$, produced little change in numbers of macrophages from controls, but the relatively insoluble compounds, Pb_2O_3 or NiO, produced marked decreases or increases, respectively, in the number of alveolar macrophages available by washing out the lungs. Both nickel compounds showed changes upon histopathologic examination; the concentration of nickel was approximately one-tenth the threshold limit value.[39]

Chelation of Lead

Calcium disodium ethylenediaminetetraacetate (EDTA) is widely used in the management of lead intoxication. While it has been considered that EDTA primarily removed lead from soft tissues, experiments with radiolabeled lead in rats have shown that the amount of lead removed by treatment with EDTA could be largely accounted for by depletion of lead stores in bone. Calcium trisodium diethylene triaminepentaacetate was somewhat more effective than EDTA in removing skeletal lead.[40] D-Penicillamine at equimolar doses was less effective than EDTA.[41] When EDTA was given to leaded rats with inhibition of δ-aminolevulinic acid dehydrase (ALA-D) activity, there was a rapid reactivation of ALA-D in the liver, but little effect on ALA-D inhibition in blood.[42]

Interactions or Lack Thereof

While pretreatment with lead nitrate caused some tolerance to acutely lethal doses of some divalent metals, such tolerance did not occur relative to biologic parameters of subacute lead intoxication. Pretreatment appeared instead to be additive or synergistic to the toxic effects manifested by body weight and hematocrit.[43]

When lead was given at a concentration of 200 μg/ml in drinking water in combination with trisodium nitriloacetate (NTA) at concentrations of either 0.01, 0.10, or 1%, there was no indication that NTA enhanced the pathologic effect of lead on the renal system. NTA alone resulted in a decrease of lead content of the kidney compared to controls and also caused elevated blood glucose levels.[44]

Organoleads Not Teratogenic to Rats

Tetraethyllead, tetramethyllead, and trimethyllead chloride were given to rats at doses that produced maternal mortality, as well as embryo or fetal toxicity in maternal rats with severe organolead toxicity. No severe teratogenic effects were observed.[45]

Abundance of Literature on Lead

The major biochemical effects of exposure to lead have been reviewed.[46,47] Emphasis was placed on the degree to which these effects might be used as predictors of potential clinical manifestations.[46] The literature pertinent to an exposure standard for inorganic lead in the workplace was published; the standard is intended to allow for a margin of safety to prevent adverse effects on health of adults.[48] Numerous papers from major conferences and comprehensive summaries on lead in the environment and its toxic hazards are available.[30,49-54]

MERCURY AND ITS COMPOUNDS

Methyl Mercury

The ability of methyl mercury chloride to affect the human nervous system, particularly during perinatal development, has been well recognized as an aftermath of exposure to high concentrations. Extensive experimental investigations have produced a great deal of information on dose–response relationships and basic mechanisms of action for methyl mercury and other mercury compounds; these studies have included in small part: short-term oral administration,[55,56] teratogenicity,[57] dominant lethal assay,[58] mercury contamination of food,[59] transport of mercury into fetal tissues,[60] biliary excretion,[61] behavioral changes in young rats,[62] fatal poisonings in Iraq,[63] a pharmacologic review,[64] a biochemical review,[47] a comprehensive review,[65] and a mini-review.[66]

Studies in rats exposed to methyl mercury chloride showed that excretion of mercury via bile into the gastrointestinal tract was predominantly as methyl mercury cysteine, which is rapidly reabsorbed, in contrast to complexes of inorganic mercury, which ended up in the feces.[67] These data suggested that an ion-exchange resin in the gastrointestinal tract might bind the methyl mercury cysteine and thus significantly enhance elimination of mercury from the body. It was subsequently found that a synthetic polythiol resin in food at a concentration of 1% would both increase excretion from the body and decrease absorption from food containing methyl mercury compounds.[68]

Quantitation of Hand Tremor

Two women workers exposed to mercury vapors in the course of calibrating glass pipettes developed symptoms of excessive exposure. Hand tremor was studied quantitatively by recording the attempt to maintain a force with the forefinger between the limits of 10 and 40 gm. The observations began 34 or 54 days after occupational exposure had terminated and within several months the women returned to normal.[69]

CADMIUM AND ITS COMPOUNDS

Animal Models for Cadmium Poisoning

Cadmium causes renal injury and the urinary excretion of protein. A study of the early signs produced by subcutaneous injection of cadmium chloride in male rabbits showed that loss in body weight and urinary excretion of protein, alkaline phosphatase, and acid phosphatase preceded temporal dysfunction of the distal tubules and renal dysfunction.[70]

Concentrations of 10, 50, or 300 ppm of cadmium chloride in the drinking water of rats produced renal changes in the proximal tubules when examined by electron microscopy. No remarkable changes were seen after 24 weeks at 1 ppm of cadmium.[71]

Cadmium as a cause of human hypertension and arteriosclerotic heart disease may be debatable, but animal models are available to study the relationship. Rabbits were made hypertensive by weekly intraperitoneal injections of cadmium acetate; a selective deposition of cadmium was observed in the liver and kidney.[72]

The bone changes seen in patients with Itai Itai disease have been produced in male rats and were most pronounced when rats were fed cadmium-added, calcium-deficient, low-protein diets. It was hypothesized that dietary deficiencies may explain individual susceptibilities to cadmium intoxication.[73]

Using whole-body autoradiography after intravenous injection of ^{109}Cd in mice, it was shown that cadmium in hair could be used as an indicator of whole-body accumulation in mice. Extrapolation of this technique to man must take into account such factors as different affinities for cadmium by hair of different colors, changes in hair with age, and external contamination of hair.[74,75]

Cadmium–Zinc Interactions

Cadmium can be considered as an antimetabolite of zinc in that it can adversely shift the dose–pharmacologic response curves for zinc relative to growth, hematologic functions, and body temperature control.[76] Thus cadmium may cause some of the characteristics of zinc deficiency even though zinc is present. The biochemical effects of cadmium have been recently reviewed.[47]

Although zinc and cadmium interact competitively at the biochemical level, they behave differently with regard to organ distribution in the mouse and rat. After equimolar quantities of radiolabeled zinc chloride and cadmium chloride were injected, zinc was accumulated more rapidly by erythrocytes and cadmium was more rapidly cleared from the plasma. Both isotopes concentrated primarily in the liver and kidneys, but within 2 weeks zinc was depleted from its association with cytoplasmic macromolecules while cadmium remained bound to proteins of 11,000–12,000 molecular weight.[77,78] When both isotopes were injected into pregnant rats, more cadmium than zinc was found in the placenta. Zinc was present in all tissues of the newborns, but cadmium was only detectable in liver, gastrointestinal tract, and in the brain tissue.[79] It was concluded that cadmium follows different metabolic pathways from those of zinc.[77]

OTHER METALS AND THEIR COMPOUNDS

Inhalation of Silver or Aluminum

Airborne silver particles were generated by exploding radioactive silver wires. The activity median aerodynamic diameter for the particles was near 0.5 μm, and 17% of that inhaled by dogs was deposited in the respiratory tract. Approximately 90% of that initially deposited in the lungs was absorbed into the body. Existing biologic values used by the International Commission for Radiation Protection for estimating the hazards of inhaled materials appear to be much too low for the inhalation of radiosilver.[80]

Metallic aluminum powders composed of flakelike particles caused focal pulmonary fibrosis when large doses were injected intratracheally into rats. However, when the powders were inhaled by hamsters and guinea pigs no pulmonary fibrosis was seen; rats developed scattered small scars resulting from foci of lipid pneumonitis with no relation to dust; alveolar proteinosis was seen in all species.[81]

Nickel Carbonyl Fatality

Three maintenance workers were apparently exposed to nickel carbonyl when inspecting a malfunction without fresh air masks or decontamination of the unit. One worker was hospitalized the following day and, despite treatment with sodium diethyldithiocarbamate, died 4 days after exposure. The pathologic diagnosis was pulmonary and cerebral edema due to nickel carbonyl poisoning.[82]

Feeding Studies with Tin, Selenium, or Tellurium

Rats were fed diets containing tin compounds for either 4 or 13 weeks. The tin compounds examined were stannic oxide, stannous oxide, stannous orthophosphate, stannous oxalate, stannous sulfide, stannous chloride, stannous sulfate, stannous oleate, and stannous tartrate. Some exposure conditions caused anemia and it was suggested that this may have been due to interference with the intestinal absorption of iron. The no-effect level of the active tin salts was 0.1% in the diet when liberal amounts of iron were present. Stannic oxide, stannous oxide, stannous sulfide, and stannous oleate, which are relatively insoluble tin compounds, did not evoke any noticeable effects at levels up to 1% in the diet.[83]

Selenium or tellurium, in both the tetra- and hexavalence states, were fed to mice in their drinking water at concentrations of 3 ppm or 2 ppm, respectively. The males showed no effects on growth, survival, longevity, or tumor incidences. Selenite-fed females were lighter than controls and their longevity was decreased. Tellurite-fed females showed a decrease longevity.[84]

No Effect with Calcined BeO

Dogs and monkeys were exposed for 30 min once a month for 3 months to an atmosphere containing between 3.30 and 4.38 mg of beryllium per cubic meter. Examination of their lungs 2 years later revealed no pathologic alterations. The beryllium oxide was calcinated at 1400°C and was free of other beryllium compounds. The high temperature of calcination, the purity, and the exposure conditions may have influenced the failure to find lung lesions within 2 years.[85]

Beryllium and Enzymes

Aryl hydrocarbon hydroxylases (AHH) in pulmonary tissue metabolize polycyclic hydrocarbons, some of which are pulmonary carcinogens. In contrast to nickel carbonyl, beryllium in the lungs did not markedly affect pulmonary AHH. Thus this study did not support the hypothesis that beryllium might act as a cocarcinogen in the lungs by interfering with the metabolism of carcinogenic polycyclic hydrocarbons in the lung.[86] Beryllium did interfere with the induction of enzymes in the liver, including induction of aminopyrine demethylase by phenobarbital and acetanilid hydroxylase by 3-methylcholanthrene.[87]

Inhalation of Uranium Compounds

Dogs and monkeys were exposed to 5 mg U/m^3 of a natural uranium dioxide aerosol with a mass median particle diameter of 1 μm. After 5 years of exposure there was little evidence of serious injury. Some of the animals were subsequently maintained for as long as $6\frac{1}{2}$ years following exposure. Frank neoplasms were found in the lungs of four dogs and foci of atypical epithelial proliferation in six of the thirteen dogs permitted to survive. These changes were not seen in monkeys; the monkeys, to a greater degree than the dogs, had pulmonary and tracheobranchial lymph node fibrosis, consistent with radiation effects.[88]

Injection and inhalation studies with uranium trioxide (enriched with ^{235}U) in dogs provided quantitative data to support early indications that its effects were more similar to soluble uranyl salts then to the relatively insoluble oxides, such as uranium dioxide. Uranium trioxide was rapidly removed from the lungs; systemic absorption was more than 20% of the exposure burden after inhalation. Elimination exceeded the initial lung burden by a factor of two, indicating that two-thirds of the initial deposition must have been in the upper airways rather than the lungs.[89]

Metal Carcinogenesis

The available literature attesting to the carcinogenicity of certain compounds of beryllium, cadmium, chromium, cobalt, iron, lead, nickel, selenium, zinc, and titanium has been reviewed. There was little experimental evidence that metals in food present a carcinogenic hazard to man.[90] Monographs covering animal data, extrapolation from animals to man, and evidence of carcinogenicity to humans for arsenic, beryllium, cadmium, chromium, nickel, lead, and iron compounds have been published by the International Agency for Research on Cancer of the World Health Organization.[30,91]

Effects of Metals: Reproduction and Teratology

Certain trace metals fed to mice and rats at doses that did not interfere with growth or survival were, however, intolerable for normal reproduction. Lead, cadmium, selenium, nickel, titanium, molybdenum, and arsenic were studied and it was suggested that reproduction studies provide a more rapid estimate of innate toxicities than does feeding the element for life.[92]

Dibasic sodium arsenate was injected intravenously into female hamsters on day 8 or 9 of their pregnancy at doses varying from 15 to 25 mg/kg; the embryos revealed a group of malformations that were quite different from those seen previously with cadmium injections. These experiments may provide a tool for the study of specific organogenetic processes in embryonic development.[93] Similar studies in mice given intraperitoneal injections of 45 mg/kg on one of days 6–12 of pregnancy showed maximum malformations occurring from injections on days, 7, 8, 9, and 10 with the peak effect on day 9.[94]

OZONE

Changes at the Biochemical Level

Rats exposed continuously to 0.7–0.8 ppm of ozone for several days showed increased levels of specific activities of lysosomal enzymes in their lung tissue fractions. It was hypothesized that ozone may (1) increase activity of enzymes due to infiltration of macrophages into the lungs and (2) decrease activity by direct inhibitory effect on certain enzymes in alveolar macrophages.[95]

Ozone at a concentration as low as 0.75 ppm for 4 hr caused a depression in the activity of benzpyrene hydroxylase in the tracheobronchial tissue of rats, as had previously been shown for lung parenchymal tissue. Nitrogen dioxide at concentrations of 5–50 ppm for 4 hr did not cause any change from control rats relative to benzypyrene hydroxylase activity of tracheobronchial tissue.[96]

After ozone exposures of 5 ppm to rats and 6.7 ppm to mice, for 90 min, it was possible to detect hydrogen peroxide in erythrocytes. This indicates that an ozone-induced oxidant effect can occur beyond the pulmonary epithelium.[97]

Rabbits exposed to 0.4 ppm ozone 6 hr/day, 5 days/week, for 10 months showed both emphysematous and vascular lesions.[98] The vascular damage to the small pulmonary arteries may have been reflected by the rise of serum trypsin protein esterase values.[99]

When rats were exposed to 33 ppm of ozone for 1 hr, there was congestion and subpleural hemorrhages in the lungs but there was neither histologic evidence[100] nor biochemical evidence[101] (based on the ratio $NADPH/NADP^+$) of effect on the epithelial cells of the trachea.

Male mice, 18–20 months of age, were exposed for 6 hr to ozone at concentrations of 0.5, 1.2, 2.5, or 3.5 ppm; at all exposures there was some mortality and in survivors there was a marked inhibition of cells synthesizing DNA which persisted for approximately 2 days.[102]

Protective Action of Antioxidants

Rats receiving a diet containing 100 mg of dl-α-tocopheryl acetate/kg of diet survived longer than did vitamin E depleted rats when both were exposed continuously to 1 ppm ozone. It was suggested that the cellular effect of ozone is an acceleration of the molecular events of vitamin E deficiency.[103]

Male rats continuously exposed to 0.8 ppm of ozone for 7 days showed an increased activity of lung enzymes participating in the pentose shunt and glycolysis. Dietary α-tocopherol partially retarded the elevation of some of the enzyme activities.[104]

Paraamino benzoic acid, a scavenger of hydroxy free radicals, when injected intraperitoneally into rats prolonged survival time when the rats were exposed to lethal concentrations of ozone.[105]

Ozone will cause the destruction of unsaturated fatty acids in erythrocytes under in vitro conditions.[106] In addition ozone and nitrogen dioxide both affect the alveolar wall of the lungs and their toxicity may be related to their oxidative nature. Phenolic antioxidants, including vitamin E, BHA, and BHT retard the oxidation of unsaturated fatty acids by ozone and nitrogen dioxide, but to different degrees.[107,108] Antioxidant-deficient animals are more susceptible to ozone than nitrogen dioxide.[109] The potential role for antioxidants as a fortification against inhaled oxidants deserves further study.

Other Lung Reactions

When ozone was supplied to only one lung of a rabbit, significant changes in pulmonary function did not occur until after there was evidence of lung edema.

It was concluded that the absence of pulmonary function changes was a poor indicator of the extent of ozone toxicity.[110]

An exposure to 0.38–1.59 ppm ozone for 4 hr and an inhalation dose of an aerosol infected with *Staphylococcus aureus* were superimposed upon male mice with and without silicotic lungs. It was concluded that the anatomic abnormalities due to silicosis did not enhance the ozone-induced inhibition in pulmonary bactericidal activity.[111]

Female beagle dogs were exposed to 1 ppm of ozone for 8, 16, or 24 hr/day, or 2 or 3 ppm of ozone for 8 hr/day, for up to 544 days. Although there were individual dogs in each group with little effect, morphologic changes, related to dose, were seen at all exposure levels based upon examination by light and electron microscopy.[112]

Ozone, which is classified as a primary irritant of the lower respiratory tract, was found to be removed more efficiently by the lower airways (starting at the trachea) than by the nasal and oral passages of dogs.[113]

Mouse Strain Variability

Twenty-one strains of mice were exposed to concentrations of ozone ranging from 4 to 24 ppm. The susceptibility of the mice to ozone was compared on the basis of the product of ozone concentration and time to death. There were no male–female differences in susceptibility, but pigmented strains appeared to be more resistant to ozone than albino strains. Resistance to both ozone and nitrogen dioxide appeared to be inherited as a dominant genetic characteristic. Further studies may provide information concerning the mechanism of action of these pulmonary irritants.[114]

NITROGEN DIOXIDE

Variable Interaction with Infection

Dose-response relationships for the effect of nitrogen dioxide on alveolar macrophages in rabbits have been developed for exposures of 5, 15, 25, or 50 ppm for 3 hr. Responses measured included phagocytic activity for killed BCG vaccine, parainfluenza 3 virus-induced resistance to rabbit pox virus, oxygen consumption, and glucose metabolism; the first two responses were the most sensitive, showing effects at 15 ppm and above.[115]

When squirrel monkeys were exposed continuously to 1 ppm of nitrogen dioxide for 493 days along with periodic challenges with a monkey-adapted influenza virus, they developed serum neutralization antibody titers earlier and greater than monkeys exposed to filtered air and similarly challenged with virus. However, only the monkeys exposed to nitrogen dioxide and virus showed slight pathologic findings in the pulmonary tissues.[116]

Male mice exposed to 2.3 or 6.6 ppm of nitrogen dioxide for 17 hr prior to staphylococcal infection showed a decrease in bacteriocidal activity; mice exposed similarly to 1 ppm showed no difference from controls.[117]

Exposure to Mixtures

An investigation of severe pulmonary damage to two silver brazers has provided warning that nitrogen dioxide will often be the cause of such pulmonary effects, since many solders do not contain cadmium. It was also noted that the possibility for synergistic action between cadmium oxide, nitrogen dioxide, and fluoride has not been studied sufficiently.[118]

Continuous exposure of monkeys and rats to 2 ppm of nitrogen dioxide with or without aerosolized sodium chloride for 14 months did not produce any enhancement or dimunition of effects attributable to the presence of the sodium chloride. The concentration of sodium chloride was approximately $330 \mu g/m^3$.[119]

Rats were exposed to diluted automobile exhaust for 6 hr/day, 5 days/week, for up to 2 years. Engine characteristics and dilution air were varied to provide exposure to an emissions mixture containing 23 ppm of nitrogen oxides (NO_x). Biologic effects consisting of body weight decrease, diminution of the sound-avoiding reflexes, and increase in the number of spontaneous tumors were observed.[120]

Biochemical, Physiologic, Morphologic Changes

Male rats were exposed to 2.9 ppm of nitrogen dioxide for 24 hr/day, 5 days/week, for 9 months. A significant reduction of the surface-active properties of the lung fluid was observed in association with a decreased percentage of palmitic acid in the phospholipid fatty acids of the lungs. It is believed that lung surfactant may consist largely of dipalmitoyl lecithin and that it may be involved in the integrity of the alveolar membrane.[121]

When rats were continuously exposed to approximately 6 ppm of nitrogen dioxide for 6 weeks, only part of them showed a reversible slowdown in mucociliary clearance. Measurements were made with a new technique using ^{99m}Tc which allowed repeated observations on the same animal. The rats that were affected did not show any apparent abnormalities of the airways and the mechanism for the change in mucociliary clearance is not known.[122]

Guinea pigs were continuously exposed to 0.4 ppm of nitrogen dioxide for 1 week. Fluid obtained by lung lavage had an increased content of protein which was believed to be due to both protein leakage from the capillary bed and increased turnover of lung cells.[123] In addition, increased levels of D-2,3-diphosphoglycerate in erythrocytes presumably indicated some effect on the hemoglobin–oxygen dissociation.[124]

Guinea pigs exposed continuously to 10 ppm nitrogen dioxide for 6 weeks developed an increased number of type 2 cells (cuboidal or columnar) in the alveolar wall relative to the thin type 1 cells normally present.[125] Continuous exposures to 2 ppm for 1, 2, 3, or 4 weeks resulted in observations that were suggestive of similar changes[126]; a significant increase in the average area of an alveolar wall cell was found.[127]

Self-protection by the Lungs

The ability of pulmonary cells to defend themselves against persistent attack was illustrated by serial observations during early response to nitrogen dioxide exposure by rats. With continuous exposure to 2 ppm of nitrogen dioxide, changes appeared after 3–7 days including loss of cilia and hypertrophy and focal hyperplasia in the epithelium of the terminal bronchiole; after 21 days of continuing exposure, the tissue recovered substantially so that for several months it was difficult to distinguish it from normal epithelium. At the higher concentration of 17 ppm, injury occurred as early as 2–4 hr; after 1–2 days of continuing exposure, repair with a low cuboidal cell type took place. This repair tolerated nitrogen dioxide but resulted in a thickened air–blood barrier and some permanent histologic aberrations.[128] With both exposures cell proliferation increased, as measured by labeling with tritiated thymidine, but returned to normal within 3–5 days.[129]

SULFUR OXIDES

Fate of Inhaled SO_2

Sulfur dioxide, long known as an irritant of the upper airways, will also rapidly enter into the body from these airway surfaces. Dogs with surgical isolation of the upper airways were exposed to radiolabeled sulfur dioxide. Blood levels of ^{35}S rose steadily during respiratory exposure and decreased only slowly over several hours postexposure. Concentrations in the plasma, two-thirds of which was dialyzable, were always higher than those in erythrocytes. One to six percent of the total amount of ^{35}S which entered the upper airways was excreted in the urine as inorganic sulfate during the several hours of the experiment.[130]

Physiologic and Morphologic Changes

Male mice originating from defined flora conditions were divided into two groups and raised either in an isolation room or in conventional mouse rooms with other mice. When both groups of mice were about 40 days old they were exposed to 10 ppm of sulfur dioxide from 4 hr to 3 days. The mice raised in conventional facilities had more severe lesions of the upper respiratory tract; these mice had also developed a mild upper-respiratory-tract infection.[131]

Experimental papain-induced emphysema in rats did not appear to affect the quantity of titanium oxide particles deposited in the lungs, but did reduce the clearance rate.[132,133] Exposure to sulfur dioxide at concentrations of 1 or 10 ppm for 7 hr/day, 5 days/week, for from 2 to 5 weeks, caused a depression in clearance of particles. Exposure to 0.1 ppm of sulfur dioxide caused stimulation or no effect on pulmonary clearance.[134]

Young cynomolgus monkeys were continuously exposed to concentrations of sulfur dioxide of approximately 0.14, 0.64, or 1.28 ppm for eighteen months and no deleterious effects were found based upon pulmonary function, hematologic and clinical biochemical measurements, or histologic examination. Monkeys similarly exposed to 4.69 ppm for 7 months followed by a 1-hr overexposure of between 200 and 1000 ppm developed deterioration of their pulmonary function and, when sacrificed 48 weeks later, histologic changes in pulmonary tissue were observed.[135]

Twenty ppm of sulfur dioxide in air was required to evoke a significant change in pulmonary flow resistance in cats, and this change was see in only 2 of 20 animals. It was suggested that the results with the cat may mirror the experience with "human reactors" and that the guinea pig which responds at 0.16 ppm may be an animal model for this "reactive" segment of the population.[136]

Exposure to Mixtures

No adverse effects were observed in cynomolgus monkeys or guinea pigs continuously exposed to 0.5 mg/m^3 of fly ash in combination with 0.1, 1.0, or 5 ppm of sulfur dioxide. The monkeys were exposed for 78 weeks and the guinea pigs for 1 year. The mass median diameter of the fly ash particles was about 3 μm.[137]

Young piglets, 1 week of age, were continuously exposed to approximately 35 ppm of sulfur dioxide in combination with either corn dust or corn starch for 6 weeks. The dust exposures were at concentrations of approximately 1 mg/ft^3, and the smallest particle diameters were in the range of 3–5 μm. With this particle size the piglets showed respiratory tract changes similar to that seen with SO_2 alone.[138]

Beagle dogs were exposed to 13.4 mg/m^3 of sulfur dioxide and 0.9 mg/m^3 of sulfuric acid alone or in combination for 21 hr/day for 620 days. One-half of the dogs for each exposure had pulmonary impairment caused by prior exposure to nitrogen dioxide. Sulfuric acid exposures produced the most serious pulmonary impairment. It was noted that the prior impairment with nitrogen dioxide did not make the lungs more susceptible to the subsequent low-level airborne toxicants.[139]

Beagle dogs were exposed for 6 hr/day for 5 years to raw auto exhaust (RAE), irradiated auto exhaust (IAE), oxides of sulfur (SO$_x$), RAE + SO$_x$, IAE + SO$_x$, low NO plus high NO$_2$, or high NO plus low NO$_2$. A detailed examination of the cardiovascular status of the dogs led to the suggestion that some of the abnormalities might have a causative association with the exposures to air pollutants.[140]

SO$_2$ Oxidation Products

Sulfur dioxide emitted into the air may be oxidized to sulfuric acid and particulate sulfates. Some of these aerosols are more irritating than sulfur dioxide itself. Air quality standards should take into account the toxicology of these oxidation products in combination with sulfur dioxide gas.[141]

Guinea pigs were continuously exposed to sulfuric acid mist at concentrations of 0.08 or 0.1 mg/m^3 for 52 weeks without observation of deleterious effect. Cynomolgus monkeys continuously exposed at concentrations ranging from 0.38 to 4.79 mg/m^3 for 78 weeks showed definite deleterious effects on pulmonary structures and deterioration in pulmonary function.[142]

PESTICIDES

DDT Ingestion by Humans

DDT was ingested for 21.5 months by human volunteers at dose rates up to 35 mg/man/day, which is approximately 555 times the average intake of all DDT-related compounds by 19-year-old men in the general population. No definite clinical or laboratory evidence of injury by DDT was found during a 5-year following period.[143] The toxicology and impact on human health of organochlorine pesticides has been reviewed.[144]

Interesting Findings with DDT in Rodents

While DDT has been reported to cause hepatomas in mice fed high doses for a prolonged period, one study found that 7 of 89 C$_{57}$B1 mice did not develop tumors following a subcutaneous injection of the Zimmerman ependymoma. One hundred percent of 87 control mice did take the tumor transplant. These data are difficult to extrapolate to the human situation.[145]

Injection of 10–20 mg/kg of DDT into guinea pigs prior to and following immunization with diphtheria toxin did not have any effect on antibody levels.[146] Furthermore the anaphylactic shock induced in the same animals by a challenge with diphtheria toxoid was markedly reduced, apparently due to the reduction of histamine content of mast cells caused by DDT[147]

The dominant lethal test has been proposed as one indicator of *in vivo* mutagenic activity. Male rodents are given the compound to be tested and then repeatedly mated with untreated females; the females are subsequently examined for failures in implantations. A statistically significant effect was found in the proportion of females with one or more dead implantations only in rats mated during the postmeiotic stage of spermatogenesis (week 3) following oral treatment with 100 mg/kg of *p,p'*-DDT. It was concluded that DDT was only marginally positive with respect to the dominant lethal test.[148] The dominant lethal assay in the mouse has been investigated with studies on 174 chemicals or chemical mixtures.[149]

2,4-D and Teratogenicity?

Rats were given 2,4-dichlorophenoxyacetic acid (2,4-D) up to the maximally tolerated dose of 87.5 mg/kg/day on days 6–15 of gestation. Embryotoxic and fetotoxic effect, but no teratogenicity, was observed. Similar results were obtained with equimolar doses of the propylene glycol butyl ether ester and the isooctyl ester. It was noted that some earlier studies with 2,4-D in mice had used dimethylsulfoxide (DMSO) as a solvent and DMSO itself has been shown to be a teratogen in several species of laboratory animals.[150] In a separate three-generation reproduction study, no deleterious effect was seen at 500 ppm of 2,4-D in the diet, but 1500 ppm, while apparently affecting neither fertility nor litter size, did sharply reduce the percent of pups born surviving to weaning and the weights of weanlings.[151]

2,4,5-T Teratogenic?

In contrast with previous reports of teratogenic and fetocidal effects of 2,4,5-trichlorophenoxyacetic acid (2,4,5-T), studies in Sprague-Dawley rats and New Zealand white rabbits failed to reveal any teratogenic or embryotoxic effects. Rats were given oral doses as high as 24 mg/kg on days 6–15 of gestation and rabbits were given oral doses up to 40 mg/kg on days 6–18 of gestation.[152] It was suggested that the effects observed in the previous reports may have been caused by the contaminant, 2,3,7,8-tetrachlorodibenzo-*p*-dioxin, which was present at a concentration of 30 ppm in the sample of herbicide tested, while only 0.5 ppm was present in the later study.[153] Studies at higher doses of the same sample of 2,4,5-T did not produce a teratogenic response in rats at 50 mg/kg/day. A dose of 100 mg/kg/day administered on days 6 through 10 of gestation caused a high incidence of maternal deaths. Of four surviving pregnant rats, three had complete early resorptions and one had a litter of viable fetuses that showed toxic effect but no terrata,[154] although another study in rats given 100 mg/kg/day showed an increased incidence of skeletal anomalies.[155] A further study in mice using 2,4,5-T (with the dioxin content below 0.1 ppm) found no teratogenic effect at an oral dose of 20 mg/kg/day given on days 6–15 of pregnancy, but doses of 35–130 mg/kg/day caused embryotoxicity and a significant increase in cleft palate.[156] This difference between the mouse and the rat has been confirmed in another laboratory.[157] Pregnant and nonpregnant rats appear to eliminate 2,4,5-T at similar rates in the urine and feces, but the biologic half-time was 3.4 hr in adult rats and 97 hr in newborn rats.[158]

2,4,5-T Metabolism

The rat and dog showed considerable difference in metabolism of 2,4,5-T at the same dose level of 5 mg/kg. Metabolism in the rat was altered at higher doses. Elimination in rats was primarily the urinary excretion of unchanged 2,4,5-T, while appreciable excretion in feces occurred with dogs and three unidentified metabolites were detected in the urine of dogs. Half-live values for elimination from the body were approximately 86.6 hr for the dog and 13.6 hr for the rat, possibly explaining why 2,4,5-T is more effective in dogs than rats.[159] In man, a dose of 5 mg/kg resulted in a half-life of 23.1 hr for clearance from the plasma and body; essentially all of the 2,4,5-T was excreted in the urine. Thus metabolism of 2,4,5-T in man is more similar to the rat than the dog.[160]

Dieldrin: Tumor Incidence, Fat Storage

The long-term study of Dieldrin fed to mice showed liver lesions, including tumors, with an increased incidence in treated groups compared to controls. Considerable discussion about the classification and diagnosis of the liver lesions was presented. The role of microsomal enzyme induction in the evolution of liver cell tumors was discussed but has yet to be established.[161,162]

Dieldrin, like other lipid-soluble compounds, is stored in body fat at relatively high concentrations. Littermate male rats were fed either a high-fat ration or a low-fat grain ration. After approximately 1 year the high-fat-fed rats weighed twice as much as their littermates and all of them were then given Dieldrin in their diets at 0.8 mg/kg/day for 7 days. The groups were then subdivided and one subgroup was given half-rations for 6 weeks to produce weight reduction. Both the "obese" and normal rats lost weight and the Dieldrin stores in the fat of the normal rats was reduced while very little change in Dieldrin concentration took place in the fat stores of the "obese" rats. The blood level of Dieldrin in the "obese" rats did rise with weight reduction, but the brain levels of Dieldrin did not increase.[163]

Interactions with Organophosphorus Pesticides

Many organophosphorus pesticides that inhibit cholinesterase activity will also inhibit aliesterase activity; in most cases the aleisterase inhibition will occur at lower doses. Any chemical or drug, including other pesticides like Malathion, which depends upon aliesterases for detoxification will have its toxic action potentiated. A procedure was developed to detect the potential for this interaction without extensive toxicity testing. The chemical of interest is fed to rats for 1 week at various dietary levels; then serum and liver aliesterase activity is measured using diethyl succinate and tributyrin as substrates.[164]

Five ppm of Abate, an organophosphate pesticide, in the drinking water of rats produced marked depression of liver carboxylesterase activity, but the animals showed normal growth rates, general appearance of good health and no appreciable effect on brain cholinesterase activity. When Malathion, another anticholinesterase pesticide, but one that is detoxified by liver carboxylesterases, was injected into the same rats, there was a significant potentiation of the anticholinesterase action at a dose of 400 mg/kg, but not at 200 mg/kg. These data suggested that the possibility of adverse interactions should be considered when there is exposure to Abate and Malathion at high concentrations.[165]

Multistudies on Carbaryl

Carbaryl, 1-naphthyl methylcarbamate, is a widely used insecticide. Previous reports on reproduction and teratogenicity have used various methods of testing. Additional studies were undertaken and the results have been evaluated following guidelines for estimating a level of Carbaryl residue intake in the diet without effect upon human reproduction or teratogenesis. A three-generation rat reproduction study resulted in no statistically significant, dose-related effect upon fertility, gestation, viability of pups, or lactation at doses up to 10 mg/kg/day of Carbaryl. A rat teratogenic study at doses up to 500 mg/kg/day of Carbaryl resulted in no teratogenic anomalies and no effect on fertility or gestation; however, survival of pups at the high dose prior to weaning was affected.[166] Differences in toxic effects were observed depending upon whether or not administration of Carbaryl was by peroral intubation or by dietary admix.[167]

Fungicides and Herbicides

Teratogenicity studies with two dithiocarbamate fungicides, manganese ethylenebis (dithiocarbamate) or Maneb and zinc ethylenebis (dithiocarbamate) or Zineb, revealed no effect on intrauterine development of the progeny with the following exposures to rats: 0.5 gm/kg for Maneb and 1.0 gm/kg for Zineb administered as a single dose on day 11 or 13 of organogenesis, or as a daily dose throughout pregnancy; or daily 4 hr periods of inhalation of 100 mg Zineb/m^3 from day 5 to the end of pregnancy. Congenital anomalies were induced when single oral doses of 1–4 gm Maneb/kg or 2–8 gm Zineb/kg were given on day 11 or 13 of organogenesis; these doses were estimated to be at least 1000 times higher than the daily human intake that could result from the consumption of foods containing the maximum residues of these compounds.[168]

Teratogenicity studies on three fungicides, Captan, Folpet, and Difolatan, were conducted in rhesus monkeys or stump-tailed macaques. The three fungicides contain the o-dicarboximido structure and are related to thalidomide. These nonhuman primates are susceptible to thalidomide-induced deformities, but there was no evidence that Captan, Folpet, and Difolatan possessed teratogenic potential.[169]

Paraquat, a dipyridylium herbicide, is absorbed through the intact skin of rabbits in quantities sufficient to produce systemic toxicity and death. When the site of application was free to the air, the toxic effects were greatly reduced. When grooming was not rigidly prevented, the rabbits developed severe tongue ulceration even though the area of application had been routinely decontaminated with water.[170] Paraquat had been characterized as a "hit-and-run" poison, but this was not supported by studies that showed accumulation of Paraquat in the lung, lung pathology, a long secondary half-life in plasma and tissues, and a correlation between tissue concentrations and degree of toxic response.[171]

2-sec-Butyl-4,6-dinitrophenol, or Dinoseb, is the active ingredient in some herbicides. It appeared to have a low potential for producing teratogenic effects in mice. The no-effect dose level of Dinoseb given throughout days 8–16 of pregnancy was 20 mg/kg/day by the oral route.[172] Dinoseb was shown to cross the placenta but embryo levels never exceeded 2.5% of maternal plasma levels.[173]

Piperonyl Butoxide in Mouse, Rat, and Man

Piperonyl butoxide has been used as a synergist with pyrethrin-containing insecticides. It is a potent inhibitor of microsomal enzyme function in mice, but rats require a 100-fold greater dose than mice for inhibition of antipyrine metabolism. The oral administration of 50 mg of piperonyl butoxide (0.71 mg/kg) did not influence antipyrine metabolism in man; this dose is 50 times the dose likely to be received by pesticide sprayers.[174]

Toxicity Variation among Bird Species

Oral LD_{50} values were determined for 16 common pesticides on mallard ducks, ring-necked pheasants, chukar partridges, *Coturnix* quail, common pigeons, and house sparrows. The doses of pesticides were administered by intubation of capsules into the proventriculus. The average range of LD_{50} values was approximately 10-fold. Although the *Coturnix* (Japanese quail) has gained wide acceptance as a species "representative" of native upland game birds, it was in fact no better as a "representative" species than any other. It was recommended that in wildlife work the species of interest should be used, at least for short-term toxicity studies.[175]

The oral LD_{50} value was obtained for 369 chemicals in a wide variety of species of wild birds, always including red-winged blackbirds and starlings. The redwings were more sensitive to lethal doses of chemicals than starlings and both were more sensitive than rats.[176] In a study with 14 pesticides in mallard ducks of ages 36 hr to 6 months, the young were not always more susceptible than adults.[177]

HYDROCARBONS

Enzyme Induction and Metabolism: Benzene, Toluene, Styrene

Benzene injected into male rats induced proliferation of smooth endoplasmic reticulum of liver cells and stimulated the metabolism of itself and some, but not all, drugs tested. It was concluded that benzene, and not its hydroxylated metabolites, was responsible for the microsomal stimulation.[178] Mouse liver microsomes metabolized benzene more rapidly than did rat and rabbit liver microsomes. Benzene metabolism appeared to be mediated by the mixed function oxidase system and binding of benzene to cytochrome P-450 was a significant rate-determining factor.[179]

Pretreatment of rats with phenobarbital stimulates the *in vitro* activities of side-chain hydroxylase and aromatic hydroxylase. *In vivo* metabolism of toluene and benzene is also enhanced and results in increased tolerance of rats to the narcotic action of toluene and the leukopenic action of benzene.[180]

Styrene appears to be metabolized in the rat to styrene oxide, styrene glycol, mandelic acid, and then to phenylglyoxylic acid or hippuric acid. Pretreatment with phenobarbital enhanced the metabolism to styrene oxide and SKF 525-A inhibited metabolism. The intraperitoneal LD_{50} for styrene oxide was about one-fourth that of styrene, indicating that metabolism is a toxification rather than detoxification mechanism.[181]

Effects of Hexane, Dicyclopentadiene, Terphenyls

Female rats were exposed to approximately 50,000 ppm of hexane up to 10 hr. Most organs reached a steady-state concentration within 4 or 5 hr, except that the concentration in the liver increased linearly over the exposure period. It was found that hexane induced accumulation of triglycerides in the liver. The concentration of total lipids in the liver doubled, but did not change in blood, brain, adrenals, kidneys, or spleen.[182]

The 4-hr LC^{50} values for dicyclopentadiene varied from 771 ppm for male rabbits to 145 ppm for male mice. Vapors were detectable by humans at 0.003 ppm. Based upon the results of repeated 7 hr/day exposures for 89 days, it was recommended that 5 ppm should be a ceiling level for exposure of workers.[183]

Hydrogenated terphenyls may be used as coolants for nuclear reactors. Mice were exposed to an aerosol of irradiated terphenyls at five times the concentration actually present around the reactor for 4 hr/day, 5 days/week, up to 8 weeks. Only slight reversible changes occurred in the lungs and liver as studied by both light and electron microscopy.[184] With chronic ingestion only electron microscopic changes were seen in the liver, but irreversible nephritis followed 16 weeks at 600 mg/kg/day of the irradiated terphenyls or 1200 mg/kg/day of the nonirradiated terphenyls; the LD_{50} for the irradiated terphenyls was also lower.[185]

HALOGENATED HYDROCARBONS

PCB's and Liver Damage

Sherman strain rats were fed the polychlorinated biphenyl (PCB) compounds, Aroclor 1260 or Aroclor 1254, at 20, 100, 500, or 1000 ppm as a dietary admix for up to 8 months. Deaths occurred among the higher dose groups including one female rat receiving 100 ppm of Aroclor 1260. Effects on the liver were seen in all dose groups with the effect of Aroclor 1254 being more pronounced than that of Aroclor 1260.[186] Rats fed Aroclor 1254 at a concentration of 500 ppm for 6 months and then examined 10 months after exposure had ceased, showed that a high concentration of PCB's in the adipose tissue and livers, as well as liver lesions, persisted throughout this period.[187] Rats intubated with Aroclor 1242 at a dose level of 100 mg/kg every other day for 3 weeks exhibited histopathologic changes in the liver and kidneys, but no other signs of toxicity.[188] A conference on the toxicologic and environmental impact of PCB's illustrated the complexities and unknowns of the problem.[189]

AOL and Poly Cleaners

The relatively new industrial disease, occupational acroosteolysis (AOL), has been clearly associated with the hand cleaning of polymerizers in the polyvinyl chloride industry.[190] The disease, which appears to be systemic rather than local, is characterized by osteolytic lesions and Raynaud's phenomenon.[191] Twenty-five definite cases and 16 suspicious cases were identified among 5011 employees in the United States and Canada. Although these workers had engaged in vinyl chloride and polyvinyl chloride manufacturing, neither the specific etiologic agent nor its portal of entry is known.

Aerosol "Sniffing"

The "sniffing," actually deep inhalation of highly concentrated vapors, of aerosol products has resulted in human fatalities. Halogenated hydrocarbons, as well as hydrocarbons themselves, used as solvents and propellants in aerosol cans, have been shown to sensitize cardiac muscle to epinephrine resulting in ventricular fibrillation, cardiac arrest, and death. Experiments with beagle dogs exposed to high concentrations of various fluorocarbons showed that stress factors, such as noise causing fright, could effect marked cardiac arrhythmias without the administration of exogenous epinephrine.[192] After exercise to increase their level of circulating epinephrine, dogs inhaling difluorodichloromethane (fluorocarbon 12) and 1,1,2,2-tetrafluoro-1,2-dichloroethane did show cardiac sensitization, but higher concentrations were required compared to studies with injected epinephrine. No cardiac sensitization was produced with inhalation of fluorotrichloromethane at concentrations as high as 1 vol %.[193] The effects of bromotrifluoromethane on rat myocardial glycolysis showed an induction of respiratory depression and hypoxia, resulting in the mobilization and intracellular accumulation of free fatty acids.[194] When fluorocarbon propellants were administered to mice, rats, and dogs as aerosols, no significant changes in heart rate or electrocardiogram tracings were observed.[195,196] Dogs developed cardiac sensitization after exposure to 50,000 ppm of fluorocarbon 12 and 5000 ppm of fluorocarbon 11 (trichlorofluoromethane). Despite the 10-fold difference in the exposure concentration, the blood concentrations associated with sensitization were similar.[197]

Human Exposures to Fluorocarbons

Human volunteers were exposed to 1,1,2-trichloro-1,2,2-trifluoroethane (fluorocarbon 113) for two 3 hr periods/day for 5 days/week for 2 weeks at concentrations of 500 and 1000 ppm. Clinical observations, laboratory tests, subjective impressions, and measurement of psychomotor performance did not reveal evidence of any detrimental effects resulting from the exposures. Analysis of breath samples indicated that a significant body buildup of fluorocarbon 113 did not occur, but further studies will be needed to determine if a slow buildup of this compound will occur in tissues.[198] Two human volunteers were exposed to dichlorodifluoromethane (flurocarbon 12) at concentrations of 1000 and 10,000 ppm for 2.5 hr. Clinical observations, laboratory tests, subjective impressions, continuous electrocardiograpm monitoring, and tests of psychomotor performance did not reveal any detrimental effects from exposure to 1000 ppm, and exposures to 10,000 ppm resulted only in a 7% reduction in the standardized psychomotor test score.[199]

Barbiturates and Solvent Toxicity

Barbiturates may have considerable use among workers and, since they are known to be able to stimulate liver-metabolizing enzymes, they may influence the toxicity of some industrial chemicals. In rats pretreatment with phenobarbital markedly potentiated the toxicity of carbon tetrachloride and chloroform as measured by the hepatoxic response of elevated levels of serum glutamic oxaloacetic transaminase. However, methylene chloride, methyl chloroform, trichloroethylene, and perchloroethylene did not have any potentiating effect with phenobarbital pretreatment. It was suggested that differences in the metabolic pathway of solvents may provide an explanation for the observations.[200]

Hazardous Decomposition at TLV of CCl_4

The industrial threshold limit value (TLV) for repeated daily exposures without adverse effects is 10 ppm for carbon tetrachloride (CCl_4). Under appropriate conditions of exposure to hot surfaces, vapors of CCl_4 may decompose to phosgene, chlorine, chlorine dioxide, and hydrogen chloride at concentrations in excess of the TLV's for these lung irritants. Following exposures of rats to various combinations of the thermal decomposition products of CCl_4, no marked potentiation of the effects of respiratory impairment were observed.[201]

COHb from CH_2Cl_2

Eleven male human volunteers, all nonsmokers and in good health, inhaled methylene chloride (CH_2Cl_2) vapors at concentrations from 500 to 1000 ppm for 1–2 hr. The industrial threshold limit value (TLV) for repeated 8 hr/day exposures is currently set at 500 ppm. The volunteers experienced some signs and symptoms of central nervous system depression and they all developed elevated carboxyhemoglobin (COHb) saturation levels. This suggested that methylene chloride may be metabolized to carbon monoxide and that a greater COHb level is produced by exposure to the TLV for methylene chloride than to the TLV for carbon monoxide.[202] Mice have been continuously exposed to 5000 ppm methylene chloride for up to 7 days, but COHb measurements were not made; partially reversible fatty changes in the liver occurred.[203]

Toxic Effects for Several Chlorinated Hydrocarbons

A 14-year-old boy attempted to get "high" by drinking about 15 ml of 1,2-dichloroethane. Despite sophisticated treatment, he died after 5 days with necrosis in the liver, kidney, and adrenal glands.[204]

Several human fatalities have been attributed to the formation of dichloro-acetylene (DCA) when trichloroethylene was passed over soda lime used as a carbon dioxide absorbent. Since pure DCA is spontaneously explosive in air, its toxicity was studied in mixtures with various organic solvents. The mixtures produced a more toxic effect by several orders of magnitude compared to the solvents themselves.[205]

Carbon tetrachloride, chloroform, and 1,1,2-trichloroethane produce renal dysfunction. Studies in mice showed that under certain circumstances pre-treatment with one of the solvents protected against the nephrotoxicity of subsequent treatment. The mechanism for the nephrotoxic effect is unclear. While carbon tetrachloride appears to be metabolized to a product that in turn causes hepatotoxicity, the nephrotoxicity may result from the parent compound or other mechanisms.[206]

CHEMICAL CARCINOGENS

Coal-Tar Pitch Tumorigenicity

Benzene solutions of various coal tar pitches and petroleum asphalts were painted on the skin of mice twice weekly. Mean survival time for mice painted with coal-tar pitch was 31 weeks and 90% had epidermal carcinomas and papillomas. Mean survival times for asphalt-painted and control mice were 81 and 82 weeks, respectively; only one carcinoma and five papillomatous growths were observed in 218 mice treated with asphalts; one papillomatous growth was seen in 26 control mice. The polynuclear hydrocarbon content of the coal-tar pitches was several orders of magnitude greater than that of the petroleum asphalts.[207] Monographs on the evaluation of carcinogenic risk of coal-tar pitch and certain polycyclic aromatic hydrocarbons and heterocyclic compounds are available.[208]

Bladder Tumors in Benzidine Workers

Thirteen of 25 exposed men employed in the manufacture of benzidine developed bladder tumors. While the men were exposed to other highly suspect chemicals, benzidine was common to all of the exposures and was considered to be the most likely carcinogen.[209]

Haloethers and Lung Tumors

An increase in the spontaneous incidence of pulmonary adenomas in strain A mice was observed after exposure for 6 hr/day, 5 days/week, for 82 days at 1 ppm of bis(chloromethyl) ether or for 101 days at 2 ppm of chloromethyl-methyl ether. It was noted additionally that the lack of irritant warning properties and high toxicity renders these compounds extremely hazardous in industrial handling.[210]

When 30 Sprague-Dawley rats, having a very low, if any, incidence of spontaneous lung tumors, were exposed to only 0.1 ppm of bis(chloromethyl) ether for 6 hr/day, 5 days/week, for 101 exposures, they all died within 659 days. A startling tumor yield was observed, including squamous cell carcinomas of the lung and esthesioneuroepitheliomas arising from the olfactory epithelium and invading the sinuses, cranial vault, and brain.[211]

Antioxidant Protection

The antioxidant butylated hydroxytoluene (BHT) fed to male mice at a concentration of 0.75% for 4 weeks gave significant protection against lethal doses of some mutagenic and carcinogenic chemicals, but not against x rays. The protective action may have been related to the induction of drug-metabolizing enzymes.[212] Rats fed BHT at a concentration of 6600 ppm for 24 (males) or 32 (females) weeks developed fewer tumors due to the carcinogens N-2-fluorenyl-acetamide and its N-hydroxy derivative. The antioxidant, diphenyl-p-phenylenediamine, failed to alter cancer induction by these agents.[213] It was concluded that BHT increases the detoxification metabolites of the carcinogens and this lowers the amount of a given dose available for activation reactions.[214]

CARBON MONOXIDE

CO and Reaction Time

Exposures of young male students to 650 or 950 ppm of carbon monoxide for 45 min caused blood carboxyhemoglobin (COHb) levels of 7.6 or 11.2%, respectively. There was no impairment of performance in depth perception, visual discrimination for brightness, and flicker fusion discrimination. There was a statistically significant decrement in reaction time to a visual stimulus; however, the decrement was not dose related nor did it correlate with COHb levels; at the high dose 5 of 20 subjects actually did better in reaction time. Conclusions about the observations warrant some caution.[215] A separate investigation with human volunteers inhaling up to 250 ppm of carbon monoxide (12.37% COHb) for 3 hr showed no decrements in performance as measured by tests for time estimation and tracking.[216]

High-Level, Short-Term CO

Male human volunteers inhaled carbon monoxide at concentrations from 1000 ppm for 10 min to 35,600 ppm for 45 sec. Measurements of carboxyhemoglobin in venous blood provided the basis for a predictive equation that should be useful for brief exposures to high concentrations of carbon monoxide.[217,218]

CO and the Impaired Heart

Individuals with coronary heart disease may have serious impairment of the mechanism for increasing blood flow to the myocardium. Thus there is a dependence on increased oxygen extraction from the blood to satisfy oxygen needs of the myocardium; carbon monoxide inhalation may limit the availability of oxygen to the myocardium through extraction because of the reaction with blood oxygen-carrying hemoglobin to form carboxyhemoglobin. Cynomolgus monkeys with induced myocardial infarction (injection of latex microspheres into coronary arteries) were exposed to 100 ppm of carbon monoxide for 23 hr/day up to 6 months. Electrocardiograms showed a higher incidence of T wave inversion in infarcted compared to noninfarcted monkeys, suggesting a greater degree of myocardial ischemia due to breathing carbon monoxide by the infarcted monkeys.[219]

Long-Term Study with CO

Cynomolgus monkeys were exposed to approximately 20 or 85 ppm of carbon monoxide for 22 hr/day, 7 days/week, for 2 years. While there were slight dose-related increases in blood carboxyhemoglobin (COHb) values, there was no indication of compensation or adverse biochemical, physiologic, or pathologic effect due to the exposures.[220] In a separate study with rats, guinea pigs, dogs, and squirrel monkeys exposed continuously to 51, 96, or 200 ppm carbon monoxide for 90 days, there was the expected elevation in COHb. In addition, exposures to 96 or 200 ppm caused elevations in the mean values for hemoglobin and hematocrit in all species.[221]

TRISODIUM NITRILOACETATE (NTA)

NTA Metabolism in Man

Trisodium nitriloacetate (NTA) was radiolabeled in the carboxy position and given to man by capsule. Eight fasted subjects received 10 mg NTA (100 μCi); after 120 hr 12% was in urine, 77% in the feces, and less than 0.1% in expired air. Blood level peaks occurred 1–2 hr after dosing and approached zero after 12 hr; no biotransformation was observed. These results are similar to those obtained with rats and dogs, except that if one assumes no enterohepatic circulation in man, then man absorbs one-fourth of the amount absorbed by the rat and dog.[222]

NTA Not Found to be Teratogenic

NTA has been used in detergents as a partial replacement for phosphates. Small amounts may potentially be ingested by way of trace amounts in ground water supplies or as trace residues on eating utensils washed with a detergent containing NTA. Rats were fed NTA for two generations, either continuously or from days 6–15 of pregnancy, at dietary concentrations of 0.1 or 0.5%; the higher level had produced kidney lesions in long-term toxicity tests.[223,224] Rabbits were given doses up to 250 mg/kg/day by intubation on days 7 through 16 of pregnancy. It was concluded that NTA was neither embryotoxic nor teratogenic in these species.[225] NTA was found to store in small amounts

(0.007% of the calcium turnover per day) in the skeleton; 97% was eliminated from the body within 3 days.[226] Despite the accumulation of NTA in the fetal skeleton no teratogenic effects were obserbed when pregnant mice were given 0.2% NTA in their drinking water from day 6 to 18 of pregnancy.[227]

NTA, Cadmium, Mercury, and Zinc

NTA exerted a protective action against the toxicity of cadmium chloride in nonpregnant rats. Excretion of cadmium was increased and organ and tissue deposition of cadmium was inhibited.[228] It was also reported that NTA did not enhance the toxicity or teratogenicity of either cadmium chloride or methyl mercury chloride, in contrast to an earlier report that was considered ambiguous because of variations in solvents and routes of administration.[229] In long-term studies, zinc concentration in bones of rats was noted but was not considered to be an adverse effect[224]; urinary zinc excretion in dogs was increased but this did not produce zinc deficiency.[230]

MISCELLANEOUS COMPOUNDS OF SPECIAL INTEREST

Aflatoxin Toxicity

Male rats were fed either a complete synthetic diet or a synthetic diet marginally deficient in lipotropes which induces fatty liver but not cirrhosis. Aflatoxin B_1 was administered intragastrically as a single dose or repeated doses. Deficient rats were resistant to single doses in that none died within 2 weeks, while there was 60–100% mortality among rats fed the complete diet. However, the deficient rats were more susceptible to repeated doses of aflatoxin as indicated by both toxicity and carcinogenicity. The latter susceptibility was explained by the failure of the drug-metabolizing enzymes in the liver to be increased by aflatoxin administration.[231] Other studies in male rats have suggested that testicular androgens in some way influence the effects of dietary intake of aflatoxin.[232] The lack of evidence of percutaneous absorption of aflatoxin in rats was reported.[233]

Single- and multiple-dose studies with various aflatoxins indicated that the furofuran moiety is essential for toxic and carcinogenic activity. Another structure–activity relationship (SAR) is the presence of the double bond in the terminal furan ring in relation to potency.[234] The toxic and carcinogenic activity was also related to the ability to inhibit RNA polymerase activity and decrease the RNA content in rat liver cell nuclei.[235] A monograph on the evaluation of carcinogenic risk of aflatoxin to man is available.[91]

Nitrosamines: A Human Health Hazard

While there are no known cases of cancer in man caused by nitrosamines, many of these N-nitroso compounds are potent carcinogens in experimental animals and the biochemical potential for their action in man exists. Nitrosamines can form from nitrite and secondary amines under the acid conditions prevailing in the mammalian stomach. In addition, there appears to be the potential for nitrates to be reduced to nitrites in the mammalian stomach. Nitrosamines have been reported to be present in some smoked meats, bacon, and tobacco smoke in very low concentrations. Regulatory agencies have been struggling with the very difficult assessment of the reality of hazards to man from nitrosamines in the environment.[236] A monograph on the evaluation of carcinogenic risk of several nitrosamines and nitrosamides to man is available.[91]

Nitrites and Nitrates in Food

Since nitrates may be reduced to nitrites under certain conditions in the human gastrointestinal tract, both of these chemicals may be related to methemoglobinemia reported in infants. In view of an apparent sensitivity of young infants, it was suggested that foods, such as spinach and beets, containing high levels of nitrate should not be given to children below 3 months of age.[237]

Cyclamate Metabolism

When cyclohexylamine (CHA), a metabolite of cyclamate, was tested with the dominant lethal assay for mutagenicity, a significant preimplantation loss in females occurred. However, since lower doses of CHA did not result in postimplantation loss and since a high percentage of ova were apparently not fertilized, it was concluded that the loss of fertility resulted from some mechanism other than that of dominant lethal mutation.[238]

CHA was found in the urine of human volunteers ingesting 5 gm of sodium cyclamate daily for 7 or 8 days; excretion was approximately 1% or less of the cyclamate intake. In contrast to cyclamate, CHA is pharmacologically active; however in these experiments no pharmacologically active concentrations of CHA were reached.[239]

The mechanism of lethality from CHA in mice has been investigated.[240]

Saccharin Not Metabolized

Studies with nonisotopic saccharin many years ago had indicated no metabolic transformation. Recent studies with ^{14}C labeled saccharin revealed the presence of two metabolites at low levels.[241] However, additional studies with radioactive saccharin in rats and monkeys failed to detect any metabolism. It was suggested that radiolabeled contaminants were present in the ^{14}C-saccharin, but similar contaminants were not present in unlabeled saccharin, which was used for identification of chromatograph fractions.[242] When saccharin was administered in 0.5–1 gm doses to human subjects, the dose was not quantitatively excreted as saccharin within 72 hr. However, no metabolite was identified.[243]

Hexachlorophene and Brain Damage

The widespread use of hexachlorophene as an antibacterial agent has been curtailed because of its association with toxicity in humans. Large doses of hexachlorophene affect the central nervous system of rats, pigs, and humans.[244] When female rats were fed hexachlorophene in their diet at a dose of 25 mg/kg/day for 10 weeks, the lesions produced in the brains represented cerebral edema limited to the white matter which was considered to resemble the diffuse spongy degeneration of the white matter of the brain described in infants.[245] The acute oral LD_{50} of hexachlorophene in the rat was 9 mg/kg at 10 days of age, 111 mg/kg at 32 days of age, and then dropped to about 60 mg/kg in adult rats. The toxic effect on the brain began when the rats were between the ages of 8 and 14 days.[246] Dermal application of hexachlorophene in propylene glycol or as a 3% commercial soap preparation at doses of 24 and 48 mg/kg/day for 30 days on the intact skin of rats produced ulceration of the treated skin and status spongiosus of the white matter of the brain. Doses of 12 mg/kg/day produced only erythema and desquamation of the treated skin.[247]

Convulsant Activity of Substituted Benzenes

The doses that induced convulsions in one-half the mice tested (CD_{50}) were determined for monosubstituted benzenes, monochloro, methyl- and amino-substituted phenols, mono-, di-, and trihydroxybenzenes, and dihydroxynaphthalenes. Phenol was the only monosubstituted benzene that caused convulsant activity. Catechol was the most potent compound tested. A quantitative assessment of motor activity was made which was in close agreement with the CD_{50} values.[248]

Chlorinated Dibenzo-(furans and dioxins)

The technical grade of various chlorinated compounds such as the polychlorinated biphenyls (PCB), 2,4,5-trichlorophenoxyacetic acid (2,4,5-T), and

2,4,5-trichlorophenol may contain small amounts of chlorinated dibenzofurans or chlorinated dibenzodioxins. Certain diseases, such as chloracne, chick edema, and x-disease in cattle, have been associated with these contaminants. In addition, the contaminants may cause pathologic changes in the liver and teratogenic effects. It was recommended that further epidemiologic and experimental animal studies are needed to clarify problems possibly related to the combined effect of a chemical compound and its contaminants.[249] This recommendation was supported by the results of dermal toxicity studies with Aroclor 1260, Clophen A 60, and Phenoclor DP6.[250] Current knowledge available about these contaminants was presented at a recent 2-day conference.[251]

Embryotoxicity and Food Contaminants

The potential for embryotoxicity or teratogenicity due to food contaminants was reviewed. Contaminants included mycotoxins, metals, nitrosamines, pesticides, and polychlorinated biphenyls. While the claim for the absolute safety of any chemical contaminant is not scientifically justified, the only contaminant of major concern as a cause of embryotoxicity was mercury, especially methylmercury; the collection of data on this problem is underway.[252]

Phthalate Esters Toxicity

Dimethyl terephthalate (DMT) was subjected to extensive toxicologic study including subacute feeding and inhalation studies and a single-generation reproduction study. DMT in the diet at 10,000 ppm for 96 days caused a reduced body weight gain in male rats; 5000 ppm caused a reduction in weight gain at weaning in the reproduction study. No effects were seen in the inhalation studies with the highest concentrations of 86.4 mg/m^3 for 4 hr/day for 58 days.[253]

A 2-day conference exploring the environmental health impact of phthalate esters, especially when used as plasticizers, focused attention on the widespread use of these compounds.[254]

Parakeets and Hot Fry Pans

Birds are more susceptible than mammals to fumes from fry pans overheated under abuse conditions. Butter or corn oil in the fry pans was equally or more hazardous than Teflon finish in that pyrolysis products were generated at lower temperatures. There was no hazard from fumes when fry pans were used according to conventional kitchen use.[255]

Organic Dinitrates

Organic dinitrates have been implicated as a cause of sudden, fatal circulatory collapse among workers in the explosives industry. Triethylene glycol dinitrate and propylene glycol dinitrate, despite their chemical similarity, showed some markedly different toxic effects.[256] Extensive studies on the effect of vapors of propylene glycol dinitrate on rats, guinea pigs, rabbits, squirrel monkeys, and dogs, including avoidance behavior of trained rhesus monkeys, have been reported.[257]

Accident with DMF

Dimethylformamide (DMF) is a widely used solvent in the chemical industry. A worker in a urethan fabric coating plant, accidentally splashed by DMF over 20% of his body surface, was also exposed to the inhalation of the concentrated vapor. The exposure caused hyperemia of the skin, severe abdominal pain, hypertension, leukocytosis, and hepatic damage. Elevated levels of porphobilinogen were detected in his urine. The worker was hospitalized and was asymptomatic approximately 2 weeks after the exposure.[258]

Metabolism of Carbon Disulfide

The sodium azide–iodine reaction has been recommended as a reliable test with urine samples for early diagnosis of carbon disulfide intoxication. Three urinary metabolites giving a positive reaction have been isolated. The greatest quantity of the metabolites has been identified as thiocarbamide. Small quantities of 2-mercapto-2-thiazolinone-5 and a third unidentified metabolite were present.[259]

Ethylene Oxide Reaction Products

Ethylene chlorohydrin and ethylene glycol may be reaction products from ethylene oxide sterilization. Ethylene glycol and ethylene chlorohydrin were not irritating to rabbit eyes after topical application at a concentration of 0.4% and 1.0%, respectively. At higher concentrations ocular toxicity occurred.[260] Ethylene oxide was, in general, a more intense eye irritant than its reaction products.[261] Details of the morphologic alterations caused by ethylene chlorohydrin on the skin of rabbits have been presented at both the light and electron microscope levels.[262]

Propylene Glycol in the Diet

Dogs were fed propylene glycol in their diets at dose levels of either 2 or 5 gm/kg/day for 2 years. Since these concentrations of propylene glycol (20% of the diet) represent a significant caloric addition to the diet, equicalorific quantities of dextrose were added to diets of controls. It was concluded that 2 gm/kg/day (approximately 8% of the diet) of propylene glycol was utilized as a carbohydrate energy source without any adverse effect. At the higher dose there was evidence of slight erythrocyte hemolysis and increases in serum total bilirubin.[263] Rats fed propylene glycol up to concentrations of 50,000 ppm in the diet (approximately 2.5 gm/kg/day) for 2 years showed no adverse effect including no increase in tumor incidence.[264] The toxicology, metabolism, and biochemistry of propylene glycol has recently been reviewed.[265]

Vapor Hazard of Trimethyl Phosphite, Caprolactam, Ether

Inhalation exposure of rats to trimethyl phosphite at a concentration of 500 ppm for 7.5 hr/day, 5 days/week, for 8 weeks affected body weight and produced severe pulmonary and cutaneous pathology. The odor threshold was reported to be 0.1 ppb under laboratory test conditions and 1 ppb in the work environment.[266]

Healthy male volunteer workers were exposed to vapors of caprolactam for several minutes at low concentrations and up to 30 sec at 100 ppm. With relatively unacclimatized subjects the irritant response threshold was approximately 10 ppm at low relative humidities. A time-weighted average threshold limit value of 5 ppm was suggested.[267]

When neonate and adult rats were exposed to approximately 15,000 ppm of diethyl ether, the neonates survived 5–6.5 times as long as the adults. This was despite a more rapid absorption by the neonates as indicated by blood ether concentrations 2.5–3 times greater for neonates than adults. It was suggested that the immature central nervous system of the neonates may be less sensitive to the depressant action of high concentration of diethyl ether.[268]

Skin Absorption of Hair Dye

HC Blue No. 1, a nitrophenylenediamine derivative, is a major color component in semipermanent hair-dying preparations. Percutaneous absorption was examined by comparative studies using topical application and injections intradermally, subcutaneously, and intraperitoneally in rats and rabbits. The dye, which is water soluble, was capable of diffusing through the skin. There was no evidence of significant metabolism, the intact compound being found in both urine and bile.[269]

The hair dye, p-toluenediamine, was applied twice weekly to the shaved dorsal skin of mice for 2 years. The exposure exceeded that likely to be encountered in practice and no adverse effects were seen over the life span of the mice.[270]

Dermal Toxicity of Cyclohexenone

Toxicologic testing of 2-cyclohexen-1-one revealed moderate acute dermal toxicity with significant eye and skin irritation. An accidental skin exposure without prompt washing with water resulted in tenderness and reddish purple discoloration which began approximately 2 days after exposure; the moderate skin injury was completely recovered approximately 1 month later.[271]

Toxicity of N,N-Dimethylamides

The toxic effects of a homologous series of N,N-dimethylamides was assessed by the intravenous, intraperitoneal, intragastric, and percutaneous routes in mice and rabbits. Precautions to prevent skin contact should be taken for safe use and handling of these compounds.[272]

Uptake of Vapors: Aldehydes, Acetone

Aldehyde vapors have been classified as primary irritants of the upper respiratory tract on the basis of their relatively high solubility in water. This classification was substantiated by studies in dogs in which most of the retention in the total respiratory tract could be accounted for by the retention in the upper tract. The approximate uptake by the total respiratory tract varied with formaldehyde at 100%, acetaldehyde at 50–54%, propionaldehyde at 74–82%, and acrolein at 81–84%. Based upon comparison of some observations with acetaldehyde in man, it seems reasonable to assume that human retention would be similar.[273,274]

Comparative studies between man and the dog exposed to vapors of acetone at 100 and 500 ppm for 2 or 4 hr demonstrated that the dog is an adequate animal model for studies of absorption, distribution, and elimination of inhaled acetone. (The current threshold limit value for acetone is 1000 ppm.) The half-life of acetone in the blood was approximately 3 hr.[275] Uptake of acetone by the total respiratory tract of the dog ranged between 65 and 70%. Simultaneous exposure to acetone and acetaldehyde caused an increased retention of acetaldehyde.[276]

Isocyanates: Sensitization versus Direct Irritation

Workers exposed to isocyanate compounds may develop symptoms of chest tightness, substernal burning, shortness of breath, and wheezing, which may be related to respiratory sensitization in some cases and, in others, to a direct irritant effect on the respiratory tract. It was suggested that measurements of forced expiratory volume in 1 sec may be helpful in differentiating sensitization from direct irritant effect.[277]

Revised EEL for Nitrogen Trifluoride

The National Academy of Science–National Research Council Committee on Toxicology has established an emergency exposure limit (EEL) of 100 ppm for 30 min and 50 ppm for 60 min inhalation exposure to nitrogen trifluoride (NF_3). The effect of actue exposures to NF_3 was studied in rats, mice, dogs, and monkeys, with dogs being most sensitive, exhibiting an anemia characterized by the presence of Heinz bodies after exposures of 7000 ppm for 15 min, 3500 ppm for 30 min, or 2000 ppm for 60 min, or approximately 120,000 ppm-minutes. With exposures to 30,000 ppm-minutes for 15, 30, or 60 min, there were no detectable effects. It was recommended that the EEL for NF_3 be revised upward from 3000 to 30,000 ppm-minutes.[278]

Inhalation Toxicity of Chlorine Pentafluoride

Chlorine pentafluoride is used as a fluorinated oxidizing propellant for rocket engines. The LC_{50} values (in ppm) for rats were 257, 194, and 122; for mice 144, 105, and 7; for dogs 298, 156, and 122; and for monkeys 249, 218, and 173, for 15-, 30-, and 60-min exposures, respectively. Mortality was related to the production of chemical pneumonia.[279]

Cyanuric Fluoride Toxicity

The effects of acute inhalation of 2,4,6-trifluoro-s-triazine, $(FCN)_3$ (also named cyanuric fluoride), and of 2,4,6-tris (trifluoromethyl)-s-triazine, $(CF_3CN)_3$, on male albino rats resulted in 4-hr LC_{50} values of 3 ppm and 1400 ppm, respectively. Acute dermal application studies gave LD_{50} values of 100 μl/kg of body weight for cyanuric fluoride and >100 μl/kg of body weight for $(CF_3CN)_3$. Cyanuric fluoride at concentrations as low as 5 ppm can be detected from its pungent odor before the other body senses respond; at higher concentrations, burning of the eyes and breathing discomfort are readily apparent.[280]

Cyanide Poisoning Treated with Cobalt

Studies in mice showed that intraperitoneal injections of cobaltous chloride could protect against the lethal effects of potassium cyanide. Combinations with sodium thiosulfate were more effective than either alone. It was suggested that the synergistic antidotal effect of cobaltous chloride may be related to the ability to chelate both cyanide and thiocyanate ions.[281]

Effects of Hydrazine

Increased interest has been shown in the usefulness of behavior methods as a measure of effect of hazardous compounds. Hydrazine sulfate was administered to rats by intraperitoneal injection at doses of 1–52 mg/kg. The following behavioral situations were studied: spontaneous motor activity, fixed ratio-20 water reinforcement, differentiated reinforcement at low rates, and free-operant shock avoidance. Some behavioral effects were seen at doses as low as 3.3 mg/kg, which is lower than doses used in toxicity studies.[282]

Hydrazine was readily absorbed through the skin of dogs. The blood concentration of hydrazine rose initially, indicating that the rate of absorption must have exceeded the rate of detoxication and excretion. Three of four dogs receiving 15 mmoles/kg died within 3.5 hr. Edema and skin discoloration occurred at the site of application.[283]

Eye Injury from Detergents

The banning of phosphates in detergents in several large municipalities has prompted the marketing of nonphosphate detergents, some of which contain sodium carbonate/metasilicates. Typical phosphate detergents caused transient irritation of the ocular tissues of rabbits. Typical carbonate detergent formulations caused considerable ocular irritation followed by opacity and corrosion of the cornea of rabbits. Metasilicates enhanced this corrosive action. Protection by washing was not effective unless performed within 1 min of exposure. The alkalinity content of the detergents was directly related to eye injury.[284]

Aniline in Man and Rat

Twenty male and female human volunteers, ages 22–45 years, were given total oral doses of 5, 15, and 25 mg aniline over 3 successive days. It was found that doses of 15 mg or below did not produce increased methemoglobinemia or Heinz bodies; doses of 25 mg produced increased methemoglobinemia but no

Heinz bodies. Humans were more sensitive to aniline than rats; the no-effect single oral dose in rats was 20 mg/kg.[285]

Methyl Amyl Ketone Ingestion

Methyl n-amyl ketone is a widely used flavoring constituent in food. The oral LD_{50} in rats is 1.67 gm/kg. At dose levels of 500 or 100 mg/kg/day given by oral intubation to rats for 13 weeks, the only adverse effects related to treatment were kidney and liver changes that were not associated with histopathologic damage. The no-effect level was estimated to be 20 mg/kg/day; it is calculated that the intake for a 60-kg man would be between 0.07 and 0.21 mg/kg/day.[286]

Branched-Chain Alcohols: Acute Toxicity

Branched-chain primary aliphatic alcohols containing 5, 6, 8, 9, 10, 13, and 16 carbon atoms were investigated. Oral LD_{50} values in rats ranged from 1.5 to greater than 8.4 gm/kg. Although percutaneous absorption was noted, all dermal LD_{50} values in rabbits were greater than 2.6gm/kg. Dermal irritation was slight to severe in general inverse relationship to molecular weight. Eye irritation was severe with the C_5, C_6, C_8, and C_{10} alcohols. Inhalation toxicity was low, but all alcohols produced some local irritation during single 6-hr exposures.[287]

Ethanol More Hazardous for Old Rats

Young and old rats metabolized ethanol at about the same rate; young rats eliminated more ethanol by pulmonary ventilation but the total was less than 10% of the dose. Nevertheless, the LD_{50} value following intraperitoneal injection was 5.1 gm/kg for older rats and 6.7 gm/kg for young rats. It was suggested that whereas the body water content is lower in old rats, the moisture content of blood and brain is similar for old and young rats, and therefore the older rats will have significantly higher blood and brain levels of ethanol, accounting for the differences in LD_{50} values.[288]

GENERAL TOPICS OF SPECIAL INTEREST

Trace Elements: Recondite Toxicity

Recondite toxicity, defined by Schroeder as a subtle metabolic change consistent with reasonable survival, may not catch on as an everyday term, but in some circles it will be preferable to the term often used, "subclinical toxicity." Schroeder has carefully reviewed the recondite toxicity of important trace elements in the environment, including the deficiency conditions of essential trace elements.[289]

A worldwide scientific effort is underway to investigate a possible connection between cardiovascular diseases and elements in drinking water and food in the natural environment. While negative associations have been reported, there is a suggestion that in areas where water is hard the death rate tends to be lower than in soft-water areas.[290]

Permissible Single Oral Doses

A comparison of oral LD_{50} values for 16 solvents was made in neonate (5–8 gm), immature (16–50 gm), young adult (80–160 gm), and older adult (300–470 gm) rats. Neonates were uniformly and exceedingly sensitive to all of the solvents. The solvents studied were acetone, acetonitrile, benzene, chloroform, cyclohexane, diethyl ether, dimethylformamide, ethanol, hexane, isopropanol, isopropyl ether, methanol, methylene chloride, methyl ethyl ketone, tetrahydrofuran, and toluene. Suggested maximum permissible single oral dose limits based upon $\frac{1}{1000}$ or $\frac{1}{10,000}$ of the dose giving the first observable gross sign of toxic action in adult rats were presented.[291]

Liquid Chemical Diet for Rats

Rats were able to obtain all of their apparent physiologic needs from a chemical diet supplied as a 33% aqueous solution for at least 8 weeks.[292] The toxicologist is increasingly concerned about trace contamination and variable composition of nutrients in commercial laboratory animal diets, since these factors may influence enzyme induction and tumorigenicity.

Changes with Decreased Body Weight Gain

Treated animals frequently decrease their food consumption for reasons of taste, or otherwise, and consequently show an inhibition of body weight gain. The toxicologist must then assess other toxic signs as related to decreased food consumption alone, or to the test compound. Rats were given quantities of food equal to 50, 75, or 87.5% of the amount consumed by a control group fed *ad libitum*. Other than decreased weight gain, the principal changes occurred in the group at the 50% feeding level and consisted of an increase in erythrocyte count, hemoglobin, hematocrit; elevated serum glucose, urea nitrogen, glutamic-pyruvic transaminase, and alkaline phosphatase; increased organ-to-body-weight ratios for brain, uterus, testes, epididymides, and adrenals; increase in hepatic fat; and an increase in iron-laden macrophages in the liver and spleen.[293]

Factors Influencing Placental Transfer

The disposition of a variety of drugs in pregnant rats and their fetal tissues was studied. The results indicated that the placenta behaves like a lipoid barrier toward cationic and neutral compounds, while it is quite permeable to anionic compounds.[294]

Lung Clearance Mechanisms

Alveolar macrophages play an important role in alveolar clearance. If the number of alveolar macrophages was increased by pretreatment with Freund's complete adjuvant, iron oxide dust was cleared from the lungs of rats more rapidly. While increased phagocytic removal of the dust is suggested, alternative interpretations are possible.[295]

Several overall reviews of alveolar clearance mechanisms have been published recently.[296,297]

Mechanism of Sensory Irritation

It was theorized that for a group of chemicals all containing an ethylenic group, the sensory irritation reaction is initiated by association with sulfhydryl groups of a receptor molecule on the free nerve endings of the afferent trigeminal which are located at the surface of the nasal mucosa. Twenty-seven chemicals of this type were tested for their potential sensory irritation properties to the upper respiratory tract when administered in an aerosol form to mice.[298]

Molecular Aspects of Toxicants

Many questions about the mechanism of action of toxic chemicals appear to have answers related to binding of chemicals with specific proteins or nucleic acids and the induction of microsomal enzymes.[299] The extensive literature dealing with enzyme induction and interactions between chemicals has been recently tabulated,[300] and the special concern for the metabolic interactions among environmental chemicals and drugs has been emphasized.[301]

Serum Enzymes and Morphologic Damage

Carbon tetrachloride, mercuric chloride, and diethanolamine were given intraperitoneally and thioacetamide was given orally to rats at varying doses to allow comparison of serum enzymes and isozyme patterns with morphologic alterations of the liver and kidney. Glutamic oxaloacetic transaminase (GOT), lactic acid dehydrogenase (LDH), and LDH isozyme patterns were measured in serum. Morphologic damage, assessed by light and electron microscopy, occurred at dosage levels below those necessary to induce detectable serum enzyme alterations. The different toxicants had different relationships between serum levels and histologic damage.[302]

Optimal Antidotal Dose

Activated charcoal is frequently used as an antidote for the general treatment of ingested poisons. The rationale for this treatment is binding of the poison to charcoal, thereby reducing the absorption from the gastrointestinal tract. *In vivo* studies with male rats showed that the optimal charcoal-drug ratio was at least 8 : 1 for the treatment of overdoses of sodium phenobarbital, chloroquin phosphate, and isoniazid.[303]

Significance of Tumor Incidence

Regulations in the United States forbid the addition of a chemical to the food consumed by man if that chemical has caused cancer when ingested by experimental animals. Evidence has been cited to show the concordance between ingestion and pellet implantation as routes for urinary bladder tumorigenesis.[304] This topic highlights the serious dilemma of our inability to agree upon an adequate experimental procedure for firm distinctions between carcinogenicity and noncarcinogenicity. The literature available on the incidence of mammary tumors in control rats has been tabulated.[305]

Thresholds: Do They Exist?

A symposium with the above title has been published[306]; it has emphasized the controversial aspects of the use of the term threshold as applied to carcinogenesis, but as might be anticipated, no uniform answer was forthcoming. Two authors[307,308] have presented the bases for their support of the conclusion that thresholds actually exist.

Criteria for Exposure Limits

Experimental toxicologists collect animal data that are extrapolated to humans as part of the basis for establishing hazardous exposure limits. However, animal models are not generally adequate to define and duplicate the levels of vitality in aging humans. Thus, while standards to limit exposures may be satisfactorily established to prevent specific occupational diseases, their adequacy to meet criteria such as "not contributing in any way to the prevalence and severity of one or another of the chronic degenerative diseases that are common among aging individuals" is less certain. T. F. Hatch reviews this and other criteria that challenge professionals in occupational health to expand their efforts to learn more about the quantitative dose-response relationships between man and hazardous agents.[309]

Toxicology and the Environment

Alastair Worden, in a recent lecture, has reviewed, with reminiscences from his vantage point in the United Kingdom, the many toxicologic and environmental problems that society has had to deal with in recent years. His topics include the impact of "Silent Spring," Dutch Margarine Sickness, thalidomide, the great smog, mercury in fish, artificial sweeteners, Chinese Restaurant Syndrome, nitrosamines, environmental pollution with PCB, lead, and others, defoliants in Vietnam, banning of organochlorine insecticides, and hexachlorophene in human neonates.[310]

Toxicologist–Physician Interactions

Henry F. Smyth, Jr., has described the contributions, activities, and shortcomings of the experimental toxicologist. Ways in which cooperation and communication between the toxicologist and physician can develop a needed improvement were presented. One major area of interaction would be the collection of documented evidence by the occupational physician in cooperation with the industrial hygienist to validate the safe exposure of workers to threshold limit values, or other hygienic standards, which have been estimated from toxicologic data obtained with experimental animals.[311]

The Many Faces of Toxicology

"It is sometimes said that one can tell a toxicologist by his worried look. This is understandable in view of the fact that his standard procedures often do not disclose any specific toxic action of a new drug. With such an experiment the toxicologist has done all he can to establish the new drug's safety, knowing only too well that there probably is no such thing as a safe or nontoxic drug. To deal with this difficult situation, he has created what one might call speculative toxicology." Gerhard Zbinden has identified the many faces which represent approaches by the toxicologist as formal toxicology, speculative toxicology, comparative toxicology, pharmacodynamic toxicology, symptomatic toxicology, systematic toxicology, and geographic toxicology.[312] What an exciting and challenging field this toxicology is!

The Future of Toxicology

Wayland J. Hayes, Jr., believes that training and research in toxicology suffers from a lack of identity of toxicology as a scientific discipline. He indicates that the greatest opportunities for toxicology can be seen but not yet grasped, and suggests that these opportunities will be realized while emphasizing diversity, but at the same time developing a more mature, unified discipline.[313]

Toxicology has benefited greatly by attracting scientists from many different disciplines. Its direction has taken a strong course toward knowledge of the mechanisms responsible for toxic action. This direction bodes well for the future of toxicology as a scientific discipline.

REFERENCES

1. "The Testing of Chemicals for Carcinogenicity, Mutagenicity and Teratogenicity." Department of Health and Welfare, Ottawa, Ontario, Canada, 1973.
2. Food and Drug Administration Advisory Committee on Protocols for Safety Evaluation: Panel on Carcinogenesis Report on Cancer Testing in the Safety Evaluation of Food Additives and Pesticides. *Toxicol. Appl. Pharmacol.* 20, 419 (1971).
3. Weil, C. S., Statistics versus safety factors and scientific judgment in the evaluation of safety for man. *Toxicol. Appl. Pharmacol.* 21, 454 (1972).
4. Golberg, L., Trace chemical contaminants in food: Potential for harm. *Food Cosmet. Toxicol.* 9, 65 (1971).
5. Golberg, L., Safety of environmental chemicals—the need and the challenge. *Food Cosmet. Toxicol.* 10, 523 (1972).
6. Panel on Chemicals and Health of the President's Science Advisory Committee, "Chemicals & Health." National Science Foundation, Washington, D.C., 1973.
7. Weil, C. S., Guidelines for experiments to predict the degree of safety of a material for man. *Toxicol. Appl. Pharmacol.* 21, 194 (1972).
8. Ad Hoc Committee of the Environmental Mutagen Society and the Institute for Medical Research, Chromosome methodologies in mutation testing. *Toxicol. Appl. Pharmacol.* 22, 269 (1972).
9. Phillips, L., II, Steinberg, M., Maibach, H. I., and Akers, W. A., A comparison of rabbit and human skin response to certain irritants. *Toxicol. Appl. Pharmacol.* 21, 369 (1972).

10. Lansdown, A. B. G., An appraisal of methods for detecting primary skin irritants. *J. Soc. Cosmet. Chem. 23*, 739 (1972).
11. Burton, A. B. G., A method for the objective assessment of eye irritation. *Food Cosmet. Toxicol. 10*, 209 (1972).
12. Hickey, T. E., Beck, G. L., and Botta, J. A., Jr., Optimum fluorescein staining time in ocular irritation studies. *Toxicol. Appl. Pharmacol. 26*, 571 (1973).
13. Weil, C. S., and Scala, R. A., Study of intra- and interlaboratory variability in the results of rabbit eye and skin irritation tests. *Toxicol. Appl. Pharmacol. 19*, 276 (1971).
14. Barrow, R. E., Vorwald, A. J., and Domier, E., The measurement of small animal respiratory volumes by capacitance respirometry. *Amer. Ind. Hyg. Ass., J. 32*, 593 (1971).
15. Adler, K. B., Wooten, O., and Dulfano, M. J., Mammalian respiratory mucociliary clearance. *Arch. Environ. Health 27*, 364 (1973).
16. Berke, H. L., and Roslinski, L. M., The roentgenographic determination of tracheal mucociliary transport rate in the rat. *Amer. Ind. Hyg. Ass., J. 32*, 174 (1971).
17. Creasia, D. A., Nettesheim, P., and Hammons, A. S., Impairment of deep lung clearance by influenza virus infection. *Arch. Environ. Health 26*, 197 (1973).
18. Creasia, D. A., Nettesheim, P., and Hammons, A. S., Impairment of lung clearance mechanisms by respiratory infection. *Health Phys. 23*, 865 (1972).
19. Jaunarajs, K. L., and Liebling, R. S., The digestion of lung tissue for mineral dust recovery. *Amer. Ind. Hyg. Ass., J. 33*, 535 (1972).
20. Raabe, O. G., Bennick, J. E., Light, M. E., Hobbs, C. H., Thomas, R. L., and Tillery, M. I., An improved apparatus for acute inhalation exposure of rodents to radioactive aerosols. *Toxicol. Appl. Pharmacol. 26*, 264 (1973).
21. Wehner, A. P., Craig, D. K., and Stuart, B. O., An aerosol exposure system for chronic inhalation studies with rodents. *Amer. Ind. Hyg. Ass., J. 33*, 483 (1972).
22. Drew, R. T., and Laskin, S., A new dust-generating system for inhalation studies. *Amer. Ind. Hyg. Ass., J. 32*, 327 (1971).
23. Borowitz, J. L., Moore, P. F., Yim, G. K. W., and Miya, T. S., Mechanism of enhanced drug effects produced by dilution of the oral dose. *Toxicol. Appl. Pharmacol. 19*, 164 (1971).
24. Baetjer, A. M., Dehydration and recovery of free alveolar macrophages. *Arch. Environ. Health 22*, 28 (1971).
25. Baetjer, A. M., Dehydration and susceptibility to toxic chemicals. *Arch. Environ. Health 26*, 61 (1973).
26. Hayes, W. J., Jr., Tests for detecting and measuring long-term toxicity. *Essays Toxicol. 3*, 65–77 (1972).
27. Weil, C. S., Condra, N. I., and Carpenter, C. P., Correlation of 4-hour versus 24-hour contact skin penetration toxicity in the rat and rabbit and use of the former for predictions of relative hazard of pesticide formulations. *Toxicol. Appl. Pharmacol. 18*, 734 (1971).
28. Feron, V. J., De Groot, A. P., Spanjers, M. T., and Til, H. P., An evaluation of the criterion "organ weight" under conditions of growth retardation. *Food Cosmet. Toxicol. 11*, 85 (1973).
29. "Criteria for a Recommended Standard . . . Occupational Exposure to Asbestos." National Institute for Occupational Safety and Health, Rockville, Maryland, 1972.
30. "IARC Monographs on the Evaluation of Carcinogenis Risk of Chemicals to Man. Some Inorganic and Organometallic Compounds," Vol. 2. Int. Agency Res. Cancer, Lyon, 1973.

31. Gross, P., and Harley, R. A., Jr., The locus of pathogenicity of asbestos dust. A theory. *Arch. Environ. Health 27,* 240 (1973).

32. Leadbetter, M. R., and Corn, M., Particle size distribution of rat lung residues after exposure to fiberglass dust clouds. *Amer. Ind. Hyg. Ass., J. 33,* 511 (1972).

33. Hitchcock, M., Piscitelli, D. M., and Bouhuys, A., Histamine release from human lung by a component of cotton bracts. *Arch. Environ. Health 26,* 177 (1973).

34. Haeger-Aronsen, B., Abdulla, M., and Fristedt, B. I., Effect of lead on δ-aminolevulinic acid dehydrase activity in red blood cells. *Arch. Environ. Health 23,* 440 (1971).

35. Maxfield, M. E., Stopps, G. J., Barnes, J. R., D'Snee, R., and Azar, A., Effect of lead on blood regeneration following acute hemorrhage in dogs. *Amer. Ind. Hyg. Ass., J. 33,* 326 (1972).

36. Hernberg, S., Tola, S., Nikkanen, J., and Valkonen, S., Erythrocyte δ-aminolevulinic acid dehydratase in new lead exposure. A longitudinal study. *Arch. Environ. Health 25,* 109 (1972).

37. El-Dakhakhny, A.-A., and El-Sadik, Y. M., Lead in hair among exposed workers. *Amer. Ind. Hyg. Ass., J. 33,* 31 (1972).

38. Stanković, M. K., Biochemical tests for the appraisal of exposure to lead. *Arch. Environ. Health 23,* 265 (1971).

39. Bingham, E., Barkley, W., Zerwas, M., Stemmer, K., and Taylor, P., Responses of alveolar macrophages to metals. I. Inhalation of lead and nickel. *Arch. Environ. Health 25,* 406 (1972).

40. Hammond, P. B., The effects of chelating agents on the tissue distribution and excretion of lead. *Toxicol. Appl. Pharmacol. 18,* 296 (1971).

41. Hammond, P. B., The effects of D-penicillamine on the tissue distribution and excretion of lead. *Toxicol. Appl. Pharmacol. 26,* 241 (1973).

42. Hammond, P. B., The relationship between inhibition of δ-aminolevulinic acid dehydratase by lead and lead mobilization of ethylenediamine tetraacetate (EDTA). *Toxicol. Appl. Pharmacol. 26,* 466 (1973).

43. Garber, B., and Wei, E., Adaptation to the toxic effects of lead. *Amer. Ind. Hyg. Ass., J. 33,* 756 (1972).

44. Mahaffey, K. R., and Goyer, R. A., Trisodium nitrilotriacetate in drinking water. Metabolic and renal effects in rats. *Arch. Environ. Health 25,* 271 (1972).

45. McClain, R. M., and Becker, B. A., Effects of organolead compounds on rat embryonic and fetal development. *Toxicol. Appl. Pharmacol. 21,* 265 (1972).

46. de Bruin, A., Certain biological effects of lead upon the animal organism. *Arch. Environ. Health 23,* 249 (1971).

47. Vallee, B. L., and Ulmer, D. D., Biochemical effects of mercury, cadmium, and lead. *Annu. Rev. Biochem. 41,* 91 (1972).

48. "Criteria for a Recommended Standard . . . Occupational Exposure to Inorganic Lead." National Institute for Occupational Safety and Health, Rockville, Maryland, 1972.

49. "Lead. Airborne Lead in Perspective." National Academy of Sciences, Washington, D.C., 1972.

50. Proceedings, International Symposium, Amsterdam, "Environmental Health Aspects of Lead." Commission of the European Communities, Directorate General for Dissemination of Knowledge, Centre for Information and Documentation, Luxembourg, 1973.

51. Goyer, R. A., and Rhyne, B. C., Pathological effects of lead. *Int. Rev. Exp. Pathol. 12,* 1 (1973).

52. Task Group on Metal Accumulation, Subcommittee on the Toxicology of Metals,

Permanent Commission and International Association on Occupational Health, Accumulation of toxic metals with special reference to their absorption, excretion and biological half-times. *Environ. Physiol. Biochem. 3,* 65 (1973).

53. Joint FAO/WHO Expert Committee on Food Additives, Evaluation of certain food additives and the contaminants mercury, lead, and cadmium. *World Health Organ., Tech. Rep. Ser. 505,* 5 (1972).

54. Teisinger, J., Xintaras, C., and Pfitzer, E., Prague International Lead Panel: Effects of atmospheric lead on biological systems. *Science 179,* 197 (1973).

55. Chang, L. W., Ware, R. A., and Desnoyers, P. A., A histochemical study on some enzyme changes in the kidney, liver and brain after chronic mercury intoxication in the rat. *Food Cosmet. Toxicol. 11,* 283 (1973).

56. Diamond, S. S., and Sleight, S. D., Acute and subchronic methylmercury toxicosis in the rat. *Toxicol. Appl. Pharmacol. 23,* 197 (1972).

57. Khera, K. S., and Tabacova, S. A., Effects of methylmercuric chloride on the progeny of mice and rats treated before or during gestation. *Food Cosmet. Toxicol. 11,* 245 (1973).

58. Khera, K. S., Reproductive capability of male rats and mice treated with methyl mercury. *Toxicol. Appl. Pharmacol. 24,* 167 (1973).

59. Clarkson, T. W., Epidemiological and experimental aspects of lead and mercury contamination of food. *Food Cosmet. Toxicol. 9,* 229 (1971).

60. Clarkson, T. W., Magos, L., and Greenwood, M. R., The transport of elemental mercury into fetal tissues. *Biol. Neonate 21,* 239 (1972).

61. Magos, L., and Clarkson, T. W., Effect of phenobarbitone on the biliary excretion of methylmercury in rats and mice. *Nature (London), New Biol. 246,* 123 (1973).

62. Post, E. M., Yang, M. G., King, J. A., and Sanger, V. L., Behavioral changes of young rats force-fed methyl mercury chloride. *Proc. Soc. Exp. Biol. Med. 143,* 113 (1973).

63. Bakir, F., Damluji, S. F., Amin-Zaki, L., Murtadha, M., Khalidi, A., Al-Rawi, N. Y., Tikriti, S., Dhahir, H. I., Clarkson, T. W., Smith, J. C., and Doherty, R. A., Methylmercury poisoning in Iraq. *Science 181,* 230 (1973).

64. Clarkson, T. W., The pharmacology of mercury compounds. *Annu. Rev. Pharmacol. 12,* 375 (1972).

65. Friberg, L., and Vostal, J., eds., "Mercury in the Environment. An Epidemiological and Toxicological Appraisal." CRC Press, Cleveland, Ohio, 1972.

66. Vostal, J. J., and Clarkson, T. W., Mercury as an environmental hazard. *J. Occup. Med. 15,* 649 (1973).

67. Norseth, T., and Clarkson, T. W., Intestinal transport of ^{203}Hg-labeled methyl mercury chloride. Role of biotransformation in rats. *Arch. Environ. Health 22,* 568 (1971).

68. Clarkson, T. W., Small, H., and Norseth, T., Excretion and absorption of methyl mercury after polythiol resin treatment. *Arch. Environ. Health 26,* 173 (1973).

69. Wood, R. W., Weiss, A. B., and Weiss, B., Hand tremor induced by industrial exposure to inorganic mercury. *Arch. Environ. Health 26,* 249 (1973).

70. Nomiyama, K., Sato, C., and Yamamoto, A., Early signs of cadmium intoxication in rabbits. *Toxicol. Appl. Pharmacol. 24,* 625 (1973).

71. Nishizumi, M., Electron microscopic study of cadmium nephrotoxicity in the rat. *Arch. Environ. Health 24,* 215 (1972).

72. Fischer, G. M., and Thind, G. S., Tissue cadmium and water content of normal and cadmium hypertensive rabbits. *Arch. Environ. Health 23,* 107 (1971).

73. Itokawa, Y., Abe, T., and Tanaka, S., Bone changes in experimental chronic cadmium poisoning. Radiological and biological approaches. *Arch. Environ. Health 26,* 241 (1973).

74. Norberg, G. F., and Nishiyama, K., Whole-body and hair retention of cadmium in mice. *Arch. Environ. Health 24,* 209 (1972).

75. Nishiyama, K., and Nordberg, G. F., Adsorption and elution of cadmium on hair. *Arch. Environ. Health 25,* 92 (1972).

76. Petering, H. G., Johnson, M. A., and Stemmer, K. L., Studies of zinc metabolism in the rat. I. Dose-response effects of cadmium. *Arch. Environ. Health 23,* 93 (1971).

77. Shaikh, Z. A., and Lucis, O. J., Biological differences in cadmium and zinc turnover. *Arch. Environ. Health 24,* 410 (1972).

78. Shaikh, Z. A., and Lucis, O. J., Cadmium and zinc binding in mammalian liver and kidneys. *Arch. Environ. Health 24,* 419 (1972).

79. Lucis, O. J., Lucis, R., and Shaikh, Z. A., Cadmium and zinc in pregnancy and lactation. *Arch. Environ. Health 25,* 14 (1972).

80. Phalen, R. F., and Morrow, P. E., Experimental inhalation of metallic silver. *Health Phys. 24,* 509 (1973).

81. Gross, P., Harley, R. A., Jr., and deTreville, R. T. P., Pulmonary reaction to metallic aluminum powders. An experimental study. *Arch. Environ. Health 26,* 227 (1973).

82. Jones, C. C., Nickel carbonyl poisoning. Report of a fatal case. *Arch. Environ. Health 26,* 245 (1973).

83. De Groot, A. P., Feron, V. J., and Til, H. P., Short-term toxicity studies on some salts and oxides of tin in rats. *Food Cosmet. Toxicol. 11,* 19 (1973).

84. Schroeder, H. A., and Mitchener, M., Selenium and tellurium in mice. Effects on growth, survival, and tumors. *Arch. Environ. Health 24,* 66 (1972).

85. Conradi, C., Burri, P. H., Kapanci, Y., Robinson, F. R., and Weibel, E. R., Lung changes after beryllium inhalation. Ultrastructural and morphometric study. *Arch. Environ. Health 23,* 348 (1971).

86. Jacques, A., and Witschi, H. R., Beryllium effects of aryl hydrocarbon hydroxylase in rat lung. *Arch. Environ. Health 27,* 243 (1973).

87. Witschi, H. P., and Marchand, P., Interference of beryllium with enzyme induction in rat liver. *Toxicol. Appl. Pharmacol. 20,* 565 (1971).

88. Leach, L. J., Yuile, C. L., Hodge, H. C., Sylvester, G. E., and Wilson, H. B., A five-year inhalation study with natural uranium dioxide (UO_2) dust. II. Postexposure retention and biologic effects in the monkey, dog and rat. *Health Phys. 25,* 239 (1973).

89. Morrow, P. E., Gibb, F. R., and Beiter, H. D., Inhalation studies of uranium trioxide. *Health Phys. 23,* 273 (1972).

90. Sunderman, F. W., Jr., Metal carcinogenesis in experimental animals. *Food Cosmet. Toxicol. 9,* 105 (1971).

91. "IARC Monographs on the Evaluation of Carcinogenic Risk of Chemicals to Man," Vol. 1. Int. Agency Res. Cancer, Lyon, 1972.

92. Schroeder, H. A., and Mitchener, M., Toxic effects of trace elements on the reproduction of mice and rats. *Arch. Environ. Health 23,* 102 (1971).

93. Ferm, V. H., Saxon, A., and Smith, B. M., The teratogenic profile of sodium arsenate in the golden hamster. *Arch. Environ. Health 22,* 557 (1971).

94. Hood, R. D., and Bishop, S. L., Teratogenic effects of sodium arsenate in mice. *Arch. Environ. Health 24,* 62 (1972).

95. Dillard, C. J., Urribarri, N., Reddy, K., Fletcher, B., Taylor, S., de Lumen, B., Langberg, S., and Tappel, A. L., Increased lysosomal enzymes in lungs of ozone-exposed rats. *Arch. Environ. Health 25,* 426 (1972).

96. Palmer, M. S., Exley, R. W., and Coffin, D. L., Influence of pollutant gases on benzpyrene hydroxylase activity. *Arch. Environ. Health 25,* 439 (1972).

97. Goldstein, B. D., Hydrogen peroxide in erythrocytes. Detection in rats and mice inhaling ozone. *Arch. Environ. Health 26*, 279 (1973).

98. P'an, A. Y. S., Béland, J., and Jegier, Z., Ozone-induced arterial lesions. *Arch. Environ. Health 24*, 229 (1972).

99. P'an, A. Y. S., and Jegier, Z., Trypsin protein esterase in relation to ozone-induced vascular damage. *Arch. Environ. Health 24*, 233 (1972).

100. Nasr, A. N. M., Dinman, B. D., and Bernstein, I. A., An experimental approach to study the toxicity of nonparticulate air pollutants. I. Rationale and methods. *Arch. Environ. Health 22*, 538 (1971).

101. Nasr, A. N. M., Dinman, B. D., and Bernstein, I. A., Nonparticulate air pollutants. II. Effect of ozone inhalation on nadide phosphate levels in tracheal mucosa. *Arch. Environ. Health 22*, 545 (1971).

102. Evans, M. J., Mayr, W., Bils, R. F., and Loosli, C. G., Effects of ozone on cell renewal in pulmonary alveoli of aging mice. *Arch. Environ. Health 22*, 450 (1971).

103. Roehm, J. N., Hadley, J. G., and Menzel, D. B., The influence of vitamin E on the lung fatty acids exposed to ozone. *Arch. Environ. Health 24*, 237 (1972).

104. Chow, C. K., and Tappel, A. L., Activities of pentose shunt and glycolytic enzymes in lungs of ozone-exposed rats. *Arch. Environ. Health 26*, 205 (1973).

105. Goldstein, B. D., Levine, M. R., Cuzzi-Spada, R., Gardenas, R., Buckley, R. D., and Balchum, O. J. *p*-Aminobenzoic acid as a protective agent in ozone toxicity. *Arch. Environ. Health 24*, 243 (1972).

106. Balchum, O. J., O'Brien, J. S., and Goldstein, B. D., Ozone and unsaturated fatty acids. *Arch. Environ. Health 22*, 32 (1971).

107. Roehm, J. N., Hadley, J. G., and Menzel, D. B., Oxidation of unsaturated fatty acids by ozone and nitrogen dioxide. *Arch. Environ. Health 23*, 142 (1971).

108. Menzel, D. B., Roehm, J. N., and Lee, S. D., Vitamin E: The biological and environmental antioxidant. *J. Agr. Food Chem. 20*, 481 (1972).

109. Roehm, J. N., Hadley, J. G., and Menzel, D. B., Antioxidants versus lung disease. *Arch. Intern. Med. 128*, 88 (1971).

110. Alpert, S. M., and Lewis, T. R., Unilateral pulmonary function study of ozone toxicity in rabbits. *Arch. Environ. Health 23*, 451 (1971).

111. Goldstein, E., Eagle, M. C., and Hoeprich, P. D., Influence of ozone on pulmonary defense mechanisms of silicotic mice. *Arch. Environ. Health 24*, 444 (1972).

112. Freeman, G., Stephens, R. J., Coffin, D. L., and Stara, J. F., Changes in dogs' lungs after long-term exposure to ozone. Light and electron microscopy. *Arch. Environ. Health 26*, 209 (1973).

113. Yokoyama, E., and Frank, R., Respiratory uptake of ozone in dogs. *Arch. Environ. Health 25*, 132 (1972).

114. Goldstein, B. D., Lai, L. Y., Ross, S. R., and Cuzzi-Spada, R., Susceptibility of inbred mouse strains to ozone. *Arch. Environ. Health 27*, 412 (1973).

115. Acton, J. D., and Myrvik, Q. N., Nitrogen dioxide effects on alveolar macrophages. *Arch. Environ. Health 24*, 48 (1972).

116. Fenters, J. D., Findlay, J. C., Port, C. D., Ehrlich, R., and Coffin, D. L., Chronic exposure to nitrogen dioxide. Immunologic, physiologic, and pathologic effects in virus-challenged squirrel monkeys. *Arch. Environ. Health 27*, 85 (1973).

117. Goldstein, E., Eagle, M. C., and Hoeprich, P. D., Effect of nitrogen dioxide on pulmonary bacterial defense mechanisms. *Arch. Environ. Health 26*, 202 (1973).

118. Mangold, C. A., and Beckett, R. R., Combined occupational exposure to silver brazers to cadmium oxide, nitrogen dioxide and fluorides at a naval shipyard. *Amer. Ind. Hyg. Ass., J. 32*, 115 (1971).

119. Furiosi, N. J., Crane, S. C., and Freeman, G., Mixed sodium chloride aerosol and nitrogen dioxide in air. Biological effects on monkeys and rats. *Arch. Environ. Health* 27, 405 (1973).

120. Stupfel, M., Magnier, M., Romary, F., Tran, M.-H., and Moutet, J.-P., Lifelong exposure of SPF rats to automotive exhaust gas. Dilution containing 20 ppm of nitrogen oxides. *Arch. Environ. Health 26,* 264 (1973).

121. Arner, E. C., and Rhoades, R. A., Long-term nitrogen dioxide exposure. *Arch. Environ. Health 26,* 156 (1973).

122. Giordano, A. M., Jr., and Morrow, P. E., Chronic low-level nitrogen dioxide exposure and mucociliary clearance. *Arch. Environ. Health 25,* 443 (1972).

123. Sherwin, R. P., and Carlson, D. A., Protein content of lung lavage fluid of guinea pigs exposed to 0.4 ppm nitrogen dioxide. Disc-gel electrophoresis for amount and types. *Arch. Environ. Health 27,* 90 (1973).

124. Mersch, J., Dyce, B. J., Haverback, B. J., and Sherwin, R. P., Diphosphoglycerate content of red blood cells. Measurement in guinea pigs exposed to 0.4 ppm nitrogen dioxide. *Arch. Environ. Health 27,* 94 (1973).

125. Yuen, T. G. H., and Sherwin, R. P., Hyperplasia of type 2 pneumocytes and nitrogen dioxide (10 ppm) exposure. A quantitation based on electron photomicrographs. *Arch. Environ. Health 22,* 178 (1971).

126. Sherwin, R. P., Dibble, J., and Weiner, J., Alveolar wall cells of the guinea pig. Increase in response to 2 ppm nitrogen dioxide. *Arch. Environ. Health 24,* 43 (1972).

127. Sherwin, R. P., Margolick, J. B., and Azen, S. P., Hypertrophy of alveolar wall cells secondary to an air pollutant. A semi-automated quantitation. *Arch. Environ. Health 26,* 297 (1973).

128. Stephens, R. J., Freeman, G., and Evans, M. J., Early response of lungs to low levels of nitrogen dioxide. Light and electron microscopy. *Arch. Environ. Health 24,* 160 (1972).

129. Evans, M. J., Stephens, R. J., Cabral, L. J., and Freeman, G., Cell renewal in the lungs of rats exposed to low levels of NO_2. *Arch. Environ. Health 24,* 180 (1972).

130. Yokoyama, E., Yoder, R. E., and Frank, N. R., Distribution of ^{35}S in the blood and its excretion in urine of dogs exposed to $^{35}SO_2$. *Arch. Environ. Health 22,* 389 (1971).

131. Giddens, W. E., Jr., and Fairchild, G. A., Effects of sulfur dioxide on the nasal mucosa of mice. *Arch. Environ. Health 25,* 166 (1972).

132. Ferin, J., Emphysema in rats and clearance of dust particles. *In* "Inhaled Particles III" (W. H. Walton, ed.), Vol. 1, pp. 283–292. Unwin Brothers Ltd., The Gresham Press, Old Woking, Surrey, England, 1971.

133. Ferin, J., Papain-induced emphysema and the elimination of TiO_2 particulates from the lungs. *Amer. Ind. Hyg. Ass., J. 32,* 157 (1971).

134. Ferin, J., and Leach, L. J., The effect of SO_2 on lung clearance of TiO_2 particles in rats. *Amer. Ind. Hyg. Ass., J. 34,* 260 (1973).

135. Alarie, Y., Ulrich, C. E., Busey, W. M., Krumm, A. A., and MacFarland, H. N., Long-term continuous exposure to sulfur dioxide in cynomolgus monkeys. *Arch. Environ. Health 24,* 115 (1972).

136. Corn, M., Kotsko, N., Stanton, D., Bell, W., and Thomas, A. P., Response of cats to inhaled mixtures of SO_2 and SO_2-NaCl aerosol in air. *Arch. Environ. Health 24,* 248 (1972).

137. Alarie, Y., Kantz, R. J., II, Ulrich, C. E., Krumm, A. A., and Busey, W. M., Long-term continuous exposure to sulfur dioxide and fly ash mixtures in cynomolgus monkeys and guinea pigs. *Arch. Environ. Health 27,* 251 (1973).

138. Martin, S. W., and Willoughby, R. A., Organic dusts, sulfur dioxide, and the respiratory tract of swine. *Arch. Environ. Health 25,* 158 (1972).

139. Lewis, T. R., Moorman, W. J., Ludmann, W. F., and Campbell, K. I., Toxicity of long-term exposure to oxides of sulfur. *Arch. Environ. Health 26,* 16 (1973).

140. Bloch, W. N., Jr., Lewis, T. R., Busch, K. A., Orthoefer, J. G., and Stara, J. F., Cardiovascular status of female beagles exposed to air pollutants. *Arch. Environ. Health 24,* 342 (1972).

141. Amdur, M. O., Aerosols formed by oxidation of sulfur dioxide. Review of their toxicology. *Arch. Environ. Health 23,* 459 (1971).

142. Alarie, Y., Busey, W. M., Krumm, A. A., and Ulrich, C. E., Long-term continuous exposure to sulfuric acid mist in cynomolgus monkeys and guinea pigs. *Arch. Environ. Health 27,* 16 (1973).

143. Hayes, W. J., Jr., Dale, W. E., and Pirkle, C. I., Evidence of safety of long-term, high, oral doses of DDT for man. *Arch. Environ. Health 22,* 119 (1971).

144. Deichmann, W. B., and MacDonald, W. E., Organochlorine pesticides and human health. *Food Cosmet. Toxicol. 9,* 91 (1971).

145. Laws, E. R., Jr., Evidence of antitumorigenic effects of DDT. *Arch. Environ. Health 23,* 181 (1971).

146. Gablicks, J., Askari, E. M., and Yolen, N., DDT and immunological responses. I. Serum antibodies and anaphylactic shock in guinea pigs. *Arch. Environ. Health 26,* 305 (1973).

147. Askari, E. M., and Gabliks, J., DDT and immunological responses. II. Altered histamine levels and anaphylactic shock in guinea pigs. *Arch. Environ. Health 26,* 309 (1973).

148. Palmer, K. A., Green, S., and Legator, M. S., Dominant lethal study of *p,p'*-DDT in rats. *Food Cosmet. Toxicol. 11,* 53 (1973).

149. Epstein, S. S., Arnold, E., Andrea, J., Bass, W., and Bishop, Y., Detection of chemical mutagens by the dominant lethal assay in the mouse. *Toxicol. Appl. Pharmacol. 23,* 288 (1972).

150. Schwetz, B. A., Sparschu, G. L., and Gehring, P. J., The effect of 2,4-dichloro-phenoxyacetic acid (2,4-D) and esters of 2,4-D on rat embryonal, foetal and neonatal growth and development. *Food Cosmet. Toxicol. 9,* 801 (1971).

151. Hansen, W. H., Quaife, M. L., Habermann, R. T., and Fitzhugh, O. G., Chronic toxicity of 2,4-dichlorophenoxyacetic acid in rats and dogs. *Toxicol. Appl. Pharmacol. 20,* 122 (1971).

152. Emerson, J. L., Thompson, D. J., Strebing, R. J., Gerbig, C. G., and Robinson, V. B., Teratogenic studies on 2,4,5-trichlorophenoxyacetic acid in the rat and rabbit. *Food Cosmet. Toxicol. 9,* 395 (1971).

153. Sparshu, G. L., Dunn, F. L., and Rowe, V. K., Study of the teratogenicity of 2,3,7,8-tetrachlorodibenzo-*p*-dioxin in the rat. *Food Cosmet. Toxicol. 9,* 405 (1971).

154. Sparshu, G. L., Dunn, F. L., Lisowe, R. W., and Rowe, V. K., Study of the effects of high levels of 2,4,5-trichlorophenoxyacetic acid on foetal development in the rat. *Food Cosmet. Toxicol. 9,* 527 (1971).

155. Khera, K. S., and McKinley, W. P., Pre- and postnatal studies on 2,4,5-trichloro-phenoxyacetic acid, 2,4-dichlorophenoxyacetic acid and their derivatives in rats. *Toxicol. Appl. Pharmacol. 22,* 14 (1972).

156. Roll, R., Untersuchungen uber die teratogene Wirkung von 2,4,5-T bei Mausen. *Food Cosmet. Toxicol. 9,* 671 (1971).

157. Courtney, K. D., and Moore, J. A., Teratology studies with 2,4,5-trichloro-

phenoxyacetic acid and 2,3,7,8-tetrachlorodibenzo-P-dioxin. *Toxicol. Appl. Pharmacol. 20*, 396 (1971).

158. Fang, S. C., Fallin, E., Montgomery, M. L., and Freed, V. H., The metabolism and distribution of 2,4,5-trichlorophenoxyacetic acid in female rats. *Toxicol. Appl. Pharmacol. 24*, 555 (1973).

159. Piper, W. N., Rose, J. Q., Leng, M. L., and Gehring, P. J., The fate of 2,4,5-trichlorophenoxyacetic acid (2,4,5-T) following oral administration to rats and dogs. *Toxicol. Appl. Pharmacol. 26*, 339 (1973).

160. Gehring, P. J., Kramer, C. G., Schwetz, B. A., Rose, J. Q., and Rowe, V. K., The fate of 2,4,5-trichlorophenoxyacetic acid (2,4,5-T), following oral administration to man. *Toxicol. Appl. Pharmacol. 26*, 352 (1973).

161. Walker, A. I. T., Thorpe, E., and Stevenson, D. E., The toxicology of dieldrin (HEOD). I. Long-term oral toxicity studies in mice. *Food Cosmet. Toxicol. 11*, 415 (1973).

162. Thorpe, E., and Walker, A. I. T., The toxicology of dieldrin (HEOD). II. Comparative long-term oral toxicity studies in mice with dieldrin, DDT, phenobarbitone, β-BHC and γ-BHC. *Food Cosmet. Toxicol. 11*, 433 (1973).

163. Zabik, M. E., and Schemmel, R., Dieldrin storage of obese, normal, and semistarved rats. *Arch. Environ. Health 27*, 25 (1973).

164. Su, M.-Q., Kinoshita, F. K., Frawley, J. P., and DuBois, K. P., Comparative inhibition of aliesterases and cholinesterase in rats fed eighteen organophosphorus insecticides. *Toxicol. Appl. Pharmacol. 20*, 241 (1971).

165. Murphy, S. D., and Cheever, K. L., Carboxylesterase and cholinesterase inhibition in rats. Abate and interaction with malathion. *Arch. Environ. Health 24*, 107 (1972).

166. Weil, C. S., Woodside, M. D., Carpenter, C. P., and Smyth, H. F., Jr., Current status of testes of carbaryl for reproductive and teratogenic effect. *Toxicol. Appl. Pharmacol. 21*, 390 (1972).

167. Weil, C. S., Woodside, M. D., Bernard, J. B., Condra, N. I., King, J. M., and Carpenter, C. P., Comparative effect of carbaryl on rat reproduction and guinea pig teratology when fed either in the diet or by stomach intubation. *Toxicol. Appl. Pharmacol. 26*, 621 (1973).

168. Petrova-Vergieva, T., and Ivanova-Tchemishanska, L., Assessment of the teratogenic activity of dithiocarbamate fungicides. *Food Cosmet. Toxicol. 11*, 239 (1973).

169. Vondruska, J. F., Fancher, O. E., and Calandra, J. C., An investigation into the teratogenic potential of captan, folpet, and difolatan in nonhuman primates. *Toxicol. Appl. Pharmacol. 18*, 619 (1971).

170. McElligott, T. F., The dermal toxicity of paraquat: Differences due to techniques of application. *Toxicol. Appl. Pharmacol. 21*, 361 (1972).

171. Sharp, C. W., Ottolenghi, A., and Posner, H. S., Correlation of paraquat toxicity with tissue concentrations and weight loss of the rat. *Toxicol. Appl. Pharmacol. 22*, 241 (1972).

172. Gibson, J. E., Teratology studies in mice with 2-sec-butyl-4,6-dinitrophenol (Dinoseb). *Food Cosmet. Toxicol. 11*, 31 (1973).

173. Gibson, J. E., and Rao, K. S., Disposition of 2-sec-butyl-4,6-dinitrophenol (Dinoseb) in pregnant mice. *Food Cosmet. Toxicol. 11*, 45 (1973).

174. Conney, A. H., Chang, R., Levin, W. M., Garbut, A., Munro-Faure, A. D., Peck, A. W., and Bye, A., Effects of piperonyl butoxide on drug metabolism in rodents and man. *Arch. Environ. Health 24*, 97 (1972).

175. Tucker, R. K., and Haegele, M. A., Comparative acute oral toxicity of pesticides to six species of birds. *Toxicol. Appl. Pharmacol. 20*, 57 (1971).

176. Schafer, E. W., The acute oral toxicity of 369 pesticidal, pharmaceutical and other chemicals to wild birds. *Toxicol. Appl. Pharmacol. 21,* 315 (1972).

177. Hudson, R. H., Tucker, R. K., and Haegele, M. A., Effect of age on sensitivity: Acute oral toxicity of 14 pesticides to mallard ducks of several ages. *Toxicol. Appl. Pharmacol. 22,* 556 (1972).

178. Saito, F. U., Kocsis, J. J., and Snyder, R., Effect of benzene on hepatic drug metabolism and ultrastructure. *Toxicol. Appl. Pharmacol. 26,* 209 (1973).

179. Gonasum, L. M., Witmer, C., Kocsis, J. J., and Snyder, R., Benzene metabolism in mouse liver microsomes. *Toxicol. Appl. Pharmacol. 26,* 398 (1973).

180. Ikeda, M., and Ohtsuji, H., Phenobarbital-induced protection against toxicity of toluene and benzene in the rat. *Toxicol. Appl. Pharmacol. 20,* 30 (1971).

181. Ohtsuji, H., and Ikeda, M., The metabolism of styrene in the rat and the stimulatory effect of phenobarbital. *Toxicol. Appl. Pharmacol. 18,* 321 (1971).

182. Bohlen, P., Schlunegger, U. P., and Läuppi, E., Uptake and distribution of hexane in rat tissues. *Toxicol. Appl. Pharmacol. 25,* 242 (1973).

183. Kinkead, E. R., Pozzani, U. C., Geary, D. L., and Carpenter, C. P., The mammalian toxicity of dicyclopentadiene. *Toxicol. Appl. Pharmacol. 20,* 552 (1971).

184. Adamson, I. Y. R., Inhaled irradiated terphenyls. Reaction of murine lung and liver. *Arch. Environ. Health 26,* 192 (1973).

185. Adamson, I. Y. R., and Weeks, J. L., The LD_{50} and chronic toxicity of reactor terphenyls. *Arch. Environ. Health 27,* 69 (1973).

186. Kimbrough, R. D., Linder, R. E., and Gaines, T. B., Morphological changes in livers of rats fed polychlorinated biphenyls. Light microscopy and ultrastructure. *Arch. Environ. Health 25,* 354 (1972).

187. Kimbrough, R. D., Linder, R. E., Burse, V. W., and Jennings, R. W., Adenofibrosis in the rat liver. *Arch. Environ. Health 27,* 390 (1973).

188. Bruckner, J. V., Khanna, K. L., and Cornish, H. H., Biological responses of the rat to polychlorinated biphenyls. *Toxicol. Appl. Pharmacol. 24,* 434 (1973).

189. "Perspective on PCBs," *Environ. Health Perspect., Exp. Issue* No. 1. National Institute of Environmental Health Sciences, Research Triangle Park, North Carolina, 1972.

190. Dinman, B. D., Cook, W. A., Whitehouse, W. M., Magnuson, H. J., and Ditcheck, T., Occupational acroosteolysis. I. An epidemiological study. *Arch. Environ. Health 22,* 61 (1971).

191. Dodson, V. N., Dinman, B. D., Whitehouse, W. M., Nasr, A. N. M., and Magnuson, H. J., Occupational acroosteolysis. III. A clinical study. *Arch. Environ. Health 22,* 83 (1971).

192. Reinhardt, C. F., Azar, A., Maxfield, M. E., Smith, P. E., Jr., and Mullin, L. S., Cardiac arrhythmias and aerosol "sniffing." *Arch. Environ. Health 22,* 265 (1971).

193. Mullin, L. S., Azar, A., Reinhardt, C. F., Smith, P. E., Jr., and Fabryka, E. F., Halogenated hydrocarbon-induced cardiac arrhythmias associated with release of endogenous epinephrine. *Amer. Ind. Hyg. Ass., J. 33,* 389 (1972).

194. Rhoden, R. A., and Gabriel, K. L., Some effects of bromotrifluoromethane inhalation on myocardial glycolysis. *Toxicol. Appl. Pharmacol. 21,* 166 (1972).

195. McClure, D. A., Failure of fluorocarbon propellants to alter the electrocardiogram of mice and dogs. *Toxicol. Appl. Pharmacol. 22,* 221 (1972).

196. Smith, J. K., and Case, M. T., Subacute and chronic toxicity studies of fluorocarbon propellants in mice, rats and dogs. *Toxicol. Appl. Pharmacol. 26,* 43 (1973).

197. Azar, A., Trochimowicz, H. J., Terrill, J. B., and Mullin, L. S., Blood levels of fluorocarbon related to cardiac sensitization. *Amer. Ind. Hyg. Ass., J. 34,* 102 (1973).

198. Reinhardt, C. F., McLaughlin, M., Maxfield, M. E., Mullin, L. S., and Smith, P. E., Jr., Human exposures to flurocarbon 113 (1,1,2-trichloro-1,2,2-trifluoroethane). *Amer. Ind. Hyg. Ass., J. 32*, 143 (1971).

199. Azar, A., Reinhardt, C. F., Maxfield, M. E., Smith, P. E., Jr., and Mullin, L. S., Experimental humam exposures to fluorocarbon 12 (dichlorodifluoromethane). *Amer. Ind. Hyg. Ass., J. 33*, 207 (1972).

200. Cornish, H. H., Ling, B. P., and Barth, M. L., Phenobarbital and organic solvent toxicity. *Amer. Ind. Hyg. Ass., J. 34*, 487 (1973).

201 Noweir, M. H., Pfitzer, E. A., and Hatch, T. F., The pulmonary response of rats exposed to the decomposition products of carbon tetrachloride vapors at its industrial threshold limit concentration. *Amer. Ind. Hyg. Ass., J. 34*, 73 (1973).

202. Stewart, R. D., Fisher, T. N., Hosko, M. J., Peterson, J. E., Baretta, E. D., and Dodd, H. C., Experimental human exposure to methylene chloride. *Arch. Environ. Health 25*, 342 (1972).

203. Weinstein, R. S., Boyd, D. D., and Back, K. C., Effects of continuous inhalation of dichloromethane in the mouse: Morphologic and functional observations. *Toxicol. Appl. Pharmacol. 23*, 660 (1972).

204. Yodaiken, R. E., and Babcock, J. R., 1,2-dichloroethane poisoning. *Arch. Environ. Health 26*, 281 (1973).

205. Siegel, J., Jones, R. A., Coon, R. A., and Lyon, J. P., Effects on experimental animals of acute, repeated and continuous inhalation exposures to dichloroacetylene mixtures. *Toxicol. Appl. Pharmacol. 18*, 168 (1971).

206. Watrous, W. M., and Plaa, G. L., The nephrotoxicity of single and multiple doses of aliphatic chlorinated hydrocarbon solvents in male mice. *Toxicol. Appl. Pharmacol. 23*, 640 (1972).

207. Wallcave, L., Garcia, H., Feldman, R., Lijinsky, W., and Shubik, P., Skin tumorigenesis in mice by petroleum asphalts and coal-tar pitches of known polynuclear aromatic hydrocarbon content. *Toxicol. Appl. Pharmacol. 18*, 41 (1971).

208. "IARC Monographs on the Evaluation of Carcinogenic Risk of Chemicals to Man. Certain Polycyclic Aromatic Hydrocarbons and Heterocyclic Compounds," Vol. 3. Int. Agency Res. Cancer, Lyon, 1973.

209. Zavon, M. R., Hoegg, U., and Bingham, E., Benzidine exposure as a cause of bladder tumors. *Arch. Environ. Health 27*, 1 (1973).

210. Leong, B. K. J., Macfarland, H. N., and Reese, W. H., Jr., Induction of lung adenomas by chronic inhalation of bis(chloromethyl)ether. *Arch. Environ. Health 22*, 663 (1971).

211. Laskin, S., Kuschner, M., Drew, R. T., Cappiello, V. P., and Nelson, N., Tumors of the respiratory tract induced by inhalation of bis(chloromethyl)ether. *Arch. Environ. Health 23*, 135 (1971).

212. Cumming, R. B., and Walton, M. F., Modification of the acute toxicity of mutagenic and carcinogenic chemicals in the mouse by prefeeding with antioxidants. *Food Cosmet. Toxicol. 11*, 547 (1973).

213. Ulland, B. M., Weisburger, J. H., Yamamoto, R. S., and Weisburger, E. K., Antioxidants and carcinogenesis: Butylated hydroxytoluene, but not diphenyl-*p*-phenylenediamine, inhibits cancer induction by *N*-2-fluorenylacetamide and by *N*-hydroxy-*N*-2-fluorenylacetamide in rats. *Food Cosmet. Toxicol. 11*, 199 (1973).

214. Grantham, P. H., Weisburger, J. H., and Weisburger, E. K., Effect of the antioxidant butylated hydroxytoluene (BHT) on the metabolism of the carcinogens *N*-2-fluorenyl-acetamide and *N*-hydroxy-*N*-2-fluorenylacetamide. *Food Cosmet. Toxicol. 11*, 209 (1973).

215. Ramsey, J. M., Effects of single exposures of carbon monoxide on sensory and psychomotor response. *Amer. Ind. Hyg. Ass., J. 34,* 212 (1973).

216. O'Donnell, R. D., Mikulka, P., Heinig, P., and Theodore, J., Low level carbon monoxide exposure and human psychomotor performance. *Toxicol. Appl. Pharmacol. 18,* 593 (1971).

217. Stewart, R. D., Peterson, J. E., Fisher, T. N., Hosko, M. J., Baretta, E. D., Dodd, H. C., and Herrmann, A. A., Experimental human exposure to high concentrations of carbon monoxide. *Arch. Environ. Health 26,* 1 (1973).

218. Peterson, J. E., and Stewart, R. D., Human absorption of carbon monoxide from high concentrations in air. *Amer. Ind. Hyg. Ass., J. 33,* 293 (1972).

219. DeBias, D. A., Banerjee, C. M., Birkhead, N. C., Harrer, W. V., and Kazal, L. A., Carbon monoxide inhalation effects following myocardial infarction in monkeys. *Arch. Environ. Health 27,* 161 (1973).

220. Eckardt, R. E., MacFarland, H. N., Alarie, Y. C. E., and Busey, W. M., The biologic effect from long-term exposure of primates to carbon monoxide. *Arch. Environ. Health 25,* 381 (1972).

221. Jones, R. A., Strickland, J. A., Stunkard, J. A., and Siegel, J., Effects on experimental animals of long-term inhalation exposure to carbon monoxide. *Toxicol. Appl. Pharmacol. 19,* 46 (1971).

222. Budny, J. A., and Arnold, J. D., Nitrilotriaceate (NTA): Human metabolism and its importance in the total safety evaluation program. *Toxicol. Appl. Pharmacol. 25,* 48 (1973).

223. Nixon, G. A., Toxicity evaluation of trisodium nitrilotriacetate. *Toxicol. Appl. Pharmacol. 18,* 398 (1971).

224. Nixon, G. A., Buehler, E. V., and Niewenhuis, R. J., Two-year rat feeding study with trisodium nitrilotriacetate and its calcium chelate. *Toxicol. Appl. Pharmacol. 21,* 244 (1972).

225. Nolen, G. A., Klusman, L. W., Back, D. L., and Buehler, E. V., Reproduction and teratology studies of trisodium nitrilotriacetate in rats and rabbits. *Food Cosmet. Toxicol. 9,* 509 (1971).

226. Michael, W. R., and Wakim, J. M., Metabolism of nitrilotriacetic acid (NTA). *Toxicol. Appl. Pharmacol. 18,* 407 (1971).

227. Tjälve, H., A study of the distribution and teratogenicity of nitrilotriacetic acid (NTA) in mice. *Toxicol. Appl. Pharmacol. 23,* 216 (1972).

228. Scharpf, L. G., Jr., Ramos, F. J., and Hill, I. D., Influence of nitrilotriacetate (NTA) on the toxicity, excretion and distribution of cadmium in female rats. *Toxicol. Appl. Pharmacol. 22,* 186 (1972).

229. Nolen, G. A., Buehler, E. V., Geil, R. G., and Goldenthal, E. I., Effects of trisodium nitrilotriacetate on cadmium and methyl mercury toxicity and teratogenicity in rats. *Toxicol. Appl. Pharmacol. 23,* 222 (1972).

230. Budny, J. A., Niewenhuis, R. J., Buehler, E. V., and Goldenthal, E. I., Subacute oral toxicity of trisodium nitrilotriacetate (Na NTA) in dogs. *Toxicol. Appl. Pharmacol. 26,* 148 (1973).

231. Rogers, A. E., and Newberne, P. M., Diet and aflatoxin B toxicity in rats. *Toxicol. Appl. Pharmacol. 20,* 113 (1971).

232. Righter, H. F., Shalkop, W. T., Mercer, H. D., and Leffel, E. C., Influence of age and sexual status on the development of toxic effects in the male rat fed aflatoxins. *Toxicol. Appl. Pharmacol. 21,* 435 (1972).

233. Purchase, I. F. H., and Steyn, M., Absence of percutaneous absorption of aflatoxin. *Toxicol. Appl. Pharmacol. 24,* 162 (1973).

234. Wogan, G. N., Edwards, G. S., and Newberne, P. M., Structure-activity relationships in toxicity and carcinogenicity of aflatoxins and analogs. *Cancer Res. 31*, 1936 (1971).

235. Edwards, G. S., Wogan, G. N., Sporn, M. B., and Pong, R. S., Structure-activity relationships in DNA binding and nuclear effects of aflatoxin and analogs. *Cancer Res. 31*, 1943 (1971).

236. Magee, P. N., Toxicity of nitrosamines: Their possible human health hazards. *Food Cosmet. Toxicol. 9*, 207 (1971).

237. Phillips, W. E. J., Naturally occurring nitrate and nitrite in foods in relation to infant methaemoglobinaemia. *Food Cosmet. Toxicol. 9*, 219 (1971).

238. Green, S., Palmer, K. A., and Legator, M. S., Effects of cyclohexylamine on the fertility of male rats. *Food Cosmet. Toxicol. 10*, 29 (1972).

239. Litchfield, M. H., and Swan, A. A. B., Cyclohexylamine production and physiological measurements in subjects ingesting sodium cyclamate. *Toxicol. Appl. Pharmacol. 18*, 535 (1971).

240. Lee, I. P., and Dixon, R. L., Various factors affecting the lethality of cyclohexylamine. *Toxicol. Appl. Pharmacol. 22*, 465 (1972).

241. Kennedy, G., Fancher, O. E., Calandra, J. C., and Keller, R. E., Metabolic fate of saccharin in the albino rat. *Food Cosmet. Toxicol. 10*, 29 (1972).

242. Byard, J. L., and Golberg, L., The metabolism of saccharin in laboratory animals. *Food Cosmet. Toxicol. 11*, 391 (1973).

243. McChesney, E. W., and Golberg, L., The excretion and metabolism of saccharin in man. I. Methods of investigation and preliminary results. *Food Cosmet. Toxicol. 11*, 403 (1973).

244. Kimbrough, R. D., Review of the toxicity of hexachlorophene. *Arch. Environ. Health 23*, 119 (1971).

245. Kimbrough, R. D., and Gaines, T. B., Hexachlorophene effects on the rat brain. Study of high doses by light and electron microscopy. *Arch. Environ. Health 23*, 114 (1971).

246. Neiminen, L., Bjondahl, K., and Möttönen, M., Effect of hexachlorophene on the rat brain during ontogenesis. *Food Cosmet. Toxicol. 11*, 635 (1973).

247. Gaines, T. B., Kimbrough, R. D., and Linder, R. E., The oral and dermal toxicity of hexachlorophene in rats. *Toxicol. Appl. Pharmacol. 25*, 332 (1973).

248. Angel, A., and Rogers, K. J., An analysis of the convulsant activity of substituted benzenes in the mouse. *Toxicol. Appl. Pharmacol. 21*, 214 (1972).

249. Kimbrough, R. D., Toxicity of chlorinated hydrocarbons and related compounds. A review including chlorinated dibenzodioxins and chlorinated dibenzofurans. *Arch. Environ. Health 25*, 125 (1972).

250. Vos, J. G., and Beems, R. B., Dermal toxicity studies of technical polychlorinated biphenyls and fractions thereof in rabbits. *Toxicol. Appl. Pharmacol. 19*, 617 (1971).

251. "Perspective on Chlorinated Dibenzodioxins and Dibenzofurans," *Environ. Health Perspect., Exp. Issue* No. 5. National Institute of Environmental Health Sciences, Research Triangle Park, North Carolina, 1973.

252. Clegg, D. J., Embryotoxicity of chemical contaminants of foods. *Food Cosmet. Toxicol. 9*, 195 (1971).

253. Krasavage, W. J., Yanno, F. J., and Terhaar, C. J., Dimethyl terephthalate (DMT): Acute toxicity, subacute feeding and inhalation studies in male rats. *Amer. Ind. Hyg. Ass., J. 34*, 455 (1973).

254. "Perspectives on Phthalic Acid Esters," *Environ. Health Perspect., Exp. Issue* No. 3. National Institute of Environmental Health Sciences, Research Triangle Park, North Carolina, 1973.

255. Griffith, F. D., Stephens, S. S., and Tayfun, F. O., Exposure of Japanese quail and

parakeets to the pyrolysis products of fry pans coated with Teflon and common cooking oils. *Amer. Ind. Hyg. Ass., J. 34,* 176 (1973).

256. Anderson, M. E., and Mehl, R. G., A comparison of the toxicology of triethylene glycol dinitrate and propylene glycol dinitrate. *Amer. Ind. Hyg. Ass., J. 34,* 526 (1973).

257. Jones, R. A., Strickland, J. A., and Siegel, J., Toxicity of propylene glycol 1,2-dinitrate in experimental animals. *Toxicol. Appl. Pharmacol. 22,* 128 (1972).

258. Potter, H. P., Dimethylformamide-induced abdominal pain and liver injury. *Arch. Environ. Health 27,* 340 (1973).

259. Pergal, M., Vukojević, N., Cirin-Popov, N., Djurić, D., and Bojović, T., Carbon disulfide metabolites excreted in the urine of exposed workers. I. Isolation and identification of 2-mercapto-2-thiazolinone-5. *Arch. Environ. Health 25,* 38 (1972).

260. McDonald, T. O., Roberts, M. D., and Borgmann, A. R., Ocular toxicity of ethylene chlorohydrin and ethylene glycol in rabbit eyes. *Toxicol. Appl. Pharmacol. 21,* 143 (1972).

261. McDonald, T. O., Kasten, K., Hervey, R., Gregg, S., Borgmann, A. R., and Murchison, T., Acute ocular toxicity of ethylene oxide, ethylene glycol, and ethylene chlorohydrin. *Bull. Parenteral Drug Ass. 27,* 153 (1973).

262. Bruckner, J. V., and Guess, W. L., Morphological skin reactions to 2-chloroethanol. *Toxicol. Appl. Pharmacol. 22,* 29 (1972).

263. Weil, C. S., Woodside, M. D., Smyth, H. F., Jr., and Carpenter, C. P., Results of feeding propylene glycol in the diet to dogs for two years. *Food Cosmet. Toxicol. 9,* 479 (1971).

264. Gaunt, I. F., Carpanini, F. M. B., Grasso, P., and Lansdown, A. B. G., Long-term toxicity of propylene glycol in rats. *Food Cosmet. Toxicol. 10,* 151 (1972).

265. Ruddick, J. A., Toxicology, metabolism, and biochemistry of 1,2-propanediol. *Toxicol. Appl. Pharmacol. 21,* 102 (1972).

266. Levin, L., and Gabriel, K. L., The vapor toxicity of trimethyl phosphite. *Amer. Ind. Hyg. Ass., J. 34,* 286 (1973).

267. Ferguson, W. S., and Wheeler, D. D., Caprolactam vapor exposures. *Amer. Ind. Hyg. Ass., J. 34,* 384 (1973).

268. Schwetz, B. A., and Becker, B. A., Comparison of the lethality of inhaled diethyl ether in neonatal and adult rats. *Toxicol. Appl. Pharmacol. 18,* 703 (1971).

269. Frenkel, E. P., and Brody, F., Percutaneous absorption and elimination of an aromatic hair dye. *Arch. Environ. Health 27,* 401 (1973).

270. Kinkel, H. J., and Holzmann, S., Study of long-term percutaneous toxicity and carcinogenicity of hair dyes (oxidizing dyes) in rats. *Food Cosmet. Toxicol. 11,* 641 (1973).

271. Levin, L., Meyers, G. B., and Liddane, L., 2-cyclohexen-1-one: Toxicology and study of an occupational dermal exposure. *Amer. Ind. Hyg. Ass., J. 33,* 338 (1972).

272. Wiles, J. S., and Narcisse, J. K., Jr., The acute toxicity of dimethylamides in several animals species. *Amer. Ind. Hyg. Ass., J. 32,* 539 (1971).

273. Egle, J. L., Jr., Retention of inhaled formaldehyde, propionaldehyde, and acrolein in the dog. *Arch. Environ. Health 25,* 119 (1972).

274. Egle, J. L., Jr., Retention of inhaled acetaldehyde in the dog. *Arch. Environ. Health 24,* 354 (1972).

275. DiVincenzo, G. D., Yanno, F. J., and Astill, B. D., Exposure of man and dog to low concentrations of acetone vapor. *Amer. Ind. Hyg. Ass., J. 34,* 329 (1973).

276. Egle, J. L., Jr., Retention of inhaled acetone and ammonia in the dog. *Amer. Ind. Hyg. Ass., J. 34,* 533 (1973).

277. Lapp, N. L., Physiological changes as diagnostic aids in isocyanate exposure. *Amer. Ind. Hyg. Ass., J. 32*, 378 (1971).

278. Vernot, F. H., Haun, C. C., MacEwen, J. D., and Egan, G. F., Acute inhalation toxicology and proposed emergency limits of nitrogen trifluoride. *Toxicol. Appl. Pharmac. 26*, 1 (1973).

279. Darmer, K. I., Jr., Haun, C. C., and MacEwen, J. D., The acute inhalation toxicology of chlorine pentafluoride. *Amer. Ind. Hyg. Ass., J. 33*, 661 (1972).

280. Griffiths, J. E., Acute inhalation and dermal application screening studies of 2,4,6-trifluoro-sym-triazine and 2,4,6-tris(trifluoromethyl)-sym-triazine. *Amer. Ind. Hyg. Ass., J. 33*, 382 (1972).

281. Isom, G., and Way, J. L., Cyanide intoxication: Protection with cobaltous chloride. *Toxicol. Appl. Pharmacol. 24*, 449 (1973).

282. Pradhan, S. N., and Ziecheck, L. N., Effects of hydrazine on behaviour in rats. *Toxicol. Appl. Pharmacol. 18*, 151 (1971).

283. Smith, E. B., and Clark, D. A., Absorption of hydrazine through canine skin. *Toxicol. Appl. Pharmacol. 21*, 186 (1972).

284. Scharpf, L. G., Jr., Hill, I. D., and Kelly, R. E., Relative eye-injury potential of heavy-duty phosphate and non-phosphate laundry detergents. *Food Cosmet. Toxicol. 10*, 829 (1972).

285. Jenkins, F. P., Robinson, J. A., Gellatly, J. B. M., and Salmond, G. W. A., The no-effect dose of aniline in human subjects and a comparison of aniline toxicity in man and the rat. *Food Cosmet. Toxicol. 10*, 671 (1972).

286. Gaunt, I. F., Carpanini, F. M. B., Wright, M. G., Grasso, P., and Gangolli, S. D., Short-term toxicity of methyl amyl ketone in rats. *Food Cosmet. Toxicol. 10*, 625 (1972).

287. Scala, R. A., and Burtis, E. G., Acute toxicity of a homologous series of branched-chain primary alcohols. *Amer. Ind. Hyg. Ass., J. 34*, 493 (1973).

288. Wiberg, G. S., Samson, J. M., Maxwell, W. B., Coldwell, B. B., and Trenholm, H. L., Further studies on the acute toxicity of ethanol in young and old rats: Relative importance of pulmonary excretion and total body water. *Toxicol. Appl. Pharmacol. 20*, 22 (1971).

289. Schroeder, H. A., Recondite toxicity of trace elements. *Essays Toxicol. 4*, 107–199 (1973).

290. Water quality, trace elements, and cardiovascular disease. *World Health Organ., Chron. 27*, 534 (1973).

291. Kimura, E. T., Ebert, D. M., and Dodge, P. W., Acute toxicity and limits of solvent residue for sixteen organic solvents. *Toxicol. Appl. Pharmacol. 19*, 699 (1971).

292. Campbell, A. H., Sewell, W. R., Chudkowski, M., Willson, J. E., Lord, G. H., and Mohammed, K., The effects of feeding an elemental chemical diet to mature rats: Toxicologic and pathologic studies. *Toxicol. Appl. Pharmacol. 26*, 63 (1973).

293. Schwartz, E., Tornaben, J. A., and Boxhill, G. C., The effects of food restriction on hematology, clinical chemistry and pathology in the albino rat. *Toxicol. Appl. Pharmacol. 25*, 515 (1973).

294. Maickel, R. P., and Snodgrass, W. R., Physicochemical factors in maternal-fetal distribution of drugs. *Toxicol. Appl. Pharmacol. 26*, 218 (1973).

295. Fisher, M. V., Morrow, P. E., and Yuile, C. L., Effect of Freund's complete adjuvant upon clearance of iron-59 oxide from rat lungs. *Res. J. Reticuloendothel. Soc. 13*, 536 (1973).

296. Casarett, L. J., The vital sacs: Alveolar clearance mechanisms in inhalation toxicology. *Essays Toxicol. 3*, 1–36 (1972).

297. Morrow, P. E., Alveolar clearance of aerosols. *Arch. Intern. Med. 131,* 101 (1973).
298. Alarie, Y., Sensory irritation of the upper airways by airborne chemicals. *Toxicol. Appl. Pharmacol. 24,* 279 (1973).
299. Newburgh, R. W., Molecular aspects of toxicants. *Essays Toxicol. 3,* 79–97 (1972).
300. Sher, S. P., Drug enzyme induction and drug interactions: Literature tabulation. *Toxicol. Appl. Pharmacol. 18,* 780 (1971).
301. Conney, A. H., and Burns, J. J., Metabolic interactions among environmental chemicals and drugs. *Science 178,* 576 (1972).
302. Grice, H. C., Barth, M. L., Cornish, H. H., Foster, G. V., and Gray, R. H., Correlation between serum enzymes, isozyme patterns and histologically detectable organ damage. *Food Cosmet. Toxicol. 9,* 847 (1971).
303. Chin, L., Picchioni, A. L., Bourn, W. M., and Laird, H. E., Optimal antidotal dose of activated charcoal. *Toxicol. Appl. Pharmacol. 26,* 103 (1973).
304. Bryan, G. T., and Yoshida, O., Artificial sweeteners as urinary bladder carcinogens. *Arch. Environ. Health 23,* 6 (1971).
305. Sher, S. P., Mammary tumors in control rats: Literature tabulation. *Toxicol. Appl. Pharmacol. 22,* 562 (1972).
306. Papers from a Joint Symposium of the American Academies of Industrial Hygiene and Occupational Medicine, Cincinnati, Feb. 10, 1970. *Arch. Environ. Health 22,* 687–706 (1971).
307. Stokinger, H. E., Concepts of thresholds in standards setting. An analysis of the concept and its application to industrial air limits (TLVs). *Arch. Environ. Health 25,* 153 (1972).
308. Dinman, B. D., "Non-concept" of "no-threshold"; chemicals in the environment. *Science 175,* 495 (1972).
309. Hatch, T. F., Criteria for hazardous exposure limits. *Arch. Environ. Health 27,* 231 (1973).
310. Worden, A. N., Toxicology and the environment. *Toxicology 1,* 3 (1973).
311. Smyth, H. F., Jr., The experimental toxicologist and the occupational physician. *Arch. Environ. Health 22,* 287 (1971).
312. Zbinden, G., "Progress in toxicology. Special Topics," Vol. 1. Springer-Verlag, Berlin and New York, 1973.
313. Hayes, W. J., Jr., The discipline of toxicology: Its future in training and research. *Toxicol. Appl. Pharmacol. 25,* 502 (1973).

Noise

PAUL L. MICHAEL

INTRODUCTION

Concern about industrial noise problems has continued to grow during the past several years as a result of increased understanding of the effects of noise and because of new rules and regulations limiting noise exposures. Valuable information on various noise problems has been gained through research; however, the magnitude of this research effort remains relatively small as compared with that directed to other environmental problems.

The major effort and concern continues to be directed toward the prevention of noise-induced hearing loss, although recognition is also being given to general effects of noise exposure that include: (1) community reactions; (2) annoyance and disturbance; (3) communication through speech and warning signals; and (4) work performance. A complicating factor is the very wide differences in physiologic and psychologic reactions to noise exposure that are found in any study of environmental force or hazard effects on humans; however, these differences appear to be more significant in noise studies, perhaps because the magnitude of the various effects can be more readily measured than the effects produced by most other environmental mental stresses.

This is a review of significant developments covering the effects of noise, its measurement, and control. The review is intended primarily to cover the period 1971–1973 which follows the review published in the preceding edition.[1] No attempt will be made to include basic acoustic theory, nor to provide general teaching materials on noise, because these materials are readily available elsewhere.

129

EFFECTS OF NOISE ON MAN:
CRITERIA, GUIDELINES, STANDARDS, RULES, AND REGULATIONS

Considerable effort continues to be directed toward the development of more accurate hearing conservation criteria and more effective rules and regulations limiting noise exposures. The A-weighted sound pressure level is retained in all major documents under revision; however, there is an American National Standards Institute (ANSI) exploratory group that is considering other frequency weighting characteristics for this purpose. The exposure time and level relationships have been reviewed by several committees and some changes have been proposed during the period 1971–1973.

American National Standards Institute

The ANSI S3-40 Hearing Conservation Writing Group, which has been working on this standard for more than 10 years, finally received a marginal vote of approval from the ANSI S3 Bioacoustics Committee on the last draft submitted in 1972. However, the opposition to the form of presentation used in this document was strong enough to convince the ANSI Board to reject the document as an ANSI Standard even though it had received slightly more than the required 80% positive votes from the S3-Bioacoustics Committee. In an attempt to develop a more acceptable standard document, the membership of the S3-40 Writing Group has been changed, and a new document is being prepared.

The major problem faced by the former S3-40 Writing Group was that a significant number of negative votes would result if absolute exposure levels are specified that *are* lower than those in the present OSHA Law [i.e., 90 dB(A) for 8 hr or the equivalent thereof], and a similar significant number of negative votes would result if the exposure levels *are not* lowered below the limits. Thus, a compromise standard draft was developed in the form of a simple risk table. That is, the best available data were presented in a form that could be used to predict the number of persons who will show a hearing loss when exposed to various levels of steady state noise over different periods of time. Slightly more than 80% of the S3-Bioacoustics Committee approved of this form of presentation, if for no other reason than to make possible the acceptance of an ANSI standard in this vital area after many years of futile efforts. However, there are quite a few S3 members who voted negatively because absolute limits of exposure were not given. Thus, it does not appear likely that an ANSI standard on hearing conservation will be forthcoming in the near future.

The Occupational Safety and Health Act and the National Institutes for Occupational Safety and Health Criteria Document

The Occupational Safety and Health Act of 1970[2] was passed and signed on December 29, 1970, and became effective April 28, 1971. The acceptable noise limits specified in this law, which are similar to those in the revised Walsh–Healy Act,[3] were discussed extensively in "Industrial Environmental Health: The Worker and the Community."[1] The results of more than 2 years under this law show significant progress in hearing conservation in many areas; however, it has become obvious that more complete specifications are needed. Also, new hearing conservation data are available for consideration. Thus, a new Department of Labor (DOL) Advisory Committee has been formed to consider a revision of the Occupational Safety and Health Standards.

The broad objective of the new DOL Advisory Committee is to "establish rules and regulations that will minimize the risk of permanent hearing impairment from exposure to hazardous levels of occupational noise." In addition to specifying permissible occupational noise exposures, the new rules and regulations are to provide specific guides on such problems as:

1. Noise measurement in the occupational environment
2. Hearing threshold measurement procedures and techniques
3. The use of personal hearing protector devices
4. Monitoring requirements for noise exposures and hearing threshold levels
5. Record keeping

The noise exposure limits for the revised OSHA standard are to be based upon all available data relating hearing loss to noise exposure. However, particular attention will be paid to the Criteria for a Recommended Standard— Occupational Exposure to Noise[4] prepared by the Office of Research and Standards Development, National Institute for Occupational Safety and Health (NIOSH). This NIOSH Criteria document provides comprehensive definitions, procedures, techniques, and recommendations on all aspects of an occupational exposure standard for noise.

American Conference of Governmental Industrial Hygienists

The American Conference of Governmental Industrial Hygienists (ACGIH) has long been recognized for its important contributions in setting exposure limits to work hazards and stresses. In fact, the ACIGH Threshold Limit Values (TLV) for Noise established in 1968 were used for the most part as a basis for the noise standards adopted in the Walsh–Healy Act, and later in the OSHA Law. The ACGIH TLV for Noise was revised May 21, 1973 during a national conference held in Boston, Massachusetts. The new TLV for noise now is based upon 85 dB(A) for 8-hr daily exposure and ranges to 115 dB(A) for $\frac{1}{8}$-hr exposure in steps of 5 decibels for each halving of exposure time. The new TLV retains the limit of 140 dB for impulsive or impact noise exposures.

The Environmental Protection Agency

The Office of Noise Abatement and Control of the Environmental Protection Agency (EPA) is presently implementing the Noise Control Act of 1972.[5] This act, signed by President Nixon on October 28, 1972, authorizes the federal government to establish noise emission standards for products distributed in commerce, to provide coordination of federal research on noise control, and to distribute information on noise emission and reduction characteristics of such products. The Act provides for the establishment of federal noise control programs, the identification of major noise sources, and gives the EPA authority to set noise emission standards for construction equipment, electric and electronic equipment, and transportation and recreational vehicles.

The EPA has already published several reports on various noise problem areas.[5-27] They have held public hearings on various noise problems and are disseminating public information on effects, acceptable levels, and techniques for measurement and control of noise. Technical assistance is being provided to state and local governments in the development and enforcement of ambient noise standards; through the Committee on Hearing, Bioacoustics and Biomechanics (CHABA) the EPA have prepared a recommendation for the training of personnel. Also, proposed legislation is being developed in many areas.

In the immediate future, EPA plans to establish a Low-Noise-Emission Product Advisory Committee to assist in determining which products qualify as low-noise-emission. Product certification would be arranged in three steps: (1) EPA will determine upon receipt of certification application whether a class or model of product is low-noise-emission as defined in an applicable standard; (2) EPA will decide whether a low-noise-emission product is a suitable substitute for a product in use at that time by federal agencies, and if so, will issue a 1-year certificate for that product; (3) the administrator of general services will determine if the certified product has a price that is no more than 125% of the retail price of the least expensive type of product for which it would be substituted.

EPA released a proposed federal standard to limit noise emissions from interstate trucks and recommendations for a national effort for aircraft and airport noise control on July 31, 1973.[17] Interstate rail carriers are not included under these proposed regulations.

The Department of Transportation

The Office of Noise Abatement within the Department of Transportation (DOT) is charged with the development and recommendation of noise abatement policies and programs related to transportation. This is a very broad and complex responsibility because it deals with many different modes of transportation and encompasses economic, social, and environmental effects in many different areas. Obviously, land use planning in the form of highway and airport designs are important considerations, as well as the development of quieter modes of transportation, and the control of noise in present systems.

The Office of Noise Abatement has published several reports on transportation noise problems, some of which are listed in References 28–50. Several rules and regulations regulating the noise levels produced by various modes of transportation have appeared in the *Federal Register.*

Department of Interior

The Department of Interior (DOI) through the Bureau of Mines has adopted noise standards that are quite similar to the present OSHA law for underground coal mine operations except that the following additional comprehensive specifications are included.[51,52]

1. Any protective device or system that the mine operator wishes to use to protect the employees from noise must meet with the approval of the Secretary of the Interior.

2. The Secretary of Health, Education, and Welfare (HEW) has been called upon to establish test procedures for inspection of the noise levels in coal mines. The tests are to be conducted by the operator of each mine with the aid of a "qualified person" and the results must be conducted and reported to the Secretaries of HEW and Interior each 6 months.

3. Following a notice of violations of the standards issued by DOI, the operator of such mine has 60 days in which to submit a plan for a hearing conservation program to a joint committee of the Bureau of Mines and DHEW.

The Bureau of Mines has conducted and supported a significant research on noise-related problems.[53-56] The Bureau has also published several important papers dealing with various noise problems.[57-62]

Armed Forces

The armed forces have directed a considerable amount of effort toward the reduction of noise exposures during the past several years. Many noise regulations have been issued on various aspects of hearing conservation; however, there is not good uniformity on regulations between the services nor on the enforcement thereof. The following are brief discussions of rules and regulations currently in effect within the Air Force, Army, and Navy.

AIR FORCE

The Air Force has recently issued AF Regulation 161–35, 27 July, 1973, that is perhaps the most comprehensive of any noise regulation issued to date. It is generally similar to the OSHA Standard except that the noise exposure limit is based upon 84 dB(A) for 8-hr daily exposures *and* permits only a 4-dB increase in exposure for each halving of exposure time.

The Air Force Regulation has a particularly comprehensive section on monitoring audiometry which might well be used as a guide for other programs. In this section, such procedures and techniques necessary in a hearing testing program as (1) calibration of instruments; (2) hearing test for specific purpose (reference, 90-day, annual, follow-up, 15-hr, 40-hr, close scrutiny, and termination); (3) interpretation of audiograms; and (4) record keeping are discussed in detail. There is also a disposition flow chart included that specifies actions to be taken when a significant threshold shift is found.

ARMY

The Army has also conducted research on noise exposure problems over the past several years. Its hearing conservation program is now carried out under Executive Order 11612, AR 40–5, DA circular 40–2, TB Med 251 and Military Standard 1474. These regulations provide for an effective hearing conservation program. The noise exposure limits set forth in these regulations are similar to those specified under the OSHA Standards in most respects except that the base level is set at 85 dB(A) for 8-hr daily exposure.

NAVY

Navy Regulation OPNAVINST5100.14 is part of the Navy Shore Safety Program that is concerned with "hearing hazardous areas." These areas are to be determined by an industrial hygienist or a medical officer and reported to the commanding officer of the base who in turn has the responsibility to reduce the noise exposures to an acceptable level. At sea and in "all commands and activities having high intensity noise levels and all military and civil service personnel," noise exposures are controlled under the Bureau of Medicine and Surgery hearing conservation program, BUMEDINST 6260.6B, 73-NER-61 (5 March, 1970). The noise exposure limit for steady state noise used in this regulation is the same as that used in the OSHA law [i.e., 90 dB(A) for 8-hr daily exposures]; however, the impact noise limit is excluded.

Many research projects related to noise problems have been carried out by the Navy over the past several years. Recently, the Navy Industrial Environmental Health Center has presented three very successful seminars (during 1973) that were well attended by members of all military services and others.

Other Federal, State, and Local Legislative Activities

HEARING CONSERVATION

The Atomic Energy Commission (now designated as the Energy Commission), the General Services Administration and other federal agencies along with several states have patterned hearing conservation rules and regulations[8] after the Walsh–Healy Act.

ACOUSTIC CHARACTERISTICS OF BUILDINGS

Rules and regulations pertaining to the noise characteristics of buildings and conditions at building sites have been established by the Federal Housing Administration (FHA) under the Department of Housing and Urban Development (HUD).[63,64] Noise exposure limits for minimum property standards for multifamily dwellings were also developed.[65] The General Services Administration (GSA) also has developed rules and regulations concerning material specifications and noise ratings.[66,67]

STATE AND LOCAL ACTIVITIES

Considerable effort has been expended at the state and local level to prohibit or control excessive noise; however, there are far too many of these to be covered comprehensively in this chapter. The Environmental Protection Agency (EPA)[8] has listed many of these legislative activities and describes their pertinent features.

NOISE MEASUREMENT

A new American National Standards Institute (ANSI) Specification for Sound Level Meters, ANSI 51.4-1971,[68] has been published as a revision of the American National Standard Specification for the General Purpose Sound Level Meters, 51.4-1961. The new standard is intended to satisfy the existing diverse requirements for precision and accuracy by specifying four types of sound level meters: precision, general purpose, survey, and special purpose. ANSI writing groups are also working on the development of standard specifications for dosimeters and integrating sound level meters.

Dosimeter or integrating sound level meters should receive increasing attention during the next few years because (1) any measurement of a noise hazard must include the time of exposure as a significant parameter, along with the level and spectral content of the noise, and (2) it is extremely difficult to obtain the time-level exposure patterns with direct-heading sound level meters in many work areas where the quasi-steady state noise exposures fluctuate in an unpredictable way. Unfortunately, it is not a simple task to write standard specifications for these instruments, and this task is made even more difficult because a concise and detailed definition for a noise exposure criterion has not been established at this writing. For example, a decision must be made on how to specify the instrument's response to noise levels below 90 dB(A) if this value remains as the limiting level. The present Occupational Safety and Health Law (1970) states that noise exposure limits are 90 dB(A) for 8 hr, 95 dB(A) for 4 hr, etc., but no time limits are specified for levels below 90 dB(A). Does this mean that 85 dB(A) should correspond to 16 hr of exposure, or is there an unlimited exposure time allowed for 89.5 dB(A)? Another question concerns the weighting to be given to levels above 115 dB(A). Still another concerns the weighting to be given to short pulses of noise. All of these questions, and others, must be answered before a comprehensive standard can be written for dosimeters and integrating sound level meters.

Generally, dosimeters are designed to be worn by the person whose noise exposure is being measured. This has the obvious advantage that the person has the measuring instrument with him at all times during a specified period of time; however, there is the disadvantage that a microphone's response may be affected by several dB due to its close proximity to the body. The microphone may produce output levels that are several dB's too high if a noise with predominant high-frequency characteristics is incident upon the side of the body where the microphone is worn. On the other hand, if the high-frequency noise is incident upon the opposite side of the body from the microphone position, the microphone output may be several dB lower than it should be due to shielding.

An interesting consideration in the use of dosimeters is that the readout is generally expressed in terms of a linear percentage of the allowed daily exposure, rather than a measure of the logarithmic sound pressure level in dB(A) that has been commonly used. If inaccuracies are allowed for dosimeters that correspond to those allowed for the ANSI Type II sound level meters (now specified in the OSHA Standard), then readings from 2 dosimeters exposed to the same high frequency noise may show differences in readout values that exceed 70% even though both meet ANSI specifications. Additional, and even larger, magnitudes of variation of microphone response can result from the effects of body baffling or shielding. Thus, inaccuracies tolerated in terms of decibels from direct-reading sound level meters will become much more obvious, and perhaps will not be so easy to tolerate when expressed linearly.

To summarize, dosimeters and integrating sound level meters do offer definite advantages for measuring noise exposures in some instances. However, standards are badly needed to provide guidance for instrument specifications, Also, care and understanding in the use of these instruments and the resulting data are essential.[69-83]

HEARING MEASUREMENT

Standards

An ANSI writing group has begun the task of revising the ANSI Specifications for Audiometers. In addition to the usual tightening of specifications wherever new technology permits, there is also some consideration being given to standardizing (1) calibration procedures and (2) procedures for pure-tone threshold audiometry.

The present ANSI Audiometer Specifications do provide complete instrumentation specifications; however, calibration procedures vary widely between various calibration laboratories. For example, some check only a single test frequency at one hearing level, while others may check all test frequencies at each 5 dB hearing level. Some laboratories check distortion of the test tone, cross-talk between earphones, interruption switch operation, etc., and others do not. The ANSI writing group has proposed that a minimum procedure for the calibration of audiometers should be standardized.

Procedures used for pure-tone threshold audiometry also vary widely and, in some cases, the results of these threshold measurements do not compare closely. Thus, there is an attempt being made to standardize a procedure for clinical and field measurements so that threshold measurement data will be more consistent between testers.

Training Audiometric Technicians

Many new training courses for industrial audiometric technicians have been initiated during the past few years. Although some of these courses are conducted by well-trained persons, it is obvious that others are not. Therefore, the Intersociety Committee on Industrial Audiometric Technician Training has been reactivated and asked to prepare recommendations for assuring better and more consistent training courses.

At the first meeting of the Intersociety Committee a writing group was appointed to prepare scientific recommendations for controlling the course content and quality. After several meetings a new writing group, now called the

Council for Accreditation in Occupational Hearing Conservation, was established. The Council is made up of two representatives from each of the following organizations: the American Academy of Occupational Medicine, the American Association of Industrial Nurses, the American Council of Otolaryngology, the American Industrial Hygiene Association, the American Speech and Hearing Association, the Industrial Medical Association, and the National Safety Council.

The objectives set forth by the Council are "to set standards and establish training policies and methods for providing industry with technicians who will be able to conduct excellent hearing conservation programs in large and small plants." It appears at this time that the Department of Labor (OSHA) will recognize those persons certified by the Council as meeting DOL standards.

The following criteria have been proposed by the Council for occupational hearing conservation training programs:

1. There shall be a minimal 20-hr course given that follows the original Intersociety syllabus.[84]

2. There shall be at least one faculty member for each course who has been certified by the Council. That member is to be responsible for the selection of the balance of the faculty members for that course.

3. There shall be a ratio of at least one instructor for every six students for laboratory instruction.

4. There shall be a ratio of at least one audiometer for every three students, and ample time must be provided for practice on different audiometer models. The practice must be supervised and a final practice examination must be given.

The course director shall send a list of all persons who have successfully completed the course to the Council.* These recorded attendees may obtain a certificate in Occupational Hearing Conservation from the Council by submitting a completed application form along with a certification fee.

The Council plans to conduct other regional workshops to enlarge the nucleus of certified faculty and to continue the certification of attendees to approved courses. In addition, the council has set forth the following objectives:

1. To monitor the quality of courses by means of attendee questionnaires

2. To work with the committee on Hearing and Bioacoustics (CHABA) and the ANSI writing groups in bringing forth the best procedures and techniques for measuring pure tone acoustical thresholds

3. To develop a Refresher Course Syllabus to enable previous Intersociety certificate holders to update their knowledge and be eligible for Council certification

---

* The Council for Accreditation in Occupational Hearing Conservation, Haddon Heights, New Jersey.

It should be remembered that accuracy in the measurement of hearing thresholds requires a well-trained technician,[84] a quiet test environment,[85] and an accurately calibrated audiometer.[86] A weakness in any one of these factors will result in inaccurate hearing measurement data. Reference materials related to hearing and hearing measurement may be found in numerous scientific journals.[87-95]

NOISE CONTROL

Engineering Noise Control Procedures

Progress continues to be made on the use of known engineering control techniques and procedures for noise reduction on noise machines and processes. However, the use of these preferred methods of noise control has developed slowly in many areas because the dissemination of this knowledge has been slow, and because of the complexity and expense in many instances. It is obvious that noise control of many existing machines and processes is exceedingly difficult or impractical, and that standards are needed that will encourage more effort in noise control at the design state of noise equipment. There have been numerous articles and books published on specific noise control procedures.

Personal Protective Devices

Personal protective devices continue to be the most common means for reducing noise exposures, and the manufacturers of personal ear protectors[96-116] have continued the development of new devices. While there have been no radically new designs offered, the newer products do generally provide more consistent and comfortable performance.

The ANSI and Institute of Electrical and Electronics Engineers (IEEE) standards writing groups are concentrating on the development of new performance evaluation standards.[117-119] A new ANSI Standard Method for the Measurement of Real-Ear Protection of Hearing Protectors and Physical Attenuation of Earmuffs, ANSI S3.19-197X,[117] will be published soon. This standard will specify new and improved subjective and objective procedures for measuring the amount of protection afforded by personal ear protectors. Another ANSI Writing Group, Z-137, has developed what is thought to be the final proposed draft of a more general American National Standard for Occupational and Educational Personal Hearing Devices[118] which covers all aspects of a hearing protector's wear, storage, and durability performance. Reference is made in this standard to the ANSI S3-197X document for measuring the amount of protection afforded. Recognition should be given to the IEEE Working Group 30.10[119] that developed much of the basic information concerned with the objective test procedure for measuring the attenuation afforded by muff-type protectors.

INFORMATION SOURCES

Conferences and Short Courses

The number of conferences and short courses on various noise-related subjects has increased to the point where it is impractical to list them in this chapter. Associations, societies, and private organizations have held conferences on noise-related topics throughout the country during the past few years.

Two new very successful and informative conferences, Inter-Noise 72 (International) and Noise-Con 73 (National), have been presented by the Institute of Noise Control Engineering, and another Inter-Noise 74 meeting is planned for the fall of 1974. The Institute of Noise Control Engineering is a nonprofit membership organization that has the primary objective to advance the technology of noise control engineering with particular emphasis on engineering solutions to environmental noise problems. Proceedings of these conferences[120-122] should provide valuable reference material to industrial hygienists, safety engineers, and others who have the responsibility of hearing conservation programs in industry.

Publications

A number of worthwhile publications on noise have been made available during the past few years.

BOOKS

The book "Fundamentals of Industrial Noise Control" by Lewis H. Bell[123] is written for the plant or safety engineer responsible for noise control. It includes case histories and illustrations from the machine tool manufacturing, power plant, plastics, food processing, packaging, and petrochemical industries. Some topics covered are: acoustic materials, gear noises, silencers and mufflers, fans, enclosures, furnace noise, vibration control, instrumentation, air jet noise, reverberation control.

"Hearing Conservation" by Joseph Sataloff and Paul L. Michael[124] is written for persons responsible for the many interdisciplinary noise problems associated with hearing conservation in industry, and with the general well-being of man away from work. The purpose of the book is to provide information and to describe techniques necessary for nonexpert persons to solve the most common noise problems. Some topics covered include: causes of hearing loss, physics of sound, noise measurement, noise control, personal ear protection, hearing measurement, noise specifications for indoor spaces, community noise problems, legal aspects.

"Noise and Vibration Control"[125] edited by Leo K. Beranek is "written for the engineer who wishes to solve a noise control problem." It is a revision of the well-known earlier book "Noise Reduction." This book emphasizes the engineering aspects of noise problems; however, a chapter on damage risk criteria has been written by Aram Glorig, and Leo Beranek has written a chapter on the various methods and procedures for noise ratings. Mathematics is used at the calculus level; however, it is possible to make practical calculations from algebraic equations given.

"The Effects of Noise on Man"[126] by Karl D. Kryter includes a wealth of information on such subjects as speech interference, temporary and permanent threshold shifts, loudness and noisiness measurements, and the measurement of human response to noise. One section covers the nonauditory responses to noise. The text is obviously intended for persons with some experince in the field since many discussions use technical terminology without definitions.

The third edition of the "American Industrial Hygiene Association Industrial Noise Manual" is nearing completion.[127] This manual is highly recommended for those interested in the broad aspects of industrial noise problems. Topics include physics of sound, sound measurement, physiology of the ear, effects of noise on man, medical aspects, personal protection, engineering control, legal aspects, and the effects and measurement of vibration.

JOURNALS, NEWSLETTERS, AND OTHER SOURCES OF INFORMATION

The Institute of Noise Control Engineering (INCE) published the first issue of its new technical journal, *Noise Control Engineering,* during the summer of 1973.[128] This journal, which is published in cooperation with the Acoustical Society of America, should provide valuable technical information covering the very wide range of interests concerned with noise control problems.

INCE also publishes *Noise/News* bimonthly. *Noise/News* is intended to carry "information on people, legislation, new products, contract awards, meeting announcements, and whatever is new and of general interest in the field." Members, affiliates, and associates of INCE receive both *Noise Control Engineering* and *Noise/News* publications.*

* For more information on *Noise Control Engineering,* write to the Circulation Department, Morristown, New Jersey. For information on *Noise/News,* write to the Circulation Department, Poughkeepsie, New York.

S/V—Sound and Vibration has had some very practical noise control papers in their monthly magazine during the past few years. In addition to the full-length articles, *S/V* includes news items and engineering briefs related to sound and vibration.*

Noise Control Report, a biweekly newsletter, is an excellent source of noise news, with particular emphasis on federal and state activities.†

In addition to those papers listed earlier, the following references covering various noise-related problems may be of interest:

1. Effects of long-term steady-state noise exposures on hearing.[129-162]
2. Effects of intermittent noise exposures on hearing.[163-165]
3. Effects of airborne ultrasonic noise exposures on hearing.[166-216]
4. Effects of impulse or impact noise exposures on hearing.[217-232]
5. Miscellaneous legislative activities.[233-271]
6. Community noise activities.[272-277]
7. Noise measurement.[278-280]
8. Noise control.[281-310]
9. General.[311-321]

REFERENCES

1. Cralley, L. V., ed., "Industrial Environmental Health—The Worker and the Community." Academic Press, New York, 1972.
2. "Occupational Safety and Health Standards" (Williams—Steiger Occupational Safety and Health Act of 1970), Federal Register, vol. 36, p. 10518, U.S. Dept. of Labor, Washington, D.C., 1971.
3. "Safety and Health Standards for Federal Supply Contracts" (Walsh—Healy Public Contracts Act), Federal Register, vol. 34, p. 7948. U.S. Dept. of Labor, Washington, D.C., 1969.
4. "Criteria for a Recommended Standard—Occupational Exposure to Noise." Health Services and Mental Health Administration, National Institutes for Occupational Safety and Health, U.S. Department of Health, Education, and Welfare, Washington, D.C., 1972.

The following publications by the Environmental Protection Agency (EPA) are available from the U.S. Government Printing Office (GPO), Washington, D.C. 20402, except where noted.

5. "Noise Control Act of 1972 Highlights." EPA, Office of Public Affairs, Washington, D.C., 1972.
6. "Noise Pollution—Now Hear This." EPA, GPO Stock No. 5500—0072 (1973).

* Subscription information can be obtained from *Sound and Vibration,* Bay Village, Ohio.

† Published by Business Publishers, Inc., P.O. Box 1067, Blair Station, Silver Spring, Maryland 20910.

7. "Fundamentals of Noise: Measurement, Rating Schemes, and Standards." EPA, GPO Stock No. 5500–0054 (1972).
8. "Laws and Regulatory Schemes for Noise Abatement." EPA, GPO Stock No. 5500–0046 (1972).
9. "Noise Programs of Professional/Industrial Organizations." EPA, GPO Stock No. 5500–00053 (1973).
10. "Environmental Protection Agency: A Progress Report." EPA, GPO (1973).
11. "Public Hearings on Noise Abatement and Control." Vol. I, Construction Noise, GPO Stock No. 5500–00037 (1973).
12. "Public Hearings on Noise Abatement and Control." Vol. II, Manufacturing and Transportation Noise, GPO Stock No. 5500–00085 (1973).
13. "Public Hearings on Noise Abatement and Control." Vol. III, Urban Planning, Architectural Design, and Noise in the Home, GPO Stock No. 5500–00055 (1973).
14. "In Productive Harmony." EPA, GPO Stock No. 5500 (1973).
15. "Your World, My World." GPO Stock No. 5500–00079 (1973).
16. "Don't Leave it All to the Experts." Office of Public Affairs, EPA, Washington, D.C., 1973.
17. "Motor Carrier Noise Background Document." Office of Public Affairs, EPA, Washington, D.C., 1973.

The following publications from EPA are available from the National Technical Information Service (NTIS), 5285 Port Royal Road, Springfield, Va. 22151.

18. "Community Noise." EPA, NTIS–NTID 300.3 (1971).
19. "An Assessment of Noise Concern in Other Nations." EPA, NTIS, NTID 300.3 (1971).
20. "State and Municipal Non-Occupational Noise Programs." EPA, NTIS, NTID 300.8 (1971).
21. "Transportation Noise and Noise from Equipment Powered by Internal Combustion Engines." EPA, NTIS–NTID 300.13 (1971).
22. "Effects of Noise on People." EPA, NTIS–NTID 300.7 (1971).
23. "The Effects of Sonic Boom and Similar Impulsive Noise on Structures." EPA, NTIS–NTID 300.12 (1971).
24. "Effects of Noise on Wildlife and Other Animals." EPA, NTIS–NTID 300.5 (1971).
25. "The Economic Impact of Noise." EPA, NTIS–NTID 300.14 (1971).
26. "The Social Impact of Noise." EPA, NTIS–NTID 300.11 (1971).
27. "Noise Facts Digest." EPA, NTIS–NTID 300.15 (1972).

The following publications of the Office of Noise Abatement, Dept. of Transportation are available from the National Technical Information Service, 5285 Port Royal Road, Springfield, Va. 22151.

28. "Noise and Vibration Characteristics of High Speed Transit Vehicles." DOT Rep. No. OST–ONA–71–7 (1971).
29. "A Study of the Magnitude of Transportation Noise Generation and Potential Abatement." Vol. 1, Summary, DOT Rep. No. OST–ONA–71–1 (1970).
30. "A Study of the Magnitude of Transportation Noise Generation and Potential Abatement." Vol. II, Measurement Criteria, DOT Rep. No. OST–ONA–71–1 (1970).
31. "A Study of the Magnitude of Transportation Noise Generation and Potential Abatement." Vol. III, Airport/Aircraft System Noise, DOT Rep. No. OST–ONA–71–1 (1970).

32. "A Study of the Magnitude of Transportation Noise Generation and Potential Abatement." Vol. IV, Motor Vehicle/Highway System Noise, DOT Rep. No. OST–ONA–71–1 (1970).
33. "A Study of the Magnitude of Transportation Noise Generation and Potential Abatement." Vol. V, DOT, Train System Noise, Rep. No. OST–ONA–71–1 (1970).
34. "A Study of the Magnitude of Transportation Noise Generation and Potential Abatement." Vol. VI, Community Transportation Noise, DOT Rep. No. OST–ONA–71–1 (1970).
35. "A Study of the Magnitude of Transportation Noise Generation and Potential Abatement." Vol. VII, Abatement and Responsibility, DOT Rep. No. OST–ONA–71–1 (1970).
36. "Acoustic and Performance Test Comparison of Intial Quieted Truck with Contemporary Production Trucks." DOT Rep. No. DOT–TST–74–2 (1973).
37. "Experimental Atmospheric Absorption Coefficients." DOT Rep. No. FAA–RD–71–99 (1971).
38. "Measurement and Analysis of Noise from Four Aircraft in Level Flight." (727, KC-135, 707-320B and DC-9), DOT Rep. No. FAA–RD–71–83 (1971).
39. "Noise Measurement During Approach Operations on Runway 21R at Detroit Metropolitan Airport." DOT Rep. No. FAA–RD–71–117 (1971).
40. "Technique for Developing Noise Exposure Forecasts, Noise Exposure Forecasts for O'Hare Airport." DOT Rep. FAA–DS–67–16 (1967).
41. "Aircraft Noise Evaluation." DOT Rep. FAA–NO–68–34 (1968).
42. "Analysis of Operational Noise Measurements in Terms of Selected Human Response Noise Evaluation Measures." DOT Rep. FAA–RD–71–112 (1971).
43. "Evaluation Measures." DOT Rep. FAA–RD–71–112 (1971).
44. "Measurement and Analysis of Noise from Seventeen Aircraft in Level Flight (Military, Business Jet and General Aviation)." DOT Rep. FAA–RD–71–98 (1971).
45. "Far Field Noise Generation by Coaxial Flow Jet Exhausts." DOT Rep. FAA–RD–71–101; 1 (1971).
46. "Comparisons Between Subjective Ratings of Aircraft Noise and Various Objective Measures." DOT Rep. No. 68–33 (1968).
47. "Subjective Evaluation of General Aviation Aircraft Noise." DOT Rep. FAA–NO–68–35 (1968).
48. "Technique for Developing Noise Exposure Forecasts; Noise Exposure Forecasts for J. F. Kennedy International Airport." DOT Rep. FAA–DS–67–15 (1967).
49. "Technique for Developing Noise Exposure Forecasts." DOT Rep. FAA–DS–67–14 (1967).
50. "Transportation Noise." GPO Stock No. 5000–0057 (1973).
51. "Federal Coal Mine Health and Safety Act of 1969." Noise Standard, Sect. 206, Public Law 91–173 (1969).
52. "Code of Federal Regulations." 30 CFR 70.500, Federal Register, Vol. 35, p. 644 (1970).
53. "Response Variations of a Microphone Worn on the Human Body." Rep. RI7810. Bureau of Mines, Pittsburgh, Pennsylvania, 1973.
54. Jensen, J. W., and Visnopuu, A., "Progress in Suppressing Noise of the Pneumatic Rock Drill" (Funded by the Bureau of Mines), Proc. Inter-Noise 72. International Conference on Noise Control Engineering, Washington, D.C., 1972.
55. Gatley, W. S., and Barth, M. G., "A Practical Approach to the Exhaust Silencing of the Pneumatic Rock Drill" (Funded by the Bureau of Mines), Proc. Inter-Noise 72. International Conference on Noise Control Engineering, Washington, D.C., 1972.
56. Bureau of Mines, U.S. Dept. of Interior. "Mining Research Contract Review." Vols.

I-IV. Pittsburgh Mining and Safety Research Center, Pittsburgh, Pennsylvania, 1970–1973.

57. LaMonica, J. A., Noise levels in cleaning plants. *Mining Congr. J.,* 29–31 (1972).

58. "Fundamentals of Noise Measurement." Bureau of Mines, Pittsburgh, Pennsylvania, 1973.

59. Michael, Paul L. *et al.,* Aspects of Noise Generation and Hearing Protection in Underground Coal Mines." Bureau of Mines Grant 0122004. Environmental Acoustic Laboratory, Penn State University, University Park, 1973.

60. "Hearing Conservation for the Mineral Industry." U.S. Bureau of Mines Information Circular, Pittsburgh, Pennsylvania, 1972.

61. Noise in underground coal mines. *U.S. Bur. Mines, Rep. Invest. RI 7550* (1972).

62. LaMonica, J. A., Coal mine noise standard. *Amer. Ind. Hyg. Ass., J. 33,* 761–765 (1972).

63. "HUD Noise Assessment Guidelines." GPO No. 2300–1194 (1972).

64. "Underwriting–Home Mortgages." FHA Manual, Vol. VII, Book I, GPO No. 71453 (1970).

65. "Minimum Property Standards for Multifamily Housing." FHA Manual, GPO No. 2600–405 (1971).

66. "General Services Administration Handbook." PBS P 3410.5, Chge 1, and PBS P 3460.1C (1969).

67. Public Building Service, "Guide Specifications." PBS 4–0950: Acoustical ceiling systems (1968); PBS 4–1031: Relocatable partition systems (1968); PBS 4515–71: Vibration insulation. Washington, D.C., 1970.

68. American National Standards Institute, "American National Standards Specifications for Sound Level Meters." S1.4–1971. ANSI, New York, 1971.

69. National Machine Tool Builders Association, "NMTBA Noise Measurement Techniques." Washington, D.C., 1970.

70. Ranz, J. R., A survey of noise measurement methods. *Mach. Des. 38,* 199 (1966).

71. Skode, F., Windscreening of outdoor microphones. *Tech. Rev. 1,* 3 (1966).

72. Bauer, B. B., and Foster, E. J., Methodology for acoustical data gathering. *J. Audio Eng. Soc. 16,* 390 (1968).

73. Schneider, E. J., Microphone orientation in the sound field. *Sound and Vibration 4*(2), 20 (1970).

74. American National Standards Institute, "American National Standard for Preferred Frequencies and Band Numbers for Acoustical Measurements." S1.6–1967. ANSI, New York, 1967.

75. "Technical Review" (Quarterly). Bruel & Kjaer, Cleveland, Ohio.

76. "Noise Measurement." General Radio Company, Concord, Massachusetts, 1972.

77. "Mechanical Vibration and Shock Measurements." Bruel & Kjaer, Cleveland, Ohio, 1971.

78. "Acoustic Noise Measurements," 2nd ed. Bruel & Kjaer, Cleveland, Ohio, 1971.

79. American National Standards Institute, "American National Standard for Octave, Half-Octave, and Third-Octave Band Sets." S1.11–1066. ANSI, New York, 1961.

80. "Sound Level Calibrator." Type 1562–A. General Radio Company, West Concord, Massachusetts, 1972.

81. "Acoustics Handbook." Hewlett–Packard Company, Palo Alto, California, 1968.

82. "Handbook of Noise Measurement." General Radio Company, West Concord, Massachusetts, 1972.

83. Broch, J., "Acoustic Noise Measurements," 2nd ed. Bruel & Kjaer, p. 33, Cleveland, Ohio, 1971.

84. Intersociety Committee of Industrial Audiometric Technician Training. Guide for

training of industrial audiometric technicians. *Amer. Ind. Hyg. Ass., J. 27,* 303 (1966).

85. American National Standards Institute, "American National Standard Criteria for Background Noise in Audiometer Rooms." ANSI S3.1–1960. ANSI, New York, 1960.

86. American National Standards Institute, "American National Standard Specifications for Audiometers." ANSI S3.6–1969. ANSI, New York, 1969.

87. Michael, P. L., Standardization of normal hearing threshold. *J. Occup. Med. 10,* 67 (1968).

88. Eagles, E. L., and Doerfler, L. G., Hearing in children: Acoustic environment and audiometer performance. *J. Speech Hear. Res. 4,* 149 (1961).

89. Knight, J. J., Normal hearing threshold determined by manual and self-recording techniques. *J. Acoust. Soc. Amer. 39,* 1184 (1966).

90. Riley, E. C., Sterner, J. H., Fassett, D. W., and Sutton, W. L., Ten years experience with industrial audiometry. *Amer. Ind. Hyg. Ass., J. 22,* 151 (1961).

91. Glorig, A., "Noise and Your Ear." Grune & Stratton, New York, 1958.

92. Rosen, S., Plester, D., El-Mofty, A., and Rosen, H. V., High frequency audiometry in presbycusis: A comparative study of the Maaban tribe in the Sudan with urban populations. *Arch. Otolaryngol. 79,* 1 (1964).

93. Rice, C. G., and Coles, R. R. A., Normal threshold of hearing for pure tones by earphone listening with a self-recording audiometric technique. *J. Acoust. Soc. Amer. 39,* 1185 (1966).

94. Whittle, I. S., and Delaney, M. E., Equivalent threshold sound-pressure levels for the TDH39/MX41–AR earphone. *J. Acoust. Soc. Amer. 38,* 1187 (1966).

95. "Guide for Industrial Audiometric Technicians." Employers Insurance of Wausau, Wausau, Wisconsin, 1968.

96. American Optical Company, Safety Products Division, Southbridge, Massachusetts.

97. Bausch & Lomb, Rochester, New York.

98. Bilson International, Inc., Reston, Virginia.

99. David Clark Company, Ear Protector Department, Worcester, Massachusetts.

100. E. I. DuPont, Wilmington, Delaware.

101. Flents Products Company, New York.

102. Glendale Optical Company, Woodbury, New York.

103. H. E. Douglass Engineering Sales Company, Burbank, California.

104. Frontier Industrial Products, Los Angeles, California.

105. Marion Health and Safety, Inc., Rockford, Illinois.

106. Mediprint, Inc., St. Louis, Missouri.

107. Mine Safety Appliances Company, Safety Products Division, Pittsburgh, Pennsylvania.

108. National Research Corporation, Cambridge, Massachusetts.

109. Safety Ear Protector Company, Los Angeles, California.

110. Sigma Engineering Company, North Hollywood, California.

111. Stayrite, Inc., Long Island City, New York.

112. Surgical Mechanical Research, Los Angeles, California.

113. Rockford I. C. Webb, Inc., Rockford, Illinois.

114. Welsh Manufacturing Company, Providence, Rhode Island.

115. Willson Products Division, E.S.B., Reading, Pennsylvania.

116. United States Safety Service Company, Kansas City, Missouri.

117. American National Standards Institute, "Method for the Measurement of Real-Ear Protection of Hearing Protectors and Physical Attenuation of Earmuffs." ANSI S3.19, 197X. ANSI, New York, 1974 (draft).

118. American National Standards Institute, "American National Standard for Occupational and Educational Personal Hearing Protective Devices." Draft Z137.1–1973. ANSI, New York, 1973.

119. Institute for Electrical and Electronics Engineers, "Procedures for the Measurement of Circumaural Ear Protectors." WG30.10. IEEE, New York, 1971.

120. Institute of Noise Control Engineering, "Inter-Noise 72 Proceedings." Noise/News Circulation Department, Poughkeepsie, New York, 1972.

121. Institute of Noise Control Engineering, "Inter-Noise 72 Tutorials." Noise/News Circulation Department, Poughkeepsie, New York, 1973.

122. Institute of Noise Control Engineering, "Noise-Con 73 Proceedings." Noise/News Circulation Department, Poughkeepsie,New York, 1973.

123. Bell, L. H., "Fundamentals of Industrial Noise Controls." Harmony Publications, Trumbull, Connecticut, 1973.

124. Sataloff, J., and Michael, P. L., "Hearing Conservation." Thomas, Springfield, Illinois, 1973.

125. Beranek, L. L., "Noise and Vibration Control." McGraw-Hill, New York, 1971.

126. Kryter, K. D., "The Effects of Noise on Man." Academic Press, New York, 1970.

127. "Industrial Noise Manual," 3rd ed. Amer. Ind. Hyg. Ass., Akron, Ohio (to be completed).

128. "Noise Control Engineering." Institute of Noise Control Engineering, Bedford, Massachusetts, 1973.

129. Baughn, W. L., Noise control—percent of population protected. *Int. Audiol. J. 5,* 331 (1966).

130. Nixon, J., and Glorig, A., Noise-induced permanent threshold shift at 2000 cps and 4000 cps. *J. Acoust. Soc. Amer. 33,* 904 (1961).

131. Cohen, A., Anticaglia, J. R., and Jones, H. H., Noise-induced hearing loss—exposures to steady-state noise. *Arch. Environ. Health 20,* 614 (1970).

132. Schneider, E. J., Mutchler, J., Hoyle, H., Ode, E., and Holder, B., The progression of hearing loss from industrial noise exposures. *Amer. Ind. Hyg. Ass., J. 31,* 368 (1970).

133. Robinson, D. W., "The Relationships Between Hearing Loss and Noise Exposure," NPL Aero Rep. Ac 32. Nat. Phys. Lab. London, 1968.

134. Ward, W. D., Temporary threshold shift following monaural and binaural exposure. *J. Acoust. Soc. Amer. 38,* 121 (1965).

135. Ward, W. D., Temporary threshold shifts in males and females. *J. Acoust. Soc. Amer. 40,* 478 (1966).

136. Lawrence, M., Gonzales, G., and Hawkins, J. E., Some physical factors in noise-induced hearing loss. *Amer. Ind. Hyg. Ass., J. 28,* 425 (1967).

137. "Hazardous Noise Exposure." Air Force Regul. No. 160–3. Dept. of Air Force, Washington, D.C., 1956.

138. Botsford, J. H., Simple method for identifying acceptable noise exposures. *J. Acoust. Soc. Amer. 42,* 810 (1967).

139. Flanagan, J. J., and Guttman, N., Estimating noise hazard with the sound-level meter. *J. Acoust. Soc. Amer. 36,* 1654 (1964).

140. Karplus, H. B., and Bonvallet, G. L., A noise survey of manufacturing industries. *Amer. Inc. Hyg. Ass., Quart. 14,* 235 (1953).

141. Morse, K. M., The assessment of the work place—a prerequisite to the diagnosis of occupational chest diseases. *Amer. Ind. Hyg. Ass., J. 28,* 141 (1967).

142. Cohen, A., and Baumann, K. C., Temporary hearing losses following exposure to pronounced single-frequency components in broad-band noise. *J. Acoust. Soc. Amer. 36,* 1167 (1964).

143. Von Gierke, H. E., Effects of sonic boom on people: Review and outlook. *J. Acoust. Soc. Amer. 39,* S43 (1966).

144. Rintelman, W. F., and Borous, J. F., Noise-induced hearing loss and rock and roll music. *Arch. Otolaryngol. 88,* 377 (1968).

145. Flugrath, J. M., Modern day rock and roll music and damage-risk criteria. *J. Acoust. Soc. Amer. 45,* 704 (1969).
146. Lebo, C. P., and Oliphant, K., Music as a source of acoustic trauma. *Laryngoscope 78,* 1211 (1968).
147. Dey, F. L., Auditory fatigue and predicted permanent hearing defects from rock and roll music. *N. Engl. J. Med. 282,* 467 (1970).
148. Anderson, J. H., The effect of high intensity "rock" music on teenage hearing thresholds. Master's Thesis, North Dakota State University of Agriculture and Applied Science, Fargo (1969).
149. Lipscomb, D. M., Ear damage from exposure to rock and roll music. *Arch. Otolaryngol. 90,* 29 (1969).
150. Ayley, J., Bartlett, B., Bedford, W., Gregory, W., and Hallum, G., "Pilot Study on the Effects of 'Pop' Group Music on Hearing," I.S.V.R. Memo No. 266. Institute of Sound and Vibration, University of Southampton, Southampton, England, 1969.
151. Lipscomb, D. M., High intensity sounds in the recreational environment. *Clin. Pediat. 8,* 63 (1969).
152. Noise and Hearing Committee, "Noise Bibliography." Industrial Medical Association, Chicago, Illinois, 1972.
153. Dougherty, J. D., and Welsh, O. L., Community noise and hearing loss. *N. Engl. J. Med. 275,* 759 (1966).
154. Tobias, J. V., Noise in light twin-engine aircraft. *Sound and Vibration 3,* 16 (1969).
155. Somerville, G. W., and Kronoveter, K. J., "Cockpit Noise-Induced Hearing Loss in Pilots." Bureau of Occupational Safety and Health, Western Area Occupational Health Laboratory, Salt Lake City, Utah, 1968.
156. Tobias, J. V., Cockpit noise intensity: Fifteen single-engine light aircraft. *Aerosp. Med. 39,* 963 (1969).
157. Gottlieb, P., "Anomalous Hearing Loss and Jet Noise Exposures" (unpublished report available from the author, 11339 Gladwin St., Los Angeles, Calif. 90049, 1969.
158. Harris, J. D., Hearing loss trend curves and the damage-risk criterion in diesel-engineroom personnel. *J. Acoust. Soc. Amer. 37,* 444 (1965).
159. Botsford, J. H., Predicting hearing impairment from a-weighted sound levels. *J. Acoust. Soc. Amer. 42,* 1151 (1967) (abstr.).
160. LaBenz, P., Cohen, A., and Pearson, B., A noise and hearing survey of earth-moving equipment operators. *Amer. Ind. Hyg. Ass., J. 28,* 117 (1967).
161. Ottoboni, F., and Milby, T. H., Occupational disease potentials in heavy equipment operators. *Arch. Environ. Health 15,* 317 (1967).
162. Smith, P. E., Jr., A test for the susceptibility of noise-induced hearing loss. *Amer. Ind. Hyg. Ass., J. 30,* 245 (1969).
163. Kryter, K. D., Ward, W. D., Miller, J. D., and Eldredge, D. H., Hazardous exposure to intermittent and steady-state noise. *J. Acoust. Soc. Amer. 39,* 451 (1966).
164. Sataloff, J., Vassallo, L., and Menduke, H., Hearing loss from exposure to interrupted noise. *Arch. Environ. Health 18,* 972 (1969).
165. Ward, W. D., Temporary threshold shift and damage risk criteria for intermittent noise exposure. *J. Acoust. Soc. Amer. 48,* 561 (1970).
166. Parrack, H. O., Effect of airborne ultrasound on humans. *Int. Audiol. J., 5,* 294 (1966).
167. Acton, W. I., A criterion for the prediction of auditory and subject effects due to air-borne noise from ultrasonic sources. *Ann. Occup. Hyg. 11,* 227 (1968).
168. Acton, W. I., A criterion for the prediction of auditory and subjective effects due to air-borne noises from ultrasonic sources. *Ann. Occup. Hyg. 11,* 227–234 (1968).
169. Acton, W. I., Private communication (1973).

170. Acton, W. I., "The Effects of Airborne Ultrasound and Near-Ultrasound." Text of a paper presented to international Congress on Noise as a Public Health Problem, Dubrovnik, 1973.

171. Acton, W. I., and Carson, M. B., Auditory and subjective effects of airborne noise from industrial ultrasonic sources. *Brit. J. Ind. Med. 24,* 297–304 (1967).

172. Allen, C. H., Frings, H., and Rudnick, I., Some biological effects of intense high frequency airborne sound. *J. Acoust. Soc. Amer. 20,* No. 1, 62–65 (1948).

173. Begun, S. J., Special aspects of industrial ultrasonics. *J. Acoust. Soc. Amer. 26,* 142–143 (1954).

174. Cohen, A., Noise effects on health, productivity and well-being. *Trans. N.Y. Acad.* [2] *30,* 910 (1968).

175. Corliss, L. M., Doster, M. E., Simonton, J., and Downs, M. P., High frequency and regular audiometry among selected groups of high school students. *J. Sch. Health 40,* 400–404 (1970).

176. Crawford, A. E., What future for ultrasonics? High power ultrasonics. *Ultrasonics 11,* No. 1, 14 (1973).

177. Crawford, A. E., "Ultrasonic Engineering." Butterworth, London, 1955.

178. Cunningham, D. R., and Goetzinger, C. P., "Extra-High Frequency Hearing Loss and Hyperlipidemia." Kansas University Medical Center, Kansas City, Kansas, 1972.

179. Cunningham, D. R., and Goetzinger, C. P., "Extra-High Frequency Hearing Loss and Hyperlipidemia" (original data). Kansas University Medical Center, Kansas City, Kansas, 1972.

180. Dadson, R. S., and King, J. H., A determination of the normal threshold of hearing and its relation to the standardization of audiometers. *J. Laryngol. Otol. 66,* 378–388 (1952).

181. Dallos, P. J., and Linnel, C. O., Subharmonic components in cochlear microphonic potentials. *J. Acoust. Soc. Amer. 40,* 4–11 (1966).

182. Dallos, P. J., and Limmell, C. O., Even-order subharmonics in the peripheral auditory system. *J. Acoust. Soc. Amer. 40,* 561–563 (1966).

183. Davis, H., Biological and psychological effects of ultrasonics. *J. Acoust. Soc. Amer. 20,* No. 5, 605–607 (1948).

184. Davis, H., Parrack, H. O., and Eldredge, D., Hazards of intense sound and ultrasound. *Ann. Otol. 58,* 732–738 (1949).

185. Dickson, E. D. D., and Chadwick, D. L., *J. Laryngol. 65,* 154 (1951).

186. Dickson, E. D. D., and Watson, N. P., *J. Laryngol. 63,* 276 (1949).

187. Dobroserdov, V. K., Effects of low frequency ultrasonic and high frequency sound waves on workers. *Gig. Sanit. 32,* No. 2, 17–21 (1967).

188. Fletcher, J. L., Cairns, A. B., Collins, F. G., and Endicott, J., High frequency hearing following meningitis. *J. Audit. Res. 7,* 223–227 (1967).

189. Goldstein, N., and Sineskey, A., "health Hazards from Ultrasonic Energy." Massachusetts Institute of Technology, Cambridge, Massachusetts, 1969.

190. Grigor'eva, V. M., Effect of ultrasonic vibrations on personnel working with ultrasonic equipment. *Sov. Phys.–Acoust. 11,* No. 4, 426–427 (1966).

191. Grigor'eva, V. M., Ultrasound and the question of occupational hazards. *Ultrasonics 4,* 214 (1966).

192. Haeff, A. V., and Knox, C., Perception of ultrasound. *Science 139,* 590–592 (1963).

193. Harris, J. D., and Ward, M. D., High frequency audiometry to 20 kc/s in children of age 10–12 years. *J. Audit. Res. 7,* 241–252 (1967).

194. Jacobsen, E. J., Downs, M. P., and Fletcher, J. L., Clinical findings in high-frequency thresholds during known ototoxic drug usage. *J. Audit. Res. 9,* 379–385 (1969).

195. Knight, J. J., Effects of air-borne ultrasound on man. *Ultrasonics 6,* 39–41 (1968).

196. Mason, R. K., Asthma and high frequency sound perception. *Nature (London) 214,* 99–100 (1967).

197. Miasnikov, L. L., and Miasnikova, E. N., Ultrasonic speech components. *Acustica 21,* 118–120 (1969).

198. Michael, P. L., Noise. *In* "Industrial Environmental Health" (L. V. Cralley, ed.), Vol. 1, p. 146. Academic Press, New York, 1972.

199. Myers, C. K., and Harris, J. D., Comparison of Seven Systems for Air Conduction Audiometry from 8–20 kHz," Rep. No. 567. U.S. Navy Submarine Medical Center, Groton, Conn., 1969.

200. Northern, J. L., and Downs, M. P., Recommended high frequency audiometric threshold levels (8000–18,000 Hz). *J. Acoust. Soc. Amer. 52,* No. 2, Part 2, 585–595 (1972).

201. Northern, J. L., Downs, M. P., Rudmose, W., Glorig, A., and Fletcher, J. L., Recommended high frequency audiometric threshold levels (8000–18,000 Hz): 1968 Colorado high frequency hearing survey. *J. Acoust. Soc. Amer.* A prepublication copy (1971).

202. Parrack, H. O., Effect of air-borne ultrasound on humans. *Int. Audiol. J. 5,* 294–308 (1966).

203. Parrack, H. O., *Ind. Med. Surg. 21,* 156 (1952).

204. Parrack, H. O., "Proposed Standard Acceptable Levels of High Frequency (High Audio and Ultrasonic Frequencies) Airborne Sound Field Around Ultrasonic Equipment (Ultrasonic Cleaners, Shaper, Drills, and other Industrial or Laboratory Equipment)." Memo., MRBM, Air Material Command, Wright–Patterson Air Force Base, Ohio, 1–3 (1968).

205. Parrack, H. O., "The Effects of Airborne Ultrasound on Humans." Tech. Memo., MRBAM, Air Material Command, Wright–Patterson Air Force Base, Ohio, 1–5 1968.

206. Institute of Electrical and Electronics Engineers, "Proceedings of 1970 Ultrasonics Symposium," pp. 65–72. IEEE, New York, 1971.

207. Rudmose, W., "Data Collected on the Standardization of the Tracor, Incorporated ARJ–4HF and RA–114HF Extra-High Frequency Audiometers." Tracor, Incorporated, Austin, Texas, 1961.

208. Sataloff, J., and Michael, P. L., "Hearing Conservation." Thomas, Springfield, Illinois, 1973.

209. Sataloff, J., Vassallo, L., and Menduke, H., Occupational hearing loss and high frequency thresholds. *Arch. Environ. Health 14,* 832–836 (1967).

210. Sivian, L. J., and White, S. D., On minimum audible sound fields. *J. Acoust. Soc. Amer. 4,* 288–300 (1933).

211. Skillern, C. P., Human response to measured sound pressure levels from ultrasonic devices. *Amer. Ind. Hyg. Ass., J. 26,* 132, 136 (1965).

212. Summer, W., and Patrick, M. K., "Ultrasonic Therapy," p. 47. Elsevier, Amsterdam, 1964.

213. von Gierke, H. E., Subharmonics generated in human and animal ears by intense sound. *J. Acoust. Soc. Amer. 22,* 675 (a) (1950). [This is a summary of *Fed. Proc., Fed. Amer. Soc. Exp. Biol. 9,* 130 (A) (1950), and a proposal for further work.]

214. Wells, P. N. T., What future for ultrasonics? Biomedical ultrasonics. *Ultrasonics 11,* No. 1, 16 (1973).

215. Zislis, T., and Fletcher, J. L., Relation of high frequency thresholds to age and sex. *J. Audit. Res. 6,* 189–198 (1966).

216. Penn State University, "An Evaluation of Acoustic Radiation Above 10 kHz, Environmental Acoustics Laboratory," under Contract No. HSM 99–72–125. National

Institute for Occupational Safety and Health, Public Health Service, U.S. Department of Health, Education and Welfare, Washington, D.C., 1974.

217. Loeb, M., Fletcher, J. L., and Benson, R. W., Some preliminary studies of temporary threshold shift with an arc-discharge impulse-noise generator. *J. Acoust. Soc. Amer. 37,* 313 (1965).

218. Ward, W. D., "Proposed Damage Risk Criterion for Impulse Noise," Report of Working Group 57. NRC Committee on Hearing, Bioacoustics and Biomechanics. Washington, D.C., 1968.

219. Ward, W. D., and Glorig, A., A case of firecracker-induced hearing loss. *Laryngoscope 71,* 1590 (1961).

220. Christiansen, A., and Rojskaer, C., Audio in uries from New Yoear's eve fireworks. *Nord. Audio 13,* 33–40 (1964).

221. Taylor, G. D., and Williams, E., Acoustic trauma in the sports hunter. *Laryngoscope 76,* 863 (1966).

222. Acton, W. I., and Forrest, M. R., Hearing hazard from small-bore weapons. *J. Acoust. Soc. Amer. 44,* 817 (1968).

223. Hodge, D. C., and McCommons, R. B., Acoustical hazard of children's "toys." *J. Acoust. Soc. Amer. 40,* 911 (1968).

224. Gjaevenes, K., Measurements on the impulsive noise from crackers and firearms. *J. Acoust. Soc. Amer. 39,* 403 (1966).

225. Coles, R. R. A., and Rice, C. G., Auditory hazards of sports guns. *Laryngoscope 76,* 1728 (1966).

226. Cohen, A., Kylin, B., LaBenz, P., Temporary threshold shifts in hearing from exposure to combined impact/steady-state noise conditions. *J. Acoust. Soc. Amer. 40,* 1371 (1966).

227. Rice, C. G., and Coles, R. R. A., Impulsive noise studies and temporary threshold shift. *In* "Proceedings of the Fifth International Congress on Acoustics" (D. C. Commins, ed.), Vol. 1a, Paper B67. Georges Thoni, Liège, 1965.

228. Hodge, D. C., and McCommons, R. B., Reliability of TTS from impulse noise exposure. *J. Acoust. Soc. Amer. 40,* 839 (1966).

229. Coles, R. R. A., and Rice, G. C., Towards a criterion for impulse noise in industry. *Ann. Occup. Hyg. 13,* 43 (1970).

230. Coles, R. R. A., Assessment of risk of hearing loss due to impulse noise. *Brit. Acoust. Soc. Meet., 1970* pp. 24–25 (1970).

231. Rice, C. G., Deafness due to impulse noise. *Phil Trans. Roy. Soc. London, Ser. X 263,* 279 (1968).

232. Forest, M. R., Ear protection and hearing in high-intensity impulsive noise. *Brit. Acoust. Soc. Meet., 1970* pp. 23–24 (1970).

233. Ross, E. M., State regulation of community noise. *J. Acoust. Soc. Amer. 47,* 54 (1970) (abstr.).

234. Little, R., State regulation of motor vehicle noise. *J. Acoust. Soc. Amer. 47,* 54 (1970) (abstr.).

235. VanAtta, F. A., Federal regulation of occupational noise. *J. Acoust. Soc. Amer. 47,* 54 (1970) (abstr.).

236. Foster, C. R., Federal regulation of transportation noise. *J. Acoust. Soc. Amer. 47,* 54 (1970) (abstr.).

237. Jones, H. H., State regulation of occupational noise. *J. Acoust. Soc. Amer. 47,* 54 (1970) (abstr.).

238. Schultz, T. J., Impact-noise recommendations for the FHA. *J. Acoust. Soc. Amer. 36,* 729 (1964).

239. "Regulations Respecting Protection of Workers from Effects of Noise," *Alberta Reg.* 185/66. Provincial Board of Health, Edmonton, Alberta, Canada 1966. [Entry into force: 15 June 1966. *Alberta Gaz., Alberta, Canada, 62,* 403 (1966).]

240. "Annotated Code of Maryland" (1964 Replacement Volume), Sect. 25A, Art. 101. Workmen's Compensation, Approved April 14, 1967, Effective June 1, 1967.

241. "California Motor Vehicle Code," Divisions 11 and 12, Paragraphs 23130 and 27160 (1968). (Chapter 2, Title 13, California Administrative Code.) California Department of Motor Vehicles, Sacramento, California.

242. "Toward a Quieter City." Report of Mayor's Task Force on Noise Control, New York City, 1970.

243. Apps, D., Automobile noise. *In* "Handbook of Noise Control" (C. M. Harris, ed.), Chapter 31, p31. McGraw-Hill, New York, 1957.

244. "Objective Limits for Motor Vehicle Noise," Rep. No. 824. Bolt, Beranek, & Newman, Inc., Van Nuys, California, 1962.

245. Campbell, R. S., A survey of passby noise from boats. *Sound and Vibration 3*(9), 24 (1969).

246. Bender, E. K., and Heckl, M., "Noise Generated by Subways Aboveground and in Stations," Rep. No. OST–DNA–70–1. Bolt, Beranek & Newman, Inc., Cambridge, Massachusetts, 1970.

247. Kryter, K. D., Psychological reactions to aircraft noise. *Science 151,* 1346 (1966).

248. Nixon, C. W., and Hubbard, H. H., Results of USAF NASA–FAA flight program to study community responses to sonic booms in the greater St. Louis Area. *NASA Tech. Note, NASA TN D–2705* (1965).

249. "Airports and the Community." National Industrial Pollution Control Council for the U.S. Department of Commerce, Washington, D.C., 1972.

250. Proceedings of the sonic boom symposium. *J. Acoust. Soc. Amer. 39,* S1 (1966).

251. Kupferman, R., Noise Regulations. H. R. Bill 14608, Congressional Record, No. 8339 (1966).

252. Rosinger, G., Nixon, C. W., and von Gierke, H. E., Quantification of the noisiness of "approaching" and "receding" sounds. *J. Acoust. Soc. Amer. 48,* 843 (1970).

253. Goodfriend, L. S., The wrong road to community noise regulation. *Sound Vibration 1*(2), 7 (1967).

254. Mehling, E. A., Community noise ordinances. *ASHRAE (Amer. Soc. Heat., Refrig. Air-Cond. Eng.) J. 9,* 40 (1967).

255. Morse, K. M., Community noise—the industrial aspect. *Amer. Ind. Hyg. Ass., J. 29,* 368 (1968).

256. Donley, R., Community noise regulation. *Sound and Vibration 3*(2), 12 (1969).

257. Bragdon, C. R., Community noise and the public interest. *Sound and Vibration 3*(12), 16 (1969).

258. American National Standards Institute, "American National Standard Methods for the Calculation of the Articulation Index," ANSI, S3.5–1969. ANSI, New York, 1969.

259. Webster, J. C., SIL—past, present, and future. *Sound and Vibration 3*(8), 22 (1969).

260. Cohen, A., Noise effects on health, productivity and well-being. *Trans. N.Y. Acad. Sci.* [2] *30,* 910 (1968).

261. Anticaglia, J. R., and Cohen, A., Extra auditory effects of noise as a health hazard. *Amer. Ind. Hyg. Ass., J. 31,* 277 (1970).

262. Cohen, A., Anticaglia, J., and Jones, H., "Sociocusis"—hearing loss from non-occupational noise exposures. *Sound and Vibration 4*(11), 12 (1970).

263. "The Effects of Sonic Boom on Structural Behavior," SST Rep. No. 65–18. Prepared for Federal Aviation Agency by J. Blume & Ass., Washington, D.C., 1965.

264. "Sonic Boom Experiments at Edwards Air Force Base," Contract AF49(638)–1758. Stanford, California, 1967.

265. Hubbard, H. H., Sonic booms. *Phys. Today 21,* 31 (1968).

266. Amendment of P.L. 58 ("The Vehicle Code") House Bill No. 1660, The General Assembly of Pennsylvania, Harrisburg, Pennsylvania, 1969.

267. International Organization for Standardization, "Noise Assessment with Respect to Community Response," Draft Recommendation No. 1996. ISO, 12 pp.

268. Goodfriend, L. S., Community noise problems–origin and control. *Amer. Ind. Hyg. Ass., J. 30,* 607 (1969).

269. Kryter, K. D., Concepts of perceived noisiness, their implementation and application. *J. Acoust. Soc. Amer. 43,* 344 (1968).

270. Ostergaard, P. B., and Donley, R., Background noise levels in suburban communities. *J. Acoust. Soc. Amer. 36,* 409 (1964).

271. Buchta, E., Distribution of transportation and community noise. *J. Acoust. Soc. Amer. 47,* 60 (1970).

272. Donley, R., Measurement of community noise. *J. Acoust. Soc. Amer. 47,* 61 (1970).

273. Nelson, D. L., Gordon, C., and Galloway, W., Methodology for highway noise prediction. *J. Acoust. Soc. Amer. 47,* 111 (1970).

274. Berendt, R. D., "Airborne, Impact, and Structure-Borne Noise Control in Multifamily Dwellings." U.S. Department of Housing and Urban Development, Washington, D. C., 1967.

275. Young, R. W., Single-number criteria for room noise. *J. Acoust. Soc. Amer. 36,* 289 (1964).

276. Webster, J. C., Speech communications as limited by ambient noise. *J. Acoust. Soc. Amer. 37,* 692 (1965).

277. Botsford, J. H., Predicting speech interference and annoyance from a-weighted sound levels. *J. Acoust. Soc. Amer. 42,* 1151 (1967) (abstr.).

278. International Organization for Standardization, "General Requirements for the Preparation of Test Codes for Measuring the Noise Emitted by Machines," ISO Recommendation R495–1966(E). ISO, Geneva, Switzerland, 1966.

279. "Sound Rating of Outdoor Unitary Equipment," Standard 270. Air Conditioniong and Refrigeration Institute, Park Ridge, Illinois, 1967.

280. Groff, G. C., Schreiner, J., and Bullock, C. Centrifugal fan sound power level prediction. [A condensed version is published in *ASHRAE (Amer. Soc. Heat., Refrig. Air-Cond. Eng.) J. 9,* 71 (1967); *ASHRAE Trans. 73,* Part. II (1967).]

281. Goss, B. L., Electric motor noise: Control of noise at the source. *Amer. Ind. Hyg. Ass., J. 31,* 16 (1970).

282. Mills, R. O., Noise reduction in a textile weaving mill. *Amer. Ind. Hyg. Ass., J. 30,* 71 (1969).

283. Judd, S. H., and Soence, J. A., Noise control for electric motors. *Amer. Ind. Hyg. Ass., J. 30,* 588 (1969).

284. Torpey, P. J., Noise control of emergency power generating equipment. *Amer. Ind. Hyg. Ass., J. 30,* 596 (1969).

285. Lowson, M. V., Theoretical analysis of compressor noise. *J. Acoust. Soc. Amer. 47,* 371 (1970).

286. Prillwitz, H., Mechalkg, K., Karl-Heinz, and Seyfarth, B., Soundproof compressed air machine. Patent reviewed in *J. Acoust. Soc. Amer. 47,* 990 (1970).

287. Carlson, R. O., Ventilated and sound-reducing enclosure for teleprinter. Patent reviewed in *J. Acoust. Soc. Amer. 47,* 991 (1970).

288. Cunningham, J. M., Ventilated and soundproofed enclosure for printer. Patent reviewed in *J. Acoust. Soc. Amer. 47,* 989 (1970).

289. Jacobson, G. R., Air turning vane with removable enclosure for insertion of acoustical material. Patent reviewed in *J. Acoust. Soc. Amer. 47,* 990 (1970).

290. Amlott, N. J., and Karn, J. D., Air cleaner and silencer assembly. Patent reviewed in *J. Acoust. Soc. Amer. 46,* 72 (1969).

291. Thomas, D., Exhaust muffler. Patent reviewed in *J. Acoust. Soc. Amer. 46,* 1114 (1969).

292. "Material Design Standard for Noise Levels." Human Engineering Laboratories, Aberdeen Proving Grounds, Maryland, Nat. Tech. Inform. Serv., Springfield, Virginia, 1972.

293. Cerami, V. V., and Bishop, E. S., Control of duct generated noise. *Air Cond.. Heat., Vent. 63,* 55 (1966).

294. Fenton, R. G., Reducing noise in cams. *Mach. Des. 38,* 187 (1966).

295. Quiet transit wheel. *J. Acoust. Soc. Amer. 41,* 537 (1967).

296. Fader, B., Practical designs for noise barriers based on lead. *Amer. Ind. Hyg. Ass., J. 27,* 520 (1966).

297. Hines, W. A., "Noise Control in Industry," p. 197. Business Applications Ltd., London, 1966.

298. Bishop, D. E., Reduction of aircraft noise measured in several schools, motel and residential rooms. *J. Acoust. Soc. Amer. 39,* 907 (1966).

299. Lynch, C. J., Noise control. *Int. Sci. Technol. 32,* 32 (1966).

300. Rosenblith, W. A., Stevens, K. N., and Staff of Bolt, Beranek & Newman, Ind., "Handbook of Acoustic Noise Control," Vol. II, WADC Tech. Rep. 52–204. Department of the Air Force, Washington, D.C., 1953.

301. G. Bradfield (reviewed by W. P. Mason), Use in industry of elasticity measurements in metals with the help of mechanical vibrations. Notes on applied science No. 30. National Physical Laboratory. *J. Acoust. Soc. Amer. 36,* 1752 (1964).

302. Jorgensen, R., "Fan Engineering." Buffalo Forge Company, Buffalo, New York, 1961.

303. Geiger, P. H., "Noise Reduction Manual." Engineering Research Institute, University of Michigan, Ann Arbor, 1953. [Prepared under the direction of the Office of Naval Research, Undersea Warfare Branch.]

304. Bolt, R. H., Beranek, L., and Newman, R., "Handbook of Noise Control," Vol. 1, WADC Tech. Rep. 52–204. Wright Air Development Center, 1952.

305. Lord, P., coordinating ed. "Applied Acoustics." Elsevier, Amsterdam. [Reviewed in *Amer. Occup. Hyg. 2,* 269 (1968).]

306. Lowson, M. V., Reduction of compressor noise radiation. *J. Acoust. Soc. Amer. 43,* 37 (1968).

307. Lucht, R. F., and Scanlan, R. H., Method of axial testing for roller bearing noise qualities. *J. Acoust. Soc. Amer. 44,* 5 (1968).

308. Plummer, W. A., Pneumatic tool muffle. Patent reviewed in *J. Acoust. Soc. Amer. 37,* 774 (1965).

309. Reed, G. A., and Rosen, D., Acoustical cabinet for office business machines. Patent reviewed in *J. Acoust. Soc. Amer. 37,* 774 (1965).

310. Dahl, C. B., Suppression of objectionable noise in rotating machinery. Patent reviewed in *J. Acoust. Soc. Amer. 36,* 1242 (1964).

311. "Industrial Noise Control and Hearing Conservation Program." International Brotherhood of Boilermakers, Iron Ship Builders, Blacksmiths, Forgers and Helpers, Brotherhood Building, Kansas City, Kansas, 1966.

312. National Center for Health Statistics. Hearing levels of adults by age and sex, United States, 1960–1962. *U.S. Pub. Health Serv., Publ. 1000,* Ser. 11, No. 11 (1965). [Available from Superintendent of Documents, U.S. Govt. Printing Office, Washington, D.C.]

313. "Industrial Noise, A Guide to its Evaluation and Control," (Hosey, A. D., and Powell, E. H., eds.), FS2.6/2:n69. DHEW, PHS (1967). [Available from Supt. of Documents, U.S. Govt. Printing Office, Washington, D.C.]

314. Bell, A., Noise, an occupational hazard and public nuisance. *World Health Organ., Publ. Health Pap. 30* (1966). [Obtainable through Columbia Univ. Press, International Documents Service, New York.]

315. Stevens, S. S., Warshofsky, F., and the Editors of Life, "Sound and Hearing." Time, New York, 1965.

316. "Industrial Noise and Hearing Protection." Employers Insurance of Wausau, Wausau, Wisconsin, 1970.

317. "Noise Information Service (NOISE)." IIT Research Institute, Chicago, Illinois, 0000.

318. "Noise as a Public Health Hazard," (Ward, W. D., and Fricke, J. E., eds.), Proc. Conf. American Speech and Hearing Association, Rep. No. 4 (1969). [Available from Director, Public Information, ASHA, Washington, D.C.]

319. Rettinger, M., "Acoustics—Room Design and Noise Control." Chemical Publ. Co., London, 1968.

320. "Industrial Noise Manual." Amer. Ind. Hyg. Ass., Southfield, Michigan, 1966.

321. "Noise Pollution." Technology Application Center, University of New Mexico, Alberquerque, 1972.

Nonionizing Radiation

DAVID H. SLINEY AND DAVID L. CONOVER

In "Industrial Hygiene Highlights" and in Edition I of "Industrial Environmental Health" the significant physiologic effects of nonionizing radiation were reviewed and commonly accepted exposure criteria presented.[1,2] The present review is intended to bring the previous physiologic reviews up to date and to emphasize new exposure criteria. Recently national consensus standards and federal rules have been published or are near publication for several types of nonionizing radiation.

STANDARDS

Exposure criteria may be reflected in two general categories of standards: occupational health and safety standards and equipment performance standards. Within the federal government, occupational exposure standards are enforced by the Occupational Safety and Health Administration (OSHA) of the U.S. Department of Labor, which derives its authority largely from the Construction Safety Amendment (83 Stat 96) to Section 107 of the Contracts, Work Hours and Safety Standards Act as Amended and Public Law 91–596, the Occupational Safety and Health Act of 1970. Federal performance standards are enforced by the Bureau of Radiological Health (BRH) of the U.S. Department of Health, Education, and Welfare under the authority of PL 90–602, the Radiation Control for Health and Safety Act of 1968. Federal standards for occupational exposure to nonionizing radiation have existed for microwave radiation and visible cw laser radiation since 1971 (29CFR 1518.54).[3] By early 1974 proposals for an ultraviolet radiation standard[4] and a laser radiation standard were under consideration within the Department of Labor. A proposed performance standard for laser products has been published in the Federal Register and could take effect as early as 1975.[5]

OPTICAL RADIATION

Ultraviolet Radiation

The proposed standard for personnel exposure to ultraviolet radiation[6] discussed in the previous volume has been placed upon the permanent list of the American Conference of Governmental Industrial Hygienists' threshold limit values (TLV's). Action has not yet been completed to adopt it as a federal standard. An ultraviolet hazard monitor has been developed to permit direct reading of hazardous irradiances of actinic ultraviolet radiation.[7] More studies are yet required to understand ultraviolet cataractogenesis and the effects of near-ultraviolet radiation upon the skin and eyes. Some progress is being made in these areas of research.[8-10]

Laser Radiation

LASER PROTECTION STANDARDS

The most familiar early laser radiation protection standards and guidelines[11] in this country were prepared by ACGIH (1968),[12] the U.S. Departments of the Army and Navy (1969),[13] and the U.S. Department of the Air Force (1969)[14] and reflected the biologic research performed through the mid 1960's. These standards were normally based upon studies of a few lasers—principally the ruby, helium–neon, argon, neodymium, and CO_2–N_2 lasers. The protection standards (TLV's) of ACGIH were most often applied in the first state codes.[15]

1. The ANSI–Z136 Standard Development. In 1969 an effort was initiated by the American National Standards Institute (ANSI) at the request of the U.S. Department of Labor to develop a consensus standard for the "Safe Use of Lasers and Masers," later redefined as "Safe Use of Lasers—Standard Z136." The Telephone Group became the sponsoring activity, and Mr. George M. Wilkening of Bell Laboratories was designated chairman. When work got underway and with subcommittees formed in 1969, the hope was expressed that a final standard could be completed in 1 year if all subcommittees worked diligently. The experienced staff at the headquarters of ANSI in New York doubted that the standard could be prepared in less than 3 years. A general consensus was not achieved, however, until a committee vote on the last official draft, dated February 29, 1972. In May 1972 the ACGIH proposed a revision of their TLV's for laser radiation, which incorporated essentially all of the ANSI–Z136 Maximum Permissible Exposures (MPE's). The ANSI standard was quite complex and because most of the ballots on the February 29th draft indicated a desire for editorial changes for clarity, the final draft was considerably revised and was issued on November 23rd as a final draft for submission to the ANSI Board of Standards Review. The document was approved on April 26, 1973 and was issued in October 1973.[16] The military services, and other federal and state agencies that make use of laser protection standards, adopted most of the new protection standards promulgated by ANSI and ACGIH.

2. Formulation of Laser Protection Standard Exposure Levels. The greatest departure in format made by the ANSI standard from previous standards is the lack of "step functions" to express the MPE levels. Previous protection standards all had values expressed as radiant exposure $(J \cdot cm^{-2})$ or irradiance $(W \cdot cm^{-2})$ for a specific range of pulse durations. Steps—typically a factor of ten—would exist between Q-switched and non-Q-switched pulse durations. With the advent of lasers having any pulse duration, it was necessary to provide a sliding scale without sudden "steps" at specific pulse durations. Indeed, such an approach permitted a closer approximation of actual biologic injury thresholds with safety factor added.

To establish a rationale for developing permissible exposure levels from biologic data required a careful analysis of the physical and biologic variables influencing the spread of the laboratory biologic data, the variables influencing the potential for injury in individuals exposed to laser radiation, the increase in severity of injury for supra-threshold exposure doses, and the reversibility of injury. Additionally, the accuracy of instruments available for radiometric measurements and the desire for simplicity in expressing the levels have influenced the protection standard levels.

It was difficult to properly weight these many factors. Interestingly enough, the authors took a poll of several specialists who have been involved in the development of the protection standard levels showing that although almost all of the specialists agreed to a certain set of MPE's or TLV's, they had a wide range of different rationales.

3. Laser Hazard Classification and Control Measures. The ANSI–Z136 standard contains a well-developed and formalized scheme of classifying lasers based upon the laser's degree of hazard. This scheme evolved from previous standards and guidelines[11] and permits rapid hazard evaluation. Specific control measures and medical surveillance requirements vary depending upon classification.

In the final analysis, the specifications that define the hazard classes will be used more often than the protection standards (MPE's) themselves. Five are defined: Class I Exempt Lasers are those lasers incapable of producing a hazardous exposure condition; such lasers are unusual and generally limited to laser diodes. Class II Low Power Lasers are visible lasers (usually He–Ne) with an output power below 1 mW which are not hazardous unless an individual looks directly into the beam against his natural aversion responses (i.e., longer than about 0.25 sec). Class III Medium Power Lasers require precautions to limit intrabeam viewing of the direct beam or a specularly reflected beam; the laser does not present a fire hazard, a skin hazard, or diffuse reflection hazard. In contrast, a Class IV High Power Laser does present a fire and skin hazard and/or a diffuse-reflection hazard, and very stringent control measures are required. Class V Enclosed Lasers, as the name implies, are those within an interlocked enclosure such that emitted laser radiation from the enclosure is not hazardous.

A SUMMARY OF THE ANSI AND ACGIH PROTECTION STANDARDS

These protection standards are for exposure to laser radiation under conditions to which nearly all personnel may be exposed without adverse effects. The values should be used as guides in the control of exposures and should not be regarded as fine lines between safe and dangerous levels. They are based on the best available information from experimental studies. Table I provides a summary of the most often used laser protection standards. Tables II-IV provide the complete list of laser protection standards. Figures 1–6 provide graphs of protection standards which may be difficult to calculate.

1. Limiting Apertures. The protection standards are expressed as radiant exposure or irradiance and are to be averaged over an aperture of 1 mm except for ocular protection standards in the retinal-hazard spectral range of 400–1400 nm, which should be averaged over a 7 mm limiting aperture (pupil). No modification of the protection standards is permitted for pupil sizes less than 7 mm.

2. Extended Sources. These protection standards for "extended sources" apply to sources that subtend an angle greater than α (Fig. 3), which varies with exposure time. This angle is not the beam divergence of the source.

3. Correction Factor A (C$_A$). All retinal-hazard protection standards in Tables II and III are intended to be used as listed for wavelengths 400–700 nm. Protection standards at wavelengths between 700 nm and 1.06 μm are increased by a uniformly extrapolated factor C_A as shown in Fig. 4.

4. Repetitively Pulsed Lasers. Since there are few experimental data for multiple pulses, caution must be used in the evaluation of such exposures. The protection standards for irradiance or radiant exposure in multiple pulse trains have the following limitations:

(i) The exposure from any single pulse in the train is limited to the protection standard for a single comparable pulse.

(ii) The average irradiance for a group of pulses is limited to the protection standard as given in Tables II, III, or IV of a single pulse of the same duration as the entire pulse group.

TABLE I

Protection Standards for Typical Lasers

Type of laser	PRF	Wavelength	Exposure duration	Protection standard for intrabeam viewing by the eye
Single-pulse ruby laser	Single pulse	694.3 nm	1 nsec–18 μsec	5×10^{-7} J cm^{-2}/pulse
Single-pulse neodymium	Single pulse	1060 nm	1 nsec–100 μsec	5×10^{-6} J cm^{-2}/pulse
CW argon lasers	CW	488 and 514.5 nm	0.25 sec	2.5 mW cm^{-2}
CW argon lasers	CW	488 and 514.5 nm	4–8 hr	1 μW cm^{-2}
CW helium-neon lasers (for alignment, etc.)	CW	632.8 nm	0.25 sec 4–8 hr	2.5 mW cm^{-2} 1 μW cm^{-2}
Erbium laser	Single pulse	1540 nm	1 nsec–1 μsec	1 J cm^{-2}/pulse
CW neodymium YAG laser	CW	1064 nm	100 sec–8 hr	0.5 mW cm^{-2}
CW carbon-dioxide laser	CW	10.6 μm	10 sec–8 hr	0.1 W cm^{-2}

TABLE II

Protection Standards for Ocular Exposure Intrabeam Viewing of a Laser Beam Single Exposure

Spectral region	Wavelength (nm)	Exposure time (t)	Protection standard	Defining aperture (mm)
UV-C	200–280	1 msec–3 × 10⁴ sec	3 mJ cm⁻²	1
UV-B	280–302	1 msec–3 × 10⁴ sec	3 mJ cm⁻²	1
	303	1 msec–3 × 10⁴ sec	4 mJ cm⁻²	1
	304	1 msec–3 × 10⁴ sec	6 mJ cm⁻²	1
	305	1 msec–3 × 10⁴ sec	10 mJ cm⁻²	1
	306	1 msec–3 × 10⁴ sec	16 mJ cm⁻²	1
	307	1 msec–3 × 10⁴ sec	25 mJ cm⁻²	1
	308	1 msec–3 × 10⁴ sec	40 mJ cm⁻²	1
	309	1 msec–3 × 10⁴ sec	63 mJ cm⁻²	1
	310	1 msec–3 × 10⁴ sec	100 mJ cm⁻²	1
	311	1 msec–3 × 10⁴ sec	160 mJ cm⁻²	1
	312	1 msec–3 × 10⁴ sec	250 mJ cm⁻²	1
	313	1 msec–3 × 10⁴ sec	400 mJ cm⁻²	1
	314	1 msec–3 × 10⁴ sec	630 mJ cm⁻²	1
	315	1 msec–3 × 10⁴ sec	1.0 J cm⁻²	1
UV-A	315–400	1 nsec–10 sec	$0.56 \sqrt[4]{t}$ J cm⁻² [a]	1
	315–400	10–10³ sec	1.0 J cm⁻²	1
	315–400	10³–3 × 10⁴ sec	1.0 mW cm⁻²	1
Light	400–700	1 nsec–18 μsec	0.5 μJ cm⁻²	7
	400–700	18 μsec–10 sec	$[1.8 \, t/\sqrt[4]{t}]$ mJ cm⁻²	7
	400–700	10–10⁴ sec	10 mJ cm⁻²	7
	400–700	10⁴–3 × 10⁴ sec	1 μW cm⁻²	7
IR-A	700–1060	1 nsec–18 μsec	$0.5 C_A$ μJ cm⁻² [b]	7
	700–1060	18 μsec–10 sec	$[1.8 \, t/\sqrt[4]{t}] \, C_A$ mJ cm⁻² [a]	7
	700–1060	10–100 sec	$10 \cdot C_A$ mJ cm⁻² [b]	7
	1060–1400	1 nsec–100 μsec	5 μJ cm⁻²	7
	1060–1400	100 μsec–10 sec	$[9 \cdot t/\sqrt[4]{t}]$ mJ cm⁻²	7
	1060–1400	10 sec–100 sec	50 mJ cm⁻²	7
	700–800	100–[10⁴/C_B] sec	$10 \cdot C_A$ mJ cm⁻² [b]	7
	700–800	[10⁴/C_B]–3 × 10⁴ sec	$C_A \cdot C_B$ μW cm⁻² [c]	7
	800–1060	100–3 × 10⁴ sec	$0.1 \cdot C_A$ mW cm⁻² [b]	7
	1060–1400	100–3 × 10⁴ sec	0.5 mW cm⁻²	7
IR-B and C	1400–10⁶	1–100 nsec	10 mJ cm⁻²	1,10 [d]
	1400–10⁶	100 nsec–10 sec	$0.56 \sqrt[4]{t}$ J cm⁻² [a]	1,10
	1400–10⁶	10–3 × 10⁴ sec	0.1 W cm⁻²	1,10

[a] These values are graphed in Figs. 1–6.

[b] $C_A = e^{(\lambda-700/224)}$.

[c] $C_B = (\lambda - 699)$.

[d] 1 mm for 1400–10⁵ nm; 10 mm for 10⁵–10⁵ nm.

TABLE III

Protection Standards for Skin Exposure to a Laser Beam

Spectral region	Wavelength	Exposure time, (t) sec	Protection standard
UV	200–400 nm	10^{-3}–3×10^{4}	Same as Table II
Light and IR-A	400–1400 nm	10^{-9}–10^{-7}	2×10^{-2} j cm^{-2}
Light and IR-A	400–1400 nm	10^{-7}–10	$1.1 \sqrt[4]{t}$ J cm^{-2} [a]
Light and IR-A	400–1400 nm	10–3×10^{4}	0.2 W cm^{-2}
IR-B and C	1.4 μm–1 mm	10^{-9}–3×10^{4}	Same as Table II

[a] These values are graphed in Fig. 6.

TABLE IV

Protection Standards for Laser Radiation Exposure of the Eye
Viewing Extended Sources and Diffuse Reflections
(400–1400 nm)

Wavelength (nm)	Exposure duration	Irradiance or radiant exposure on diffuse perfect surface	Radiance or integrated radiance from extended source
200–400	1 nsec–3×10^{4} sec	(Use values in Table II)	
400–700	1 nsec–10 sec	$10\,\pi \sqrt[3]{t}$ J cm^{-2} [a]	$10\,\sqrt[3]{t}$ J cm^{-2} sr^{-1}
	10–10^{4} sec	$20\,\pi$ J cm^{-2}	20 J cm^{-2} sr^{-1}
	10^{4}–3×10^{4} sec	$2\pi \times 10^{-3}$ W cm^{-2}	2×10^{-3} W cm^{-2} sr^{-1}
700–1060	1 nsec–10 sec	$10\,\pi C_A \sqrt[3]{t}$ J cm^{-2} [a]	$10\,C_A \sqrt[3]{t}$ J cm^{-2} sr^{-1}
700–1060	10–100 sec	$20\,\pi C_A$ J cm^{-2}	$20\,C_A$ J cm^{-2} sr^{-1}
700–800	100–$(10^{4}/C_B)$ sec	$20\,\pi C_A$ J cm^{-2}	$20\,C_A$ J cm^{-2} sr^{-1}
700–800	$(10^{4}/C_B)$ sec	$0.2\,\pi C_A C_B$ W cm^{-2}	$0.2\,C_A C_B$ W cm^{-2} sr^{-1}
800–1060	100–3×10^{4} sec	$0.2 C_A \pi$ W cm^{-2}	$0.2\,C_A$ W cm^{-2} sr^{-1}
1060–1400	1 nsec–10 sec	$50\pi \sqrt[3]{t}$ j cm^{-2} [a]	$50\,\sqrt[3]{t}$ J cm^{-2} sr^{-1}
1060–1400	10–100 sec	100π J cm^{-2}	100 J cm^{-2} sr^{-1}
1060–1400	100 sec–3×10^{4} sec	π W cm^{-2}	1.0 W cm^{-2} sr^{-1}
1400–10^{6}	10 nsec–3×10^{4} sec	(Use values in Table II)	

[a] These values are graphed in Figs. 1–6.

t is the exposure duration in seconds, λ is wavelength in nanometers, and
$C_A = e\,[(\lambda–700\ \text{nm})/22]$; $C_B = (\lambda–699\ \text{nm})$ and is unitless.

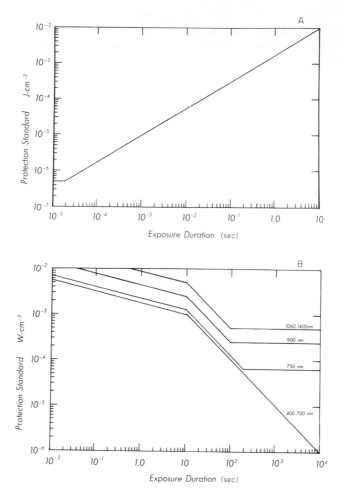

Fig. 1. (A) Protection standard for intrabeam viewing of pulses of visible (400–700 nm) laser radiation. Protection standards for intrabeam viewing of pulsed IR–A (700–1400 nm) laser radiation are obtained by multiplying values in the graph by C_A. (B) Protection standard for intrabeam viewing of CW visible (400–700 nm) and IR–A (750, 900, and 1060–1400 nm) laser radiation.

(iii) When the Instantaneous Pulse Repetition Frequency (PRF) of any pulses within a train exceeds one, the protection standard applicable to each pulse is reduced as shown in Fig. 5 for pulse durations less than 10^{-5} sec. For pulses of greater duration, the following formula should be followed:

$$\text{Protection}\atop\text{standard} \left[\begin{matrix} \text{single pulse} \\ \text{in train} \end{matrix} \right] = \frac{\text{standard (pulse } nt)}{n}$$

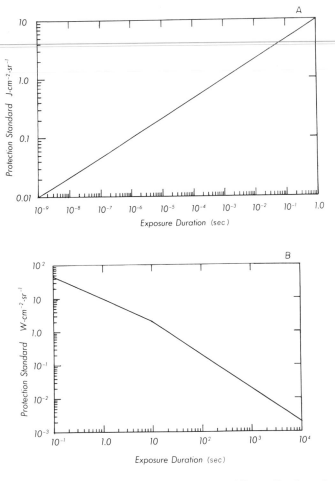

Fig. 2. (A) Protection standard for extended sources or diffuse reflections of pulses laser radiation (400–700 nm). To obtain protection standard for wavelengths 700–1400 nm, multiply by C_A. (B) Protection standard for extended sources or diffuse reflections of CW laser radiation (400–700 nm).

where n = number of pulses in train, t = duration of a single pulse in the train, and standard (nt) = protection standard of one pulse having a duration equal to nt sec.

Future Outlook

The principal protection standards for laser radiation are not likely to change for some time. However, the protection standards for repetitive exposures, long

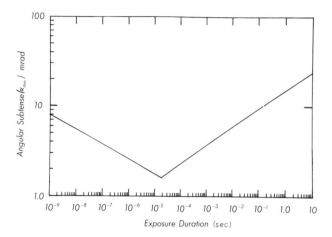

Fig. 3. Limiting Angular Subtense of an extended source (α_{min}). Sources whose angular subtense are less than α_{min} are considered collimated; those greater or equal to a α_{min} are considered extended sources.

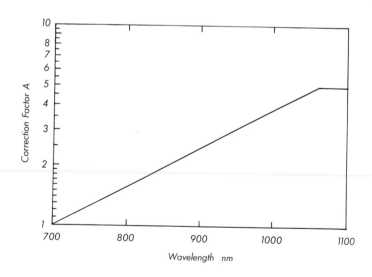

Fig. 4. Protection standard correction factor (C_A) for laser wavelengths between 700 and 1100 nm. $C_A = 5$ for wavelengths between 1100 and 1400 nm.

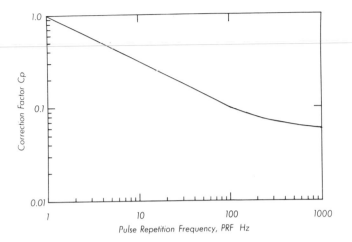

Fig. 5. Correction Factor C_p for repetitively pulsed lasers having pulse durations less than 10^{-5} sec. The protection standard for a single pulse of the pulse train is multiplied by the above correction factor. C_p for a PRF greater than 1000 Hz is 0.06.

exposure durations (greater than a few minutes), and for wavelengths outside of the visible band (i.e., infrared and ultraviolet radiation) were based upon a considerable amount of extrapolation.[17] One can expect, therefore, that progress may be forthcoming in some of these areas of biologic research. Several groups are exploring the retinal injury thresholds for groups of short pulses.[18-20] Little progress has been made recently in determing injury thresholds from ultraviolet and infrared laser radiation, with the notable exception of several U.S. Air Force studies. One theory has been proposed for the action spectrum of UV-induced cataracts, but this is yet to be proven.[9] Preliminary data for retinal burn thresholds for 30 psec (picosecond) mode-locked laser exposures obtained by Ham and co-workers showed that thresholds were reduced by a factor of at least 10 when compared with 30 ns (nanosecond) exposures to a minimal image area of the retina.[20]

Although there is still much to be learned about the biologic effects of certain types of laser exposures, most of the present standards will probably remain intact for a considerable time to come.

Laser Control Measures for the Construction Industry

By far the largest number of lasers in use today (over 100,000) are low-to-medium power He–Ne lasers used for leveling, alignment, and distance measurement in the construction industry. The output power of most of these

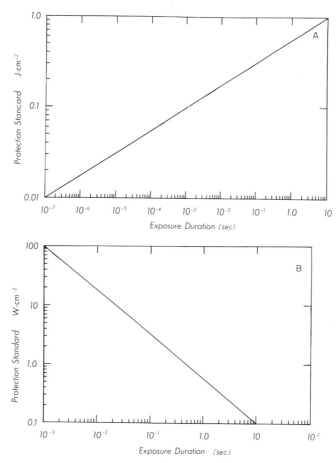

Fig. 6. (A) Protection standard for pulsed laser exposure of skin and eyes for far-infrared radiation (wavelengths greater than 1400 nm). Protection standards for skin exposure (400–1400 nm) are twice these values. (B) Protection standard for CW laser exposure of skin and eyes for far-infrared radiation (wavelengths greater than 1400 nm). Protection standards for skin exposure (400–1400 nm) are twice the values given in the graph.

lasers is 2 mW which is greater than the 1 mW limit for a Class II low-power laser. These lasers are used primarily in trenches (Fig. 7) and the beam is terminated by the trench wall. Occasionally these trench-grade lasers are used above ground, but in these cases the beam is terminated by the back hoe. Therefore, little risk is associated with these types of lasers. A set of guidelines that has been used within the U.S. Army and was more recently recommended by ACGIH[21] has been shown to be particularly useful:

1. Only qualified and trained employees shall be assigned to install, adjust, and operate laser equipment.

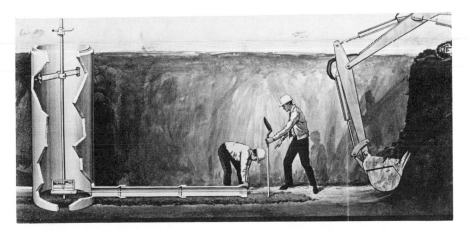

Fig. 7. Portable laser utilized for laying sewer pipe. Note location of laser at the base of manhole and location of laser beam at foot level. (Courtesy of Blount and George, Inc., Jacksonville, Arkansas.)

2. Proof of qualification of the laser equipment operator shall be available and in possession of operator at all times. This operator card may be obtained from a representative of the manufacturer when the operator has completed a minimum of 1 hr training in the safe use of this equipment by that representative.

3. Areas in which lasers are used shall be posted with standard laser warning placards if Class III.

4. When the laser is not required for a substantial period of time such as during lunch hour, overnight, or at change of shifts, beam shutters or caps shall be utilized or the laser turned off.

5. Mechanical or electronic means shall be used as a detector for guiding the alignment of the laser where feasible.

6. Precautions shall be taken to assure that persons do not look directly into the beam (intrabeam viewing is hazardous) unless the beam irradiance is below the applicable TLV at that observing location.

7. The laser beam should be terminated at the end of its useful beam path and shall in all cases be terminated if the hazardous distance exceeds the beam path beyond the controlled area (construction site).

8. Laser equipment shall bear a label to indicate maximum output and the nominal hazardous distance beyond which the laser beam irradiance does not exceed $2.5 \text{ mW} \cdot \text{cm}^{-2}$.

9. When the laser is not being used it shall be stored in a location where unauthorized personnel cannot gain access to the laser unit.

10. Placement of the laser beam path at or near eye level should be avoided whenever feasible.

11. Precautions shall be taken to assure that the laser is not pointed at mirrorlike (specular) surfaces.

MICROWAVE EXPOSURE CRITERIA

Since the publication of the last volume there has been a substantial increase in the amount of microwave/RF bioeffects research performed where effects were demonstrated in the absence of measurable temperature rise. In the past, the term "nonthermal effects" has been used to designate microwave/RF bioeffects where no measurable temperature rise was observed. However, the use of the word "nonthermal" is often a misnomer because E-M radiation is seldom absorbed in a biologic medium without some heat being produced. The terminology of nonthermal effects will not be used in this discussion. This class of bioeffects where no temperature rise was measured will be described next.

There is presently a great deal of controversy over the relative importance of effects that are accompanied by a temperature rise and those that are not. Effects due to heating have been well documented, but evidence for those occurring in the absence of a temperature rise is incomplete.[22-24] Those effects that are due to special microwave or RF receptors within the organism and cannot be induced by other factors will be referred to as specific effects in subsequent portions of this text.

Frey[25] reported an acoustic response that was postulated to be a direct auditory nerve response to microwaves. He reported that this phenomenon occurred instantaneously in human subjects at power densities as low as $100 \mu W \cdot cm^{-2}$. This specific effect was perceived as a buzz, ticking, or knocking, depending upon the pulsewidth and pulse repetition rate. The greatest sensitivity was observed in humans within the frequency range 300–1200 MHz. The area directly over the temporal lobe of the brain was identified as the most sensitive area. More recently, Labovitz[26] has proposed a mechanism for the production and detection of this audible sound. He has stated that the cochlear hair cell structures within the vestibulo–cochlear complex of the human ear could directly respond to stimulation from pulse-modulated microwave radiation. Guy[27] confirmed the reports of human auditory perception of pulse-modulated microwave radiation. He demonstrated a similar auditory response in cats which disappeared when the fluid was removed from the vestibulo–cochlear complex. These data are in agreement with the theory of Lebovitz[26] because he postulated that the cochlear hair cell structures could respond to movements of the intravestibular fluid induced by pulsed microwave radiation. Sommer and von Gierke[28] confirmed the existence of this specific effect, but stated that the effect was due to electromechanical transduction rather than direct stimulation of neural fibers or cortical neural tissue. They concluded that the cochlea was stimulated by electromechanical field forces by air or bone conduction.

The possibility that microwave radiation could interact with the central nervous system (CNS) without detectable heating has been suggested by several Eastern investigators.[29-39] Osipov[33] feels that some of the effects that have not been attributed to heating may in fact be due to "microthermal" heating. This postulated microthermal heating is very localized and the temperature rise would not be detectable by conventional temperature measurement techniques. Contrary to the subjective clinical complaints reported by Eastern research personnel in previous scientific papers, recent Polish papers, such as the work of Baranskis,[29] use more objective measurements to formulate their conclusions. Present papers that are being given by Polish authors show better controls, improved statistics, a clearer description of the experimental design, and well-documented experimental procedures. Further research is needed by Eastern and Western scientists before CNS effects can be fully understood.

Genetic and developmental effects of microwave/RF radiation are currently being investigated with renewed interest. Webb[40] has reported that irradiation with microwave frequencies from 40 to 150 GHz interferes with the syntheses of protein and DNA in *Escherichia coli*. Blackman[41] has observed enhanced cell growth of CS strain *E. coli* irradiated at 2.45 GHz with power densities not sufficient to cause detectable heating. Dietzel[42] demonstrated the production of teratologic effects such as gross malformations of limbs, head, and palate in rats. These malformations were attributed to a modification of normal DNA synthesis.

One of the more important bioeffects related to the production of heat in the biologic media by microwave radiation is cataract formation. Carpenter and his associates have done considerable work on microwave-induced cataracts in the eyes of rabbits.[43-50] On the basis of some of these studies, Carpenter suggested a "nonthermal" mechanism for cataractogenesis. However, current work by Carpenter[50] indicates that cataracts are formed in rabbit eyes only with an observable temperature rise in the intraocular fluid. Single acute doses of microwave radiation at 3 or 2.45 GHz will cause animal death if the energy is not focused on the rabbit eye.[50,51] Carpenter[50] has used a dielectric lens and Appleton and Hirsch[51] have used a parabolic dish antenna for the purpose of focusing microwave radiation at the position of the rabbit eye. Power densities of 300–500 mW · cm^{-2} caused acute ocular effects in rabbits for exposure times of 15–30 min.[51] Kramar *et al.*[52] have concluded that a temperature of at least $41°C$ within the rabbit eye behind the lens is needed for cataractogenesis. They made careful measurements of the temperature behind the lens following cessation of radiation to eliminate possible perturbation of the incident microwave field. Weiter *et al.*[53] reported that the ascorbic acid content of rabbit lenses is a good index of microwave-induced cataracts. They reported that ascorbic acid content of rabbit lenses decreased with increasing microwave irradiation. Additional research is needed to better define the possible cumulative effects of chronic microwave irradiation on cataract formation.

Present behavioral effects studies indicate that the observed modifications of normal behavior are related to the production of an increased body thermal burden. Thomas et al.[54] observed that a rat's ability to perceive a constant time interval was degraded by irradiation for times sufficient to cause whole body heating. Hunt et al.[55] found that irradiation of rats at 2.45 GHz caused a decrease in their ability to swim a water alley. The same investigators found that errors of omission for rats performing in visual discrimination tests increased immediately following microwave irradiation. Soviet investigators have concluded that behavioral effects are primarily not related to whole body heating.[56] Further behavioral research attempts to resolve the contradictions between Western and Eastern behavioral observations.

The results of the microwave/RF radiation bioeffects studies discussed above are being considered for incorporation in future E-M radiation standards. Since the results of these investigations are relatively new, appropriate regulatory agencies have not had sufficient time to modify relevant microwave/RF exposure standards. However, some new and revised standards have been promulgated.

The ANSI C95.1 standard was modified to include the specification of the TLV's in the equivalent free-space electric field strength $(200 \text{ V} \cdot \text{m}^{-1})$ RMS and the magnetic field strength $(0.5 \text{ A} \cdot \text{m}^{-1})$ RMS for CW (continuous wave) fields and in electric field strength squared $(40,000 \text{ V}^2 \cdot \text{m}^{-2})$ and magnetic field strength squared $(0.25 \text{ A}^2 \cdot \text{m}^{-2})$ for modulated fields. This revision was primarily the result of a growing realization that separate electric and magnetic field strength measurements were mandatory for meaningful and accurate characterization of RF fields below approximately 300 MHz.

Radio Frequencies below 300 MHz

The biologic effects for frequencies below 300 MHz (0.3 GHz) are currently being investigated in much greater detail. Previously, it was thought that such effects were essentially nonexistent. However, the U.S. Information Agency (USIA) and the U.S. Air Force (USAF) are funding bioeffects research within the HF (High Frequency) band which extends from 3 to 30 MHz. Both government agencies desire to evaluate the accuracy of the present standards that apply to this frequency band. The ANSI C95.1 and the OSHA regulations[57] (which were derived from the ANSI standard) specify their usable frequency range to extend from 10 MHz to 100 GHz.

In a study funded by the USAF, Bollinger[58] has found no discernible biologic effects on monkeys irradiated at 10.5, 19.3, and 26.6 MHz for 1 hr exposures to power density levels ranging from 100 to 200 mW · cm^{-2}. The cellular components of the blood were not affected by this exposure regimen. No alterations in cell-membrane integrity were detected through Serum K^{2-}, LDH, SGOT, SGPT, and CPK determinations. Serum BUN and Na+ determinations indicated no obvious damage to excretory functions. No changes in general metabolic activity could be inferred from serum glucose and protein determinations. ECG measurements and deep-body temperatures revealed no obvious sign of thermal stress. Thermal stress was noted in the monkeys during irradiation at 26.6 MHz with power densities in excess of 400 mW · cm^{-2}. As a result of these studies it has been suggested that the TLV's for the magnetic and electric field strengths could be less conservative from 3 to 30 MHz.

Kall[59,60] has studied the effects of 21 and 6 MHz RF fields on rats when exposed to dominant H (magnetic) fields, dominant E (electric) fields, and to fields where the far-field exposure conditions existed. In his more recent investigation Kall[60] detected no significant effects during the following tests: hematology, gross metabolic behavioral response, cardiovascular–respiratory system, pathology, central nervous system, gastric acid secretion, and teratology. He found that the results of the gastrointestinal motor activity and cholinesterase activity were statistically significant. The gastrointestinal activity test was significant only at 21 MHz for the dominant E and far-field exposure conditions. The cholinesterase activity test responses were significant for dominant E, dominant H, and far-field exposure conditions at 6 and 21 MHz. From the results of these studies on rats Kall[60] has recommended to the USIA that the present exposure standards should be modified to specify an electric field strength of 1500 V · m^{-1} and a magnetic field strength of 5 A · m^{-1} for the frequency range from 3 to 30 MHz. In a former study Kall[59] concluded that hazardous levels existed for electric field strengths in the range from 400 to 4000 V · m^{-1} and for magnetic field strengths ranging from 1 to 10 A · m^{-1}. The same author recommended 11 mW · cm^{-2} as being the TLV for far-field exposure situations.

The theoretical data of Lin[61] for a spherical phantom model simulating man has shown that the magnetic field component of the E-M field may be the most hazardous. For RF radiation from 1 to 20 MHz the heating within the human model due to the magnetic field component is an order of magnitude greater than that due to the electric field component during far-field exposure conditions. For RF fields in close vicinity to typical RF power sources the heating of the theoretical phantom model due to the magnetic field component can be even larger. These conditions should be carefully considered when attempting to estimate the potential hazard from an RF radiation field.

Microwave/RF Measurements

One of the areas of microwave/RF research which is constantly plagued with inaccuracies and ambiguities is that of dosimetry. This confusion is increased when the definitions of E-M field measurement quantities are not completely understood. The quantity power density or power flux $(mW \cdot cm^{-2})$ is only defined where the strictest far-field conditions exist. Consequently, exposure measurements should ideally be expressed in terms of the electric and magnetic field strengths or equivalent parameters that are defined under all exposure conditions. Measurements of power density within the near-field of a source (very close vicinity) do not express a true measure of power density.

In the RF region (specifically below 30 MHz) the potentially hazardous environments are generally within this near-field region.[62] Further ambiguity results because most survey probes respond only to the electric field. The electric field vector has no fixed relationship to the magnetic field vector. Therefore, the vector denoting power flow has no meaning and power density cannot be defined. Truly meaningful measurements of an RF field should be made in terms of electric and magnetic field strength values.

Even if the magnetic and electric field strength are correctly measured under free-space conditions (negligible reflections), they still must be related to the values that would exist in the sample to be irradiated. Probes that can measure the electric field strength within an experimental animal medium have been developed by Bassen[63] of the Bureau of Radiological Health (U.S. DHEW, FDA). These tissue implantable probes can make measurements during microwave irradiation without significantly changing the incident E-M field pattern. Further development is needed to produce a tissue implantable probe that will measure the magnetic field strength in an analogous manner.

REFERENCES

1. Matelsky, I., The non-ionizing radiations. "Industrial Hygeine Highlights," Vol. I, pp. 140–178. Industrial Hygiene Foundation of America, Pittsburgh, Pennsylvania, 1968.
2. Sliney, D. H., Nonionizing radiation. *In* "Industrial Environmental Health" (L. V. Cralley, ed.), Vol. 1, pp. 171–241. Academic Press, New York, 1972.
3. U.S. Department of Labor, Title 29, Code of Federal Regulations 1910. Occupational Safety and Health (OSHA) Standards, Washington, D.C., 1972.
4. U.S. Department of Health, Education, and Welfare, National Institute for Occupational Safety and Health, "Criteria for a Recommended Standard . . . Occupational Exposure to Ultraviolet Radiation," Publ. HSM 73–11009. U.S. Govt. Printing Office, Washington, D.C., 1972.
5. U.S. Department of Health, Education, and Welfare, Food and Drug Administration, "Laser Products, Proposed Performance Standard," Fed. Regist., Vol. 38(236):34084(21 CFR Part 1040). US Govt. Printing Office, Washington, D.C., 1973.

6. Sliney, D. H., The merits of an envelope action spectrum for ultraviolet radiation exposure criteria. *Amer. Ind. Hyg. Ass., J. 33,* 644 (1972).

7. Parr, W. A., "An Ultraviolet Hazard Monitor," presented at the American Industrial Hygiene Conference, Boston, Massachusetts, 1973 (to be published).

8. Pitts, D. G., The Ocular ultraviolet action spectrum and protection criteria. *Health Phys. 25,* 559 (1972).

9. Kurzel, R. B., Staton, G., Borkman, R. F., Wolbarsht, M. L., and Yamanashi, B. S., Excited states of tryptophan and ultraviolet induced cataracts. *Nature (London), 241,* 132 (1973).

10. Zigman, S., Eye lens color: Formation and function. *Science 171,* 807 (1971).

11. Sliney, D. H., "The development of laser safety criteria–biological considerations. *In* "Laser Applications in Medicine and Biology" (M. L. Wolbarsht, ed.), vol. 1, p. 163. Plenum, New York, 1971.

12. American Conference of Governmental Industrial Hygienists, "A Guide for Uniform Industrial Hygiene Codes or Regulations for Laser Installation." ACGIH, Cincinnati, Ohio, 1968.

13. U.S. Department of the Army, U.S. Department of the Navy, "Control of Hazards to Health from Laser Radiation," Publ. TB MED 279, NAVMED P–5052–35. US Govt. Printing Office, Washington, D.C., 1969.

14. U.S. Air Force, "Laser Health Hazards Control," Publ. AFM 161–8. US Govt. Printing Office, Washington, D.C., 1969.

15. Parker, G. S., The current status of state regulations on laser radiation. *Laser J. 2,* 17 (1970).

16. American National Standards Institute, "The Safe Use of Lasers," Standard Z–136.1, 1973. ANSI, New York, 1973.

17. Wolbarsht, M. L., and Sliney, D. H., The formulation of protection standards for lasers. *In* "Laser Applications in Medicine and Biology" (M. L. Wolbarsht, ed.), Vol. 2, pp. 303–352. Plenum, New York, 1974.

18. Skeen, C. H., Bruce, W. R., Tips, J. H., Jr., Smith, M. G., and Garza, C. G., "Ocular Effects of Repetitive Laser Pulses," Air Force Contract F41609–71–C–0018 (AD 746795). Technology Inc., San Antonio, Texas, 1972.

19. Gibbons, W. D., "Retinal Burn Thresholds for Exposure to a Frequency-Doubled Neodymium Laser," Rep. SAM–TR–73–45. USAF School of Aerospace Medicine, Brooks Air Force Base, San Antonio, Texas, 1973.

20. Ham, W. T., Mueller, H. A., and Goldman, A. A., Retinal hazards from 30-picosecond neodymium laser pulse. *Science 185,* 362 (1974).

21. American Conference of Governmental Industrial Hygienists, "A Guide for Control of Laser Hazards." ACGIH, Cincinnatti, Ohio, 1973.

22. Michaelson, S. M., Biomedical aspects of microwave exposure. *Amer. Ind. Hyg. Ass., J. 32,* 338 (1971).

23. Milroy, W. C., and Michaelson, S. M., Biological effects of microwave radiation. *Health Phys. 20,* 567 (1971).

24. Michaelson, S. M., and Dodge, C. H., Soviet views on the biological effects of microwaves–an analysis. *Health Phys. 21,* 108 (1971).

25. Frey, A. H., Human auditory system response to modulated electromagnetic energy. *J. Appl. Physiol. 17,* 689 (1962).

26. Lebovitz, R. M., Caloric vestibular stimulation via UHF-microwave irradiation. *IEEE Trans. Bio-med. Eng. 20,* 119 (1973).

27. Guy, A. W., Chou, C. K., Lin, J. C., and Christensen, D., "Microwave Induced Acoustic Effects in Mammalian Auditory Systems and Physical Materials," Conf. Biol. Effects Non-Ioniz. Radiat. N.Y. Acad. Sci., New York, 1974.

28. Sommer, H. C., and von Gierke, H. E., Hearing sensations in electrical fields. *Aerosp. Med. 35*, 834 (1964).

29. Baranski, S., and Edelwejn, Z., "Experimental Morphologic and Electroencephalographic Studies on Microwave Effects on the Nervous System," Conf. Biol. Effects Non-Ioniz. Radiat. N.Y. Acad. Sci., New York, 1974.

30. Cleary, S. F., Biological effects of microwave and radiofrequency radiation. *Crit. Rev. Environ. Contr. 1*, 257–306 (1970).

31. Dodge, C. H., and Kassel, S., "Soviet Research on the Neural Effects of Microwaves," ATD Rep. 66–133. Library of Congress, Washington, D.C., 1966.

32. Presman, A. S., The effect of microwaves on living organisms and biological structures. *Usp. Fiz. Nauk 86*, 263 (1965).

33. Osipov, Y. A., "The Health of Workers Exposed to Radio-frequency Radiation," ATD Rep. 66–133. Library of Congress, Washington, D.C., 1966.

34. Livshits, N. N., On the causes of the disagreements in evaluating the radio-sensitivity of the central nervous system among researchers using conditioned reflex and maze methods. *Radiobiology 7*, 238 (1967).

35. Vavala, D. A., "Soviet Research on the Pathophysiology of Ultrahigh Frequency Electromagnetic Fields," Rep. AMD–CR–01–03–68. Brooks Air Force Base, San Antonio, Texas, 1968.

36. Presman, A. S., "Electromagnetic Fields and Life." Nauka, Moscow, 1968.

37. Gorodetshaia, S. F., The effect of centimeter radio waves on mouse fertility. *Fiziol. Zh. 9*, 394 (1963).

38. Levitina, N. A., Effect of microwaves on cardiac rhythm of rabbits during local irradiation of body areas. *Bull. Exp. Biol. Med. (USSR) 58*, 67 (1964).

39. Gorodetshaia, N. A., The influence of an SHR electromagnetic field on reproduction, composition of peripheral blood, conditioned reflex activity, and morphology of the internal organs of white mice. *In* "Biological Action of Ultrasound and Super-high Frequency Electromagnetic Oscillations" (A. A. Gorodetskiy, ed.), pp. 80-91. Acad. Sci., Kiev, USSR, 1964.

40. Webb, S. J., "Genetic Continuity and Metabolic Regulation as Seen by the Effects of Various Frequencies of Microwaves on these Phenomena," Conf. Biol. Effects Non-Ioniz. Radiat. N.Y. Acad. Sci., New York, 1974.

41. Blackman, C. F., Benane, S. G., Weil, C. M., and Ali, J. S., "Effects of Non-Ionizing Electromagnetic Radiation on Single Cell Biological Systems," Conf. Biol. Effects Non-Ioniz. Radiat. N.Y. Acad. Sci., New York, 1974.

42. Dietzel, F., "Effects of Electromagnetic Radiation on Implantation and Intra-Uterine Development of the Rat," Conf. Biol. Effects Non-Ioniz. Radiat. N.Y. Acad. Sci., New York, 1974.

43. Carpenter, R. L., Experimental radiation cataracts induced by microwave irradiation. *Proc. 2nd Annu. Tri-Serv. Conf. Biol. Effects Microwave Energy* ASTIA Doc. AD 131–477, pp. 146–166 (1958).

44. Carpenter, R. L., Studies on the effects of 2450 MHz radiation on the eye of the rabbit. *Proc. 3rd Annu. Tri-Serv. Conf. Biol. Hazards Microwave Radiat. Equipments (Univ. Calif., Berkeley)* Tech. Rep. RADC–TR–59–140, pp. 279–290 (1959).

45. Carpenter, R. L., "An Experimental Study of the Biological Effects of Microwave Radiation in Relation to the Eye," (Tufts Univ., Midford, Mass.), Tech. Rep. RADC–TDR–62–131. U.S. Air Force Rome Air Development Center, Rome, New York, 1962.

46. Carpenter, R. L., Experimental microwave cataract: A review. *In* "Biological Effects and Health Implications of Microwave Radiation" (S. F. Cleary, ed.), Rep. PHS, BRH,

DBE 70–2, pp. 76–81. U.S. Dept. of Health, Education and Welfare, Washington, D.C., 1970.

47. Carpenter, R. L., Biddle, D. K., and Van Ummersen, C. A., Opacities in the lens of the eye experimentally induced by exposure to microwave radiation. *IRE Trans. Med. Electron. 7*, 152 (1960).

48. Carpenter, R. L., Biological effects of microwave radiation with particular reference to the eye. *Proc. Int. Conf. Med. Electron., 3rd, 1960* pp. 401–408 (1961).

49. Carpenter, R. L., and Van Ummersen, C. A., The action of microwave radiation on the eye. *J. Microwave Power 3*, 3 (1968).

50. Carpenter, R. L., Ferri, E. S., and Hagan, G. J., "Some Current Studies on Microwave Ocular Effects," Conf. Biol. Effects Non-Ioniz. Radiat. N.Y. Acad. Sci., New York, 1974.

51. Appleton, B., and Hirsch, S., "Experimental Microwave Cataractogenesis," Conf. Biol. Effects Non-Ioniz. Radiat. N.Y. Acad. Sci., New York 1974.

52. Kramar, P. O., Emery, A. F., Guy, A. W., and Lin, J. C., "The Ocular Effects of Microwaves on Hypothermic Rabbits: A Study of Microwave Cataractogenic Mechanisms," Conf. Biol. Effects Non-Ioniz. Radiat. N.Y. Acad. Sci., New York, 1974.

53. Weiter, J. J., Finch, E. D., Schultz, W., and Frattali, V., "Ascorbic Acid Changes in Cultured Rabbits Lenses Following Microwave Irradiation," Conf. Biol. Effects Non-Ioniz. Radiat. N.Y. Acad. Sci., New York, 1974.

54. Thomas, J. R., Finch, E. D., Fulk, D. W., and Burch, L. S., "Effects of Microwave Radiation on Behavioral Baselines," Conf. Biol. Effects Non-Ioniz. Radiat. N.Y. Acad. Sci., New York, 1974.

55. Hunt, E. L., King, N. W., and Phillips, R. D., "Behavioural Effects of Pulsed Microwave Irradiation," Conf. Biol. Effects Non-Ioniz. Radiat. N.Y. Acad. Sci., New York, 1974.

56. Sadchikova, A. A., and Orlova, A. A., Clinical picture of the chronic effects of electromagnetic waves. *Ind. Hyg. Occup. Dis. (USSR) 2*, 16 (1958).

57. U.S. Congress, Occupational Safety and Health Act of 1970, Nonionizing Radiation. *Fed. Regist. 37*, No. 202, 22162 (1972).

58. Bollinger, J. N., "Detection and Evaluation of Radiofrequency Electromagnetic Radiation-Induced Biological Damage in Macaca Mulatta," Final Rep. under Contract F41609–70–C–0025, SWRI 05–2808–01. U.S. Air Force, Brooks AFB, San Antonio, Texas, 1971.

59. Kall, A. R., "Final Technical Report on Research Project to Study Radiation Hazards Caused by High Power High Frequency Fields," Contract 1A–11651. United States Information Agency, Washington, D.C., 1968.

60. Kall, A. R., "Final Technical Report on Research Project to Study Radiation Hazards Caused by High Power High Frequency Fields," Contract 1A–14121, United States Information Agency, Washington, D.C., 1972.

61. Lin, J. C., Johnson, C. C., and Guy, A. W., "Power Deposition in a Spherical Model of Man Exposed to 1–20 MHz E-M Fields," IMPI Symp., 1973 (oral presentation).

62. Rogers, S. J., and King, R. S., Radio hazards in the M.F./H.F. band. *Non-Ioniz. Radiat. 1*, 178 (1970).

63. Bassen, H., and Swicord, M., "A Broadband Miniature Electric Field Probe," Conf. Biol. Effects Non-Ioniz. Radiat. N.Y. Acad. Sci., New York, 1974.

Ionizing Radiation

McDONALD E. WRENN AND HARRY F. SCHULTE

INTRODUCTION

Problems presented by the increasing use of radiation and radioactive materials are of concern to everyone, including the industrial hygienist. Public interest in the subject is high and, because of the complexity of the subject, misunderstandings frequently arise at the public level. Honest differences of opinion probably are no greater in this than in any other field of public health, but they seem to create greater public concern and perplexity. Partly as a result of this interest, developments in the field are rapid and the output of technical information is immense. Certainly, *Health Physics,* the journal of the Health Physics Society, is by far the major source of publications in the field, although by no means the only one. This journal published nearly 1400 pages of technical information from 1971 to 1973. It should be emphasized that the industrial hygienist is only concerned with part of the field of health physics, although the boundaries of his interest will vary greatly, depending on his employer and his responsibilities. In this review, an effort has been made to focus on developments that directly involve the working environment, taking into account the off-work stresses that may influence it.

Major sources of information were reviewed in "Industrial Hygiene Highlights"[1] and there have been no important changes. A new international journal, *Aerosol Science,* has appeared which will include radioactive aerosols, among the many within its scope. The English translations of *Staub* (German) and *Hygiene and Sanitation* (Russian) contain frequent articles dealing with radioactive materials. *Nuclear Safety,* published by the U.S. Atomic Energy Commission (USAEC), publishes frequent articles of interest, mostly literature reviews on specific topics. *Radiation Data and Reports* published by the U.S. Environmental Protection Agency, presents much specific information and quantitative data, although most of it is not directly related to the work of the industrial hygienist.

The International Radiation Protection Association, IRPA, which has about 6000 members worldwide, has now held three international conferences. The constitution[2] and proceedings[3] of the first Congress (held in Rome in 1966) are available. Although the second IRPA Congress (held in Brighton, England, in 1970) did not assemble the papers presented in a single publication, the abstracts have been published.[4] These are scattered throughout the literature. The third Congress was held in Washington, D.C., in the fall of 1973, and the collected papers of this conference will be available shortly.

Another source of foreign information, particularly in radiobiology, is the series of translations from the Russian published under the general title, "The Toxicology of Radioactive Substances," of which five volumes have appeared so far.[5] For popular expositions of topics related to atomic energy, the series of booklets on "Understanding the Atom," published by the U.S. Atomic Energy Commission, are truly superb.[6] Each deals with a specific topic and is written by an authority in the field. While intended for popular consumption, they contain enough technical information to make them very useful to anyone except a specialist in the particular field covered.

The topic of this review includes off-the-job stresses and it is important to consider such influences. One may speculate about a wide variety of off-the-job stresses or influences which may be important in influencing the potential effects of radiation exposure. However, three aspects can be clearly identified.

First (and least complex) is additional radiation exposure. Environmental exposures generally are less than 5% of the annual occupational dose limits in almost all areas of the world.

There are several references that relate to general environmental exposure, which can be usefully consulted by the specialists. In particular, the summaries of the United Nations Scientific Committee on the Effects of Atomic Radiation (which have been issued every 2 or 3 years since 1958)[7] make comprehensive summaries of the extant environmental levels of radioactivity, the exposure of populations of the world to natural background and fallout, periodic summaries of occupational exposures, and summaries of the literature on radiobiologic effects. The latter, of course, are more relevant to occupational than to environmental exposures. In addition, a series of conferences has been held in the United States and around the world on the environmental radioecologic aspects.[8-10] The latest UNSCEAR report in 1973 shifts attention from the environmental aspects of nuclear weapons testing to nuclear power production for peaceful means. Accordingly, these summaries will, in the future, take on greater importance as the expansion of the nuclear industry for peaceful purposes takes place. The most compact and complete description of environmental exposure is given in a book by Eisenbud.[11]

Clearly, the most important additional exposures are medical radiation exposures for diagnostic or even therapeutic means, and clearly fluoroscopic examinations and even x rays may deliver local doses well in excess of those received on the job—certainly in excess of those characteristic of the annual dose limits (i.e., 5 rems whole body or 15 rems to any organ). For example, Clemente has reported on the results of routine whole body counter examinations of nuclear workers in Italy and has shown that, in 2000 workers examined, 1 in 200 carried iodine-131 burdens in their thyroids attributable to medical diagnostic tests. The four highest doses were evaluated as ranging between 140 and 1000 rads to the thyroid. One such case (estimated thyroid dose 700 rads) has been reported from the United States in a routine whole body evaluation of 200 reactor maintenance workers.[12] These doses are consistent with what has been reported as common medical practice for ^{131}I use.[13] Doses of this magnitude have both biologic and legal significance, and perhaps also significance regarding epidemiologic research on occupationally exposed groups.

Second, exposure to agents that might act with, supplement, or produce conditions conducive to the enhancement of radiation sensitivity are clearly important. Nelson has discussed these and pointed out that "the first reasonably clear demonstration in man of interaction between radiation and a chemical carcinogen (tobacco) is seen in an enhancement of lung cancer incidence in uranium miners who smoke cigarettes." In fact, we know little about the additive or synergistic effects of radiation and chemical mutagens, and their combined ability to produce genetic and somatic mutation, although we know both are capable of activating latent viruses that may then result in the development of a tumor.[14] We must be alert for occupational opportunities for such multiple exposures to occur. Clearly, cigarette smoking is an unfavorable habit in potential exposure circumstance where lung is the critical organ at risk for radiation exposure.

Finally, age and sex are likely to be more important than previously in the workplace. The National Council on Radiological Protection (NCRP) has already identified stricter occupational dose limits for women of childbearing age one-tenth that of the other adult workers in order to limit the potential dose to the fetus.[15] Clearly, the entry of more women into jobs requiring occupational radiation exposures will present not only potential occupational health problems, but will also create scientific, ethical, and legal problems of enormous complexity.

APPLICATIONS OF RADIATION AND RADIOACTIVE MATERIALS

The nuclear industry, spurred primarily by the development and utilization of light water reactors to produce electric power, is increasing at a very rapid rate.

As of April 1974, about 6% of the installed electric-generating capacity in the United States was nuclear, whereas only a few years ago it was only 1%. Although this increase is primarily with two types of light water reactors [the pressurized water reactor (PWR) and the boiling water reactor (BWR)], other types of power reactors are being introduced in the United States, such as the high temperature gas-cooled reactor (HTGR), and advanced reactor systems are being worked on.[16,17] The enormous increase in the rate of fission in power reactors will make available large amounts of waste to be handled and controlled very carefully, and also large amounts of by-product radioactive materials, which may find substantial uses in medical therapy, space nuclear power sources, and other areas not yet thought of.

Occupationally, hospitals and nuclear medicine departments are a potential source of significant exposures, both to patients and physicians, other professional personnel, and technicians administering radioactive material and diagnostic tests. A medical physicist, who is also a specialist in radiation protection, usually is in charge at sufficiently large institutions. However, many hospitals are too small to have such persons on the staff, and consultants may provide such services in those cases. Members of the American Association of Physicists in Medicine number about 600. Many are also health physicists and perhaps a few, industrial hygienists.

NUCLEAR FUEL CYCLE

By far the most numerous reactor for the generation of commercial power in the United States is the light water reactor, composed both of the pressurized water and boiling water types. As of March 31, 1974, there were 44 commercial plants in operation with 185 additional planned, ordered, or in the construction phase.[7] New orders are being received at the rate of about 40 per year for these plants, each with capacity generally exceeding 1000 MW electric (or roughly 1/400 of the present United States generating capacity).[16]

These reactors generate energy by the fission of ^{235}U, which comprises only about 0.7% of natural uranium. Uranium used in these reactors is in the form of uranium oxide, somewhat enriched in ^{235}U content to between 2 and 3%. This, of course, requires an enrichment process which at the moment is primarily by gaseous diffusion. Several large government-owned plants produce all the enrichment for the United States economy.

Some of the uranium in these reactors absorbs neutrons and is converted into plutonium, which itself can be used as a fuel. In present LWR reactors, about 30–40% of the uranium atoms are so converted; this is called a conversion ratio when the percentage converted is less than 100. When the fraction of ^{238}U atoms converted into plutonium relative to ^{235}U atoms fissioned exceeds 1, then a reactor can produce more fuel than it burns. This means that more atoms of ^{238}U can be converted into plutonium than the original atoms fissioned. Accordingly, the energy extractable from available uranium resources can be increased roughly 100-fold above that which would be extractable if only the ^{235}U were fissioned. Thus, there is an incentive to develop reactors of this type, called breeders. There are a number of potential types of reactors that conceptually would breed. However, in the United States a major effort is being made on one particular type—the liquid metal fast breeder reactor (LMFBR). This reactor uses sodium as a coolant and heat transfer medium and plutonium for fuel.

Partly as a result of the work on the fast breeder and its important potential in future energy production, the interest in plutonium has increased greatly. It should be pointed out, however, that light water reactors make significant quantities of plutonium, so that a need already exists to process plutonium occupationally. In addition, this plutonium can also be used in the present light water reactors. This process is called recycling, and although there is no routine use of plutonium in this way at the moment, such use may become commonplace by the latter part of this decade.

Experimental Pu recycle fuel is already in use in one reactor for the production of power.

The plutonium used in power production is largely ^{239}Pu when measured by its mass. However, other isotopes are also formed and their concentrations increase with the length of time the plutonium remains in the reactor. The isotopic composition of plutonium from light water reactors under present operating conditions is expected to be similar to that of plutonium from the LMFBR. The major activity is associated in both cases with ^{238}Pu. This plutonium is roughly 6–8 times higher in specific activity than pure ^{239}Pu. Some reactors make ^{238}Pu, which is produced from neutron capture of ^{237}Np. The ^{238}Pu in pure form is of great value as a heat source. This is important both for space nuclear applications and for such esoteric projects as powering heart pacemakers and potentially also artificial hearts. The specific activity of ^{238}Pu is 270 times greater than that of ^{239}Pu, but only about 30 times greater than that of plutonium produced in present-day power reactors. It is, accordingly, more toxic per unit mass. Copious numbers of neutrons and γ-rays are produced by high specific activity Pu by α-particle interactions with nearby light elements, such as oxygen or fluoride. In many industrial processes, plutonium is present either as the oxide or fluoride. Accordingly, it is clear that fabrication plants for this new high burnup plutonium will be made in a manner uncharacteristic of the past, which was basically by a well-enclosed glovebox operation. Modern plants may indeed be completely remote in handling. This will ameliorate the problems of personnel exposure from handling of plutonium but, of course, not eliminate them. The industrial hygiene, health physics, and related aspects of plutonium have been reviewed in an IAEA monograph[18] and in a recent summary of the toxicology of Pu.[19]

A great deal of new interest is being given to thorium, which can be converted by neutron capture to the fissionable isotope, ^{233}U. There are two commercial operating gas-cooled reactors, in which helium gas extracts heat from the fission occurring in a mixture of fuel containing ^{233}U or ^{235}U with the fertile material, ^{232}Th. The reactor presently is not a breeder, although advanced gas-cooled reactors that are capable of breeding could be constructed. In the United Kingdom the gas-cooled reactor using CO_2 for coolant has been the standard power unit for many years; unfortunately, these units have developed unexpected corrosion problems and their power curtailed. However, the United Kingdom deserves the credit for producing a large portion of its baseload for electric generation earlier than other countries. The development of gas-cooled high temperature reactors using the thorium cycle will produce some radio-nuclides that are not common to the uranium–plutonium cycle. Accordingly, there may be new toxicologic problems ahead with high specific activity uranium not yet handled on any scale.

Estimates of the number of facilities required for the nuclear fuel cycle for the generation of electricity in the United States, are listed in Table I for the year 1985.[19] By far the most numerous plants are nuclear power plants, of which several hundred will be in operation. The major type of occupational radiation exposure in these plants is external exposure and is associated with

TABLE I
Fuel Cycle Plants[a]

Type	In operation	Planned or under construction
Uranium mills	20	5
UF_6 production plants	2	—
Enriched uranium processing and fabrication plants	19	6
Plutonium processing and fabrication plants	11	6
Fuel reprocessing plants	1	4
Waste burial grounds	6	—
	—	—
Total	59	21
Nuclear power plants[b]	44	185

[a] As of June 30, 1973. From Ref. 17.

[b] As of March 31, 1974.

maintenance operations and the handling of radioactive wastes. The next most numerous facilities will be uranium mills and mines. Uranium mines have been a source of grievous occupational exposure in the past, due primarily to misattention to proper ventilation practices, and this is covered thoroughly later in this section. Mills above ground are better ventilated and are not associated with any worrisome occupational exposures, although on an industrywide basis detailed assessment of internal exposure in these facilities has not been sufficiently studied. Fuel fabrication plants involve the processing of oxides either of uranium or plutonium and are a potential source of both internal exposure from inhalation or puncture wounds, or external exposure especially in the case of high α-specific active materials where α, n reactions are important in producing external exposure. Table II[199,6] shows the summary of the United States accidental experience to date much of it in one plant has been used for the production of weapons material. Accordingly, we will be dealing shortly with about 15 facilities that have various potential designs and handle a variety of different types of material—mostly consisting of uranium and plutonium, but in varying chemical compounds and isotopic compositions.

Most likely there will be three fuel processing plants in operation by 1985. These will receive spent reactor fuel, which is shipped from the power plants to the reprocessing plants where the radioactive wastes are chemically separated from the fuel and the fuel reprocessed. The wastes will then be held in storage, in liquid form, for some 5 years and subsequently will be converted to solids. Solids with then be sent to a federal repository, neither the location nor design of which is yet firm. It now appears that the interim step in the long-term storage of waste will be to store solids in retrievable cannisters in a federal repository until a suitable long-term repository has been designated and operated on a pilot scale. The most likely ultimate repository in the United States appears to be bedded salt. A major consideration associated with this deposit will be limitation of human activities nearby which might compromise the integrity of the geologic structure. There appear to be no purely technical reasons why a suitable location cannot be found and so developed.

The peaceful uses of nuclear energy are many and are distributed throughout a variety of fields. A booklet on this subject, issued by the USAEC, outlines many of these applications and gives the reader some appreciation of the possibilities.[20] The Plowshare Program is concerned with the peaceful applications of nuclear explosions, such as the stimulation of natural gas flow, by shattering underground rock structures. Many projects are under study in this program, but it has also generated much controversy, as might be expected.

In the past 3 years, there have been many advances made in the control of the radiation hazard in underground uranium mines. Nevertheless, there are still gaps in our knowledge and even more in the application of knowledge in this field. From the standpoint of making knowledge available to a wide audience, the

TABLE II

Internal Plutonium Depositions Exceeding 25% of the Occupational Permissible Body Burden among AEC Contractor Personnel during the Period 1957–1970

By year	Number of cases	By therapy employed	Number of cases
1957	12	Chelate	37
1958	6	Excision	21
1959	10	Both	10
1960	10	None	135
1961	16		
1962	20		
1963	9		
1964	29		
1965	22	By route of entry	Number of cases
1966	27		
1967	10	Inhalation	131
1968	8	Wound	48
1969	6	Both	8
1970	3	Unknown	16
?	15		
Total	203		

By activity	Number of cases	By % of permissible body burden	Number of cases
Research	25	25 to 50%	118
Production	109	50 to 75%	35
Maintenance	17	75 to 100%	13
Development	4	100 to 200%	15
Health physics	18	200 to 500%	15
Construction	2	500 to 1000%	7
Analytical	1		
Recovery	5		
Unknown	22		

special issue of *Health Physics* dedicated to Duncan Holaday is outstanding.[21] This issue is wholly devoted to this subject and contains many valuable papers. However, it is not the sole source of information and the number of publications was extremely large during this period. For those wishing to acquaint themselves with the history and background of this problem, the lead article by Holaday in the special issue is an excellent source.[22] Later a contribution from Czechoslovakia added information relating to the Joachimsthal mines.[23] Much technical information is given by Evans in a review of the physics aspect of the background.[24] Related to the latter is a plea by Morken that the working level concept is defective and not a satisfactory index of exposure or hazard.[25] This criticism has largely been ignored and practically all studies are based on measurement of working level. The difficulties in selecting a safe working level and the range of possible values has been discussed by Tompkins of the Federal Radiation Council.[26]

Since the last review, based upon epidemiologic data purporting to show the development of lung cancer in uranium miners, with exposures as low as 100 working level (WL) months, a decision was made to reduce the WL limits in mines to 4 WL months per year per man, after due study indicated that it was economically and technologically feasible to limit exposures to these levels.[27] On the other hand, the epidemiologic dose response curve in uranium miners, developed by Lundin et al.,[28,29] has been criticized.[30] The basic dose estimates on which the curve is based are not always founded on good estimates of exposure. That is to say, in the early days measurements were extremely infrequent and much of the exposure for many of the miners related to exposure incurred in the 1950's.[31] In addition, many miners worked in mines other than uranium mines, and the exposure to radon daughters which is known to occur in many other types of mines was not included. More recently, Archer and Lundin have updated their estimates of dose to include such exposures.[28] One of the most important aspects of this problem has been the observation both by Lundin et al.[29] and by Saccamanno[32,33] that lung cancer is much more frequent among miners who smoke than nonsmoking miners. As a result of this, for example, the American National Standard N-13.8 on uranium mining expressly prohibits smoking in the mines by the miners. In view of the potential relationship of smoking and radiation, this appears to be a wise course of action. Of course, the miner's smoking habits out of the mine are his own business, and although it would be prudent for uranium miners (and, for that matter, other miners) not to smoke, no effective control off the job, other than persuasion, can be exercised. Also of interest are two British papers on exposure to radon daughters and incidence of lung cancer among hematite miners (underground).[34,35] These point out the need for more studies among nonuranium miners.

Calculations of the magnitude of the radiation dose to the basal layers of the bronchial epithelium in man, which are considered the cells from which cancer in uranium miners originates, have been made by a number of investigators. The classic calculations by Altshuler[36] gave results similar to those of Jacobi,[37] although the assumptions made by both were quite at variance with respect to the reference atmospheres to which the miners were exposed and the manner in which deposition and respiratory clearance were calculated. Several other subsequent attempts at this calculation have been made.[37a] However, the biologic variables are so formidable and poorly understood that the real dose to the basal epithelium will probably not be known by better than an order of magnitude. These estimates vary between 0.1 and 20 rads/WL month. A recent

National Academy of Science committee chose 0.5 rad as the most realistic estimate.[37b] In particular, this view is espoused by Parker,[37c] who considers the biologic variables an intractable dilemma of the lung dosimetry.

This type of calculation probably has little application in deriving acceptable levels of daughter concentrations in the mines, but is very helpful in understanding the mechanisms involved and in pointing to factors to be controlled in reducing exposure. Information that may be useful in such a calculation was found in the work of Raabe, who investigated the probable particle size distribution from adsorption of the daughters on aerosols[38,39] and in the total respiratory deposition measurements made by workers at Colorado State University[40] and the USAEC Health and Safety Laboratory.[71]

Major emphasis in estimating exposure of miners has been on air sampling. Since the original Kusnetz and Tsivoglou methods[42] of measuring working level by counting a sample after a fixed sampling period followed by fixed waiting periods, there have been many significant improvements and variations. Some of these involve utilizing total counts rather than count rate measurements, other use an α spectrometer, some involve single counts, and others follow the decay curves.[43-48] While there are still controversies about these various details, and improvements are valuable, the investigator does have the means at hand now to make good estimates of the working level at any one time and place. Since it is the radon that produces the daughters, and its concentration cannot be ignored as an exposure source, there is still interest in improving methods of measuring the concentration of this gas. Use of a portable ionization chamber has been described[49] and a method of using a charge to collect the daughters from a trapped filtered sample of gas has been incorporated into a usable instrument.[50] An older idea of drawing air through two filters spaced some distance apart has been studied and made practicable for use in mines.[51] Measurement of radon daughters has recently been reviewed by Budnitz.[51a]

Such air sampling merely gives results at a single location at a single time. In order to estimate the exposure of each miner, an enormous number of individual air concentrations must be measured and these results must be related to the movements of the individual miner. A great deal of effort is now being devoted to this and much could be gained if a satisfactory device could be built to give the total daily integrated exposure at a given place or, even better, if a dosimeter device could be produced which the miner could wear. A type of film badge, utilizing a plastic plate in which α tracks are made visible by etching, has been described and tested in mines.[52,53] Most other devices are based on drawing air through a collector located close to a radiation-sensitivie material, like lithium fluoride, which serves as a thermoluminescent detector.[54] A number of these devices have been tested and none of them is quite satisfactory as yet.[55] The measurement of unattached radioactive atoms is still of interest, although no additional data have been published on work in this country. A new method of making this measurement has been described from the United Kingdom[56] and some actual measurements in mines have been reported in Japan.[57] Although widely variable results have been reported for this measurement, it is hard to see how its significance can really be appraised at the present stage. Other factors of unknown significance, but presently presumed unimportant in mine exposures, are the concentration of long-lived daughters and the intensity of direct γ radiation.

Another approach to the measurement of total individual exposure has been to measure the concentration of one of the longer-lived radon daughters in the body. Most studies have concerned the measurement of lead-210, although polonium-210 also has been looked at. Using material obtained from autopsies, several investigators have analyzed bones for lead-210 and tried to relate these to exposures in terms of working level months as obtained from other measurements.[58-60] There seems little doubt from these data that there is a correlation, although it is not an exact one. One of the factors complicating the relationship is that all lead-210 in the body does not originate from the decay of inhaled radon daughters. Inhaled radon itself is carried by the bloodstream where it decays to lead. Lead is also inhaled directly from the decay of daughter products in air and lead-210 occurs in the mine dust itself.[61-67] In any case, this approach seems very promising, especially where it can be applied *in vivo*. A sensitive method for lead-210 in urine has been reported[65] and urine assay for both lead-210 and polonium-210 has been investigated in uranium miners with somewhat discouraging results.[66] However, this approach is useful only for miners not currently receiving exposure as current exposure complicates the interpretation of bioassay results of urine or blood. On the other hand, the *in vivo* measurement of ^{210}Pb in bone, usually the skull, appears to give a reasonable long-term cumulative indication of past radon and radon daughter exposure.[31,67]

While epidemiologic and dosimetry studies continue, a great deal of useful effort is going into the reduction of exposures in the mines. It has been observed that falling barometric pressure increases the release of radon into the mine as expected.[68] A theoretical study, followed by a practical demonstration, showed that working levels can be significantly reduced by rapid mixing of the air within the working volume.[69,70] Workers at the Bureau of Mines have studied this problem and, in a booklet, have reported on the effects of pressuring, sealing, dilution, filtering, radon removal, and mine planning.[71] The most widely used method at present is dilution ventilation, but this is limited by the high air velocities required in tunnels. Careful planning of mine layout seems likely to be the most helpful technique in new mines. Respirators find some limited application and these have been the object of at least one study.[72] The Bureau of Mines has established a new amendment to Approval Schedule 21B for such respirators.[73] A powered filter respirator also has been developed for use in uranium mines.[74] Much additional work is going on in this field, but the results have not been published as yet. Application of all methods of control is producing a gradual lowering of exposure levels in most mines, but the limits that can be achieved vary from one mine to another. Complete reliance on dilution ventilation alone will be impossible in many mines, and individual exposures must be restricted or new or additional control measures introduced.

At least three problems are related to the handling of tailings from processed uranium ores which accumulate at the mills. These mills are located along waterways, and the tailings contain essentially all of the radium-226 originally present in the ore. In the past, these tailings were the source of considerable radium input to the adjacent water courses, although control practices have reduced greatly the input of radium both from leaching and immediate washoff of tailings into the streambeds. However, it is conceivable that these tailings are still the source of an amount of radium roughly equivalent to that washed in the watersheds (for example, the Colorado River watershed) from natural sources. These piles also emit radon gas and are a potential source of airborne particulates, which offer potential hazards in nearby communities. However, an evaluation of these, as such sources have indicated, that this hazard is minimal.[75,76] Finally, in Grand Junction, Colorado, a tailings pile was used as a source of fill material under and around buildings, and resulted in the accumulation of radon and its daughters. Over 11,000 buildings have been surveyed for external gamma radiation and many of these for radon daughters also, and as a result of these surveys the Surgeon General issued guidelines for remedial action. Based on these guidelines, a remedial program costing about $15 million is underway in which up to 1000 residences may require their tailings removed or their emanation controlled.

ESTIMATION OF EXPOSURE TO EXTERNAL RADIATION

This subject includes exposure to radiation from sources external to the body such as x rays, γ rays, and particulate radiation, principally electrons and neutrons. Under special circumstances, protons and heavier particles also are to be evaluated as external sources but, because of their low penetrating power, α particles are practically never considered a source of external radiation. Judging by the number of publications, this specialty is certainly one of the most active in the whole field of radiation protection, reflecting the heavy emphasis on evaluation and records-keeping in the health physics profession. The needs and problems involved in personnel radiation dosimetry were discussed in a symposium on the subject in 1967, and a summary has been published in *Health Physics.*[77] The introduction of thermoluminescent detectors (TLD) and of the radiophotoluminescent (RPL) detectors several years ago has caused a real change as these replace film badges in many applications. The principles of these detectors were discussed in the previous review in "Industrial Hygiene Highlights."[1] Since that time there have been further advances, especially in the investigation of new substances useful as detectors. Beryllium oxide,[78] strontium fluoride,[79] and aluminum oxide[80] were found useful and many others were screened. Calcium fluoride, calcium sulfate, and lithium fluoride have been incorporated in plastic to make a product capable of fabrication into a wide variety of useful forms.[81] Bibliographies on both TLD[82,83] and RPL[84] have been published. Those on TLD include 678 references and that on RPL include 150, which are in addition to the previous list that contained 253 references.[85] This topic is too large and diverse for a summary and the reader must refer to the literature. Unfortunately, there has been no recent critical review of the subject. Among newer developments are the use of TLD for high-dose-rate dosimetry,[86] for electrons,[87] and for personnel neutron dosimetry.[88] Many installations have switched to TLD in place of films, and descriptions of the complete systems have been described for the National Reactor Testing Station[89] and at Hanford,[90,91] and are used at nuclear power plants.

There are several excellent books summarizing both radiation dosimetry and instrumentation.[92-95] IRCU Report 20 on Radiation Protection Instrumentation and Its Application is both concise and relevant.

Significant, but somewhat fewer, results have been published on work with glass dosimeters using RPL. A system that is recieving increasing attention is thermally stimulated exoelectron emission (TSEE). This is similar to the TLD except that instead of measuring the light emitted when the dosimeter material is heated, emitted electrons are measured. The electrons may be measured with a Geiger tube or similar device. Emission of electrons may be stimulated by light (optical), as well as by by heat, or ultraviolet light may be emitted following optical stimulation.[96] Such detectors can be made very sensitive; they respond differently to particulate radiations of varying linear energy transfer, and they can be made very thin for microdosimetry.[97-101]

Estimation of high-level exposures received as a result of accidents is important, both in planning therapy and in documenting exposure for comparison with clinical observations. A wide variety of systems has been used, including chemical and TLD dosimeters,[102] electron spin resonance in teeth and hair,[103] and direct counting of phosphorus-32 in hair.[104]

Measurement of exposure to neutrons or to high energy particles around accelerators, or in outer space, are extremely difficult because of the complexity of the interactions of such particles with matter, such as tissue. Such measurements usually are outside the field of the industrial hygienist. A manual on neutron protection was recently issued by the National Council on Radiation Protection and Measurements.[105]

NCRP Publication No. 38 summarizes what is known about questions of neutron protection. The measurement of neutrons, however, remains a highly complex and nonroutine problem, especially if the energy-dependent spectral shape is not known. Detection of the presence of neutrons, or estimation of their flux intensity (monitoring) as distinguished from dose measurement, is closer to the industrial hygienist's field. Here, there is still a need for more satisfactory instrumentation.

ESTIMATION OF RADIATION EXPOSURE FROM INTERNAL SOURCES

Radioactive materials may be taken into the body by inhalation, ingestion, or skin penetration through wounds or the intact skin. Their biologic effect then depends on their physical and radioactive properties and also on their residence time in the body, site of deposition, and rate and path of translocation to various organs. Thus, any attempt to predict biologic effects from environmental and personnel measurements requires a detailed knowledge of the radiobiology of the substance absorbed. There are three general methods of estimating such exposure: (a) direct measurement of radiation from the material while present in the body, (b) measurement in excreta, and (c) measurement of concentrations in the environment, such as in food, air, or water. All of these are complex and based on many assumptions that are difficult to confirm. In most cases, the assumptions used necessarily apply to an average or "standard" man and numbers used may diverge considerably from those correct for the individual being studied. ICRP has long relied on a "standard" man[106] for the derivation of secondary exposure limits such as MPC's in air and water. The IRCP is in the process of issuing a new report that includes parameters for "standard" woman and child as well as the discussion of the variation of the physiologic factors that influence dose as a function of age and sex.

At first sight, it may seem that direct measurement involves no assumptions and it is true that this method probably is the most accurate where it can be applied. In this method, an instrument external to the body measures the amount of radiation being emitted from the body and so gives results that can reveal how much radioactive material is deposited in the body. For strong γ emitters and where a single isotope has been deposited the results are excellent, although there are still assumptions about the precise location in the body and the effect of shielding by body tissues. Crystal counters, which have largely replaced liquid scintillation counters for *in vivo* counting, can be used to localize the deposition site and by energy discrimination can provide a γ-ray spectrum of the radioactivity. This permits separate identification of several separate isotopes.

ICRP Publication No. 10 describes maximum permissible body burdens as well as the sensitivity of different systems of analysis for assessing the body burdens. This excellent reference relates to the estimation of occupational exposures following accidental intakes of radionuclides, which is characteristic of the manner in which occupational exposures generally occur.[107] Accordingly, internal body burdens usually take discrete jumps associated with some sort of an accidental or unusual situation, and there is a need to understand the rate of excretion subsequent to an initial measurement. An estimate of the potential dose as the result of a given internally contaminating event to be delivered over the residual expected lifespan of a worker is usually required. In the event that the half-life of the nuclide or the rate of elimination is short, or the rate of elimination from the body is rapid, this represents a dose that will be delivered in a relatively short time, but in the case of long-lived nuclides that are not excreted rapidly from the body, such as ^{239}Pu, an estimate of the potential dose delivered over the estimated residual lifespan should be made. This estimate is called the dose commitment, and is more properly referred to as the estimate of dose commitment.

The greatest need and the most significant advances have been made in the detection and analysis of emitters of low energy γ rays, such as plutonium in lungs. Use of a thin cesium iodide crystal coupled to a thick sodium iodide crystal was reported in 1967.[108] Since then, advances in this technique, which involves pulse shaping, have improved the sensitivity and reduced backgrounds, and although minimum detection levels of 4 nCi have been reported for ^{239}Pu[109] this low a detection limit is not considered reasonable by some investigators.[110] Minimum detection levels on the order of half a lung burden have been reported for ^{239}Pu, but because the x rays from this nuclide are strongly absorbed by the chest walls, the calibration remains a very difficult procedure for this nuclide and the sensitivity varies with the build and geometry of the person being counted. Accordingly, for bulky individuals, minimum detection levels may well exceed the permissible lung burden, which is generally taken as 16 nCi for occupational exposure. For ^{238}Pu, the detection limits are slightly better because of a three-fold greater x ray yield. However, using dual thin crystals for Am-241 1% of a maximum permissible lung burden may be detected.[111]

Proportional counters also have improved and in the United Kingdom and Japan a detection level of 8 nCi has been reported.[112-114] Because of the difficulty of measuring the 17 keV x ray from plutonium-239, the 60 keV radiation from americium-241 is frequently measured, if the ratio of the two isotopes in the parent material is known. A recent study on implanted material indicates that translocation from the implant site causes changes in the ratios of these isotopes.[115] Thus, an error might be introduced in estimating plutonium in organs resulting from a contaminated wound. For pure β emitters like strontium-90, measurement of bremsstrahlung can be used to detect body

burdens of about 30 nCi.[116] Simplified whole-body counters for more penetrating radiation, using shielded chairs[117,118] and a rotating unit for localization
of deposition, have been found useful.[119]

Whole-body counters are bulky and expensive and their use is limited to
certain materials and conditions. Most estimation of exposure to internal sources
is done by the analysis of excreta, particularly urine. This involves the use of
some type of mathematical model, if the urinary excretion rate is to be related
to the amount of material resident in specific tissues and organs.[120,121] Such
models must include assumptions about rates of transfer from respiratory tract
to blood by various routes and rates of transfer from one organ to another and
from blood to kidney to urine. Specific data on these, where available, have been
published by the ICRP[122] and this compendium is useful but illustrative of the
difficulties and gaps in required information. It is especially hazardous to
estimate lung exposures from urinary excretion data, particularly for insoluble
materials. Analysis of feces is more useful as an indication of such exposure but
is seldom of quantitative value. The use of lung and whole-body counters has
revealed the serious errors of such calculations from excretion data.[123-127]
However, urine assay is still very valuable as an indication of exposure and, as
such, it will continue to be used widely. In the use of urine assay, particularly
for long-lived α emitters, it is necessary to use extreme caution in the
interpretation of results since apparent excretion rates may be influenced by
many factors such as metabolic changes, contamination, sample collection
methods, and fluid intake.[128]

Lafuma *et al.* have pointed out that the presence of plutonium in the urine
reflects only its transport from one site in the body to another, so that much
additional data are needed in order to interpret this in terms of body burden. On
the other hand, if long-term measurements in the urine are available, then this
will allow one to make an assessment, for example, following an inhalation
accident, of the cumulative fraction that has been mobilized from lung to
bone.[129]

Accumulation of long-lived emitters in the body is usually the result of a
series of acute exposures rather than continuous chronic exposure, since most
operations involving these materials are carried out in almost completely closed
systems. Analysis of tissue samples available at autopsy is the only way in which
present methods of estimating deposition can be checked. Some data of this
nature already have been published and a U.S. Transuranium Registry has been
organized and funded to see that such information is obtained and made
available.[125,130,131] It is apparent that most interest has centered on the long-lived
α emitters, particularly plutonium-239, and, more recently, plutonium-238. Data
are still needed on any human exposure cases, such as the 27-day effective chest
half-time reported for seven persons exposed to ruthenium-103.[132] Obviously,
this field is closely related to radiobiology and results on animal data are
reported in that section.

The use of urine assay for the quantitative assessment of exposure to tritium oxide always has been considered the most successful application of this technique. Since the tritium is presumably in the body water and this is identical to the water in the urine, the urine assay is effectively a measure of a sample of the body. A most efficient sampling program for tritium in urine has recently been described.[132a] Recently, some concern has been expressed over the possibility of tritium entering into organic molecules where it may remain longer than the normal turnover time of body water. Measurements on deer living near a source of small amounts of tritium contamination suggest that there may, indeed, be some possibility of this, although the deviations are quite small.[133] This also should show up as a long component at the end of an excretion curve following tritium exposure.

However, for purposes of calculating radiation dose from tritium excretion data, it is assumed that the hydrogen in the body is uniformly labeled, so that a dose to the whole body is usually calculated, a procedure that overestimates the real whole-body dose. Analyses of several workers heavily contaminated have shown that the dose associated with the long-term excretion, presumably due to labeling of organic compounds with lives in the body much longer than that of body water, tends to deliver a very small percentage of the total dose.[107]

The estimation of exposure by means of environmental measurements, particularly the analysis of air samples, is almost universally used and such data usually are combined with urine assay data to produce the best estimate of exposure. However, air sampling is more closely related to monitoring or the determination of the probable upper limits of inhalation of radioactive materials. It also is closely related to the evaluation of the control system designed to prevent the release of material into the air. For these reasons, this topic is covered in the section on Hazard Evaluation. It should be remembered that the primary value of any measure or estimation of exposure, external or internal, is as a check on the control system.

HAZARD EVALUATION

Evaluation of radiation hazards is closely related to exposure estimation as previously discussed. This section deals largely with measurements in the working environment rather than laboratory studies. Measurements in or on people comprise a part, but only a part, of the evaluation process. Frequently in a single installation, a wide variety of exposure types is encountered and sometimes these are combined in a single operation. Thus, in processing the transplutonium elements operators are exposed to α, β, γ, and neutron radiation, including both internal and external exposures to materials emitting these. Interest in such materials continues to grow and the problems involved have been described in reports on two installations.[134,135] One of these materials is californium-252, which emits neutrons by spontaneous fission. This isotope then can be fabricated into a compact neutron source, useful in many applications, including therapy. Formulas for dose rate, as a function of distance and attenuation by absorbers, have been worked out for users.[136]

External radiation problems continue to arise, some from old operations or some from those which are new or newly studied. x Rays have been used for a long time for analyzing materials for various elements and this application is increasing with thousands of units in use in this country. A survey of experiences with the units indicates that overexposures and injuries continue to happen.[137-139] In fact, such operations constitute a major source of acute radiation injuries as distinct from overexposures. These exposures generally tend to be highly local, although they may be quite serious and result in the amputation or loss of digits or limbs. Very high-intensity pulsed x ray machines have been in use in research organizations for nearly 10 years, and now they are being used in industry to take flash x ray photographs. These present unique problems in measuring radiation intensity in the working area and in the design of shielding and other protection.[140] Television receivers have been noted as an x ray source but this is largely a problem of consumer exposure. This problem has been largely eliminated by the setting of standards by FDA and as a result of the 1969 Radiation Control for Health and Safety (Electronics Product) Act. However, large television projectors may be a serious source of radiation to their operators.[141] Evaluation of this hazard is straightforward but its presence may be overlooked. Another easily neglected source of radiation comes from adhesive tapes frequently used to hold objects being irradiated for neutron activation. The presence of trace materials can cause emission of appreciable induced radiation and varies considerably among various brands and types of tape.[142]

Combinations of various types of exposure are not uncommon even in relatively simple operations. As tritium has been substituted for radium in luminous dial painting, the degree of hazard from this operation has decreased considerably. However, it has not disappeared entirely and relatively few reports are available on studies of this operation. In one published report, it was noted that the most serious route of tritium into the operator is via the intact skin and that no satisfactory protective gloves are presently available.[143] Another new application of radioactive materials is as ionization sources in detectors in chromatographs. Some of these emit appreciable radiation when removed from the apparatus for repair, while others lose radioactive material into the work area.[144] A long-used method of evaluating certain hazards from radium sources is leak-testing but there are various methods of performing this test, all not equally reliable. A comparative study of eight test methods showed the charcoal method to be best and only four of the methods had the required sensitivity.[145] While this seems perfectly straightforward and much like evaluating chemical hazards, it has its own difficulties. Since the effects of inhaled radioactive materials are only apparent after long periods and since such effects are never trivial or reversible, a high degree of reliability is required. It is seldom sufficient to collect occasional air samples using a survey technique and, hence, samplers must run continuously at appropriate locations, if indeed they are required at all. The International Commission on Radiological Protection has issued a guide on monitoring the workplace which gives some suggestions on where air sampling is actually required.[146] This guide suggests that surface monitoring may be sufficient in many areas.

Surface monitoring is another technique of hazard evaluation which is seldom discussed in the literature since it appears so simple. Reports on the significance of surface monitoring and on correlation of its results with other techniques would be welcome and valuable. By means of a simple (or complex) instrument for detecting the presence of radioactive contamination on floors, furniture, or other surfaces, a great deal can be learned concerning the potentiality of an internal hazard. Except in the case of strong γ-emitting material, the mere presence of radioactive material on a surface does not present a hazard. However, the unexpected detection of such material is an indication of a failure of control methods and the material may have deposited from air or can be resuspended into the air. Thus, there is a close connection between airborne material and surface deposits. Surface monitoring usually is simple and, in the complete absence of surface contamination, an airborne hazard is unlikely. Where very hazardous material is handled, both air and surface monitoring is required.

Plutonium is an α emitter and any instrument for detecting its presence, based on this α-ray emission, must be held very close to the surface or the plutonium will not be noticed. The presence of a film of oil or water will completely block the α radiation and the deposit will escape detection. If in addition to detection it is desired to estimate the quantity present, accurate measurement of the α radiation for this purpose is nearly impossible. This was the situation that confronted the surveyors following the crash of a bomb-carrying Air Force plane near Thule AFB in Greenland in January 1968. Plutonium was scattered on the ice in a mixture of gasoline, snow, and ice. Fortunately, a newly developed meter capable of detecting low energy x rays was made available when the use of α survey meters proved impracticable under the difficult circumstances.[147] Plutonium and americium emit small quantities of such radiation, as do most α emitters, and this radiation will penetrate oil, water, and such materials. This type of meter has since proven useful in many applications.

Where air sampling is used for routine hazard evaluation, many samplers are often used and the amount of data requiring evaluation is enormous. Computers and automation have been used in an attempt to cope with this and several systems have been described.[148-149] These do not solve the basic problem since they only assist in collecting, processing, and storing data and do not give much aid in the interpretation of the assembled data. For this, more than concentration measurements are required. Workers in the United Kingdom atomic energy establishments have particularly advanced in studying all phases of the problem including particle size, presence of dominant particles, data from personal samplers, and other measurements. Reports of their work are covered in descriptions of the air-sampling programs at various locations.[150] and in several papers describing special techniques.[151-154] Descriptions of air-sampling systems and techniques of other countries and installations are described in proceedings of a symposium on Assessment of Airborne Radioactivity convened by the International Atomic Energy Agency in 1967.[149]

Some very sophisticated sampling devices have been developed.[155] Nevertheless, developments in this field are somewhat disappointing in view of the intense interest prevailing in recent years. Most emphasis is still on hardware and not enough on the interpretation of results or on defining the information required. It seems reasonable to expect that careful statistical treatment of data could lead to the collection of fewer but more significant samples. The large amounts of accumulated data are a challenge to the industrial hygienist. The results of developing a method of handling these data also should be of great value in the evaluation of airborne chemical hazards such as coal, silica, lead, beryllium, and others.

Tritium is a separate problem since it is gaseous rather than particulate. Available air-monitoring instruments are mostly flow-through ionization chambers and are not specific for tritium. By means of filters, ion traps, and compensating ion chambers, most interfering sources, except radioactive gases, can be eliminated. High sensitivity can be obtained, if necessary, by the use of large ion chambers. There have been no outstanding developments in this area.

In the case of tritium, however, assay urine remains a highly sensitive and reliable means of estimating exposure once it has occurred. Radioiodine is still sampled by means of adsorption on charcoal with few recent improvements reported.

The expansion in number and type of nuclear facilities was examined in the first part of this chapter. Power reactors were identified as potentially the most numerous and the major type of occupational exposure is most likely external rather than internal. Accordingly, control of the major part of occupational exposure is exercised by the traditional use of time, distance, and shielding once the external fields have been properly determined with instrumentation.

However, that part of the fuel cycle where fuel is processed, fabricated, or reprocessed will provide abundant opportunity for internal exposure to long-lived α-emitting members of the actinide elements, such as uranium, thorium, and plutonium. Fortunately, a remarkable book has just been published which comprehensively reviews the occupational hygiene aspects of all but thorium.[19] "The Handbook of Experimental Pharmacology" has five chapters particularly germane, and because of their relevance they are listed here: Chapter 5, Uranium: Protection Criteria; Chapter 6, Environmental Monitoring and Personnel Protection in Uranium Processing; Chapter 7, Uranium Mining Hazards; Chapter 12, Maximum Permissible Body Burdens and Concentrations of Plutonium: Biologic Basis and History of Development; and Chapter 14, Plutonium: Industrial Hygiene, Health Physics, and Related Aspects.

The industrial hygiene aspects of thorium are discussed comprehensively in an AIHA monograph by Albert.[155a]

HANDLING OF RADIOACTIVE WASTES

Liquid and solid wastes are created whenever radioactive materials are produced or processed and the amount of radioactivity per pound of waste varies widely. While numerous methods of handling, storage, and disposal are used in dealing with these wastes, nothing can be done to increase the rate at which the radioactivity diminishes. These rates vary from half-times of minutes to thousands of years and, thus, the problems created are varied. While the prospects of disposing of plutonium wastes having a half-life of 25,000 years seems incredibly difficult even to consider, it should not be forgotten that such stable materials as lead, mercury, arsenic, and cadmium have infinite life-times and we are beginning to face this implication. Reactors of all sorts generate enormous quantities of highly active wastes, and the future of nuclear power may be dependent on the solution of the waste disposal problem.

The concept of storage of highly active wastes in excavated salt formations deep underground appears to be the most attractive one at present,[156] although plans for such a facility in a specific salt mine were abandoned by the Atomic Energy Commission due to the presence of nearby human activities that might tend to compromise the integrity of the local salt formation. These are naturally dry, stable, unaffected by radiation, and located in areas of little seismic activity. They are also capable of dissipating the heat emitted as a result of radioactivity.

Gaseous or airborne wastes are more likely to concern the industrial hygienist who deals with similar air-cleaning processes for nonradioactive materials. For particulates, filtration is still used almost exclusively. High-efficiency air filters are not a recent development for this purpose, but there has been increased attention given to assuring the integrity of filter systems. Testing of filter systems "in place" after installation and at periodic intervals is a necessity in systems where efficiencies of 99.9% and higher are a requirement. Leaks in and around filters must be detected and repaired, especially where plutonium is handled. Filter banks in series are now being used to a degree almost unheard of a few years ago. Partly, this resulted from a disastrous fire in a plutonium facility which directed attention to the possibilities inherent in the loss of a single filter bank. Methods of protecting filters from fire, heat, and shock are under study. Tighter restrictions on emission limits are forcing attention on containment, recycling, total enclosure, and modification of processes to reduce airborne wastes. Recirculation of room air, which is anathema to the industrial hygienist, may be reconsidered when the air-cleaning system consists of double or triple filtration with 99.9% efficiency at each filter stage.

Gases such as tritium, krypton, and xenon still pose serious problems of removal, and research is being done on these problems. In 1968, the International Atomic Energy Agency sponsored a symposium, Treatment of Airborne Radioactive Wastes, and the proceedings of this symposium are now available as a source of much detailed information.[157] The U.S. Atomic Energy Commission and the Harvard Air Cleaning Laboratory sponsor periodic air-cleaning conferences and proceedings of these also are available.[158] The high-efficiency filter remains the mainstay of air cleaning in nuclear installations and much experience and data on such systems have been accumulated.[159] For radioiodine, activated charcoal filters usually are used and their efficiencies are tested with radioiodine. A recent paper suggests that the efficiency decreases at low iodine concentrations and, hence, filters should be tested using the same total iodine concentration that they are expected to encounter in service.[160] A manual on the "Management of Radioactive Wastes at Nuclear Power Plants," based on worldwide experience, has been published by the International Atomic Energy Agency.[161]

RADIOBIOLOGY

Radiobiology is a very large field and bears much the same relation to radiation protection as toxicology and pharmacology do to protection against chemical agents. As in the latter case, only a small part of the field of radiobiology is of concern to the industrial hygienist. The greatest need is for information on tissue distributions and effects following inhalation, and there are comparatively few such studies reported, but those that are available provide excellent information. A second need is for information on effects following wounds that may be simulated by subcutaneous administration. Studies following intravenous injection must be applied cautiously in relation to actual exposure situations or standards setting.

A considerable variety of radionuclides have been subject to radiobiologic investigation, because radioactive isotopes of almost every element can be produced by neutron activation, fission, or charged particle interactions. Accordingly, discussion of their effects is facilitated by considering important radioelements or groups in the periodic table.

Stannard has recently published an excellent concise review of the "Toxicology of Radionuclides"[162] relevant to human occupational exposure as well as being an editor of a remarkable 995-page "Handbook on Pharmacology,"[19] which comprehensively summarizes the known literature on uranium, plutonium, and the transplutonium elements. A shorter treatment of the metabolism of Pu and the actinides is given by ICRP[163] and a recent symposium on the radiobiology of Pu is available.[163a]

A classic report by Evans and his colleagues summarized the continuing results of follow-up studies of radium-burdened people.[164] This group of occupationally exposed people continues to furnish the basic evidence for the adoption of the radiation standards for radium and by analogy all bone seekers. More work on this group is continuing at Argonne National Laboratory.[165]

The late effects of ionizing radiation are discussed in a book and symposium.[166,167]

The biologic behavior of several nuclides was briefly described in the last edition of this chapter.[168-186] These included the rare earths, the alkaline metal Cs-137, radioiodine, radiostrontium, Zr-95, mercury, uranium, and plutonium.

Little additional information of use to the industrial hygienist is available with respect to radiobiologic effects of external radiation sources. The fact that such radiation produces detectable chromosome aberrations is being studied as a possible early indication of radiation damage.[187] It can be useful in detecting moderate or high exposures to γ rays and neutrons.

MEDICAL ASPECTS

No attempt is made to review the medical literature in relation to the effects, uses, and other aspects of ionizing radiation. There have been no outstanding changes in the methods of treating cases of radiation exposure, but more physicians are now trained in the field. Even in an installation where high levels of radiation can be encountered, the occupational physician finds that almost all of his work deals with nonradiation problems,[188] unless he also directs the preventive programs of health physics and radiation protection. In such installations, training and preparation for the possibility of serious radiation accidents are required but, fortunately, seldom used. Where radiation is only one hazard among many others, there is apt to be more stress on its importance than can be justified in a balanced program. To quote from a physician of a large university, "There are valid reasons for a physical examination program in the practice of modern preventive medicine but there is no specific reason why radiation exposure, when there is good environmental control, should be used as the excuse for initiating and continuing such a program."[189] The International Atomic Energy Agency has prepared a manual on "Medical Supervision of Radiation Workers."[190] It is a useful handbook for physicians in a nuclear energy industry, but only a very small fraction of the manual is devoted to medical aspects. Even there the topics covered relate to conditions that would be encountered extremely rarely.

Fortunately, there have been relatively few major radiation accidents recently where serious clinical cases demand the best in medical care and also add to the knowledge of effects of severe overexposure. Nor have there been any reports of drugs or chemicals useful in mitigating the serious course of illness from radiation exposure. Chelating agents are still used in certain cases for the accidental intake of radioactive materials. DTPA administered to dogs following inhalation of the oxides of cerium-144 and praseodynium-144 reduced the amount retained in the body as compared with controls.[191] A study on rats given plutonium oxide and DTPA intraperitoneally showed diminished phagocytic action with DTPA, suggesting a possibly adverse effect on lung clearance if DTPA is used following inhalation exposure.[192] A study of DTPA effects following implantation of plutonium and americium oxides subcutaneously in dogs revealed a reduction in body retention of the americium but little effect on the plutonium.[193] Further work is still needed in this field to assist the physician in planning therapy.

An alternative procedure in inhalation cases is suggested by experiments on rats[183] and on dogs[194] using lavage or saline washing of the lungs following inhalation of plutonium oxide dust. The animals tolerated the treatment well and the authors suggest its possible therapeutic use, although no one has applied it to humans as yet.

The physician is often called on to testify in workmen's compensation cases on the question of whether radiation was the cause of a disease of the claimant. Sagan, after reviewing all the complicating factors involved in such a judgment, concludes "that often no witness, or group of witnesses, no matter how sagacious, can offer any but highly arbitrary judgments."[195] Medicolegal problems in radiation cases remain very difficult to handle.

INSTRUMENTATION

Instruments used in detecting and controlling ionizing radiation are extremely varied and many of them are built by electronic specialists closely associated with the health physicist. Many of these are built to supply a special need such as monitoring a waste stream or checking the air around a specific operation. Most instruments have already been discussed in previous sections of this review. There are no specifically new developments in instrumentation but only gradual changes and improvements. There is increasing use of solid-state, semiconductor detectors since these lend themselves well to energy discrimination with the consequent screening out of unwanted background. It is interesting to note that improvements are still being made in the simple Geiger tube instrument, which is hand carried and used for the measurement of γ-ray intensity.[196] For x rays, a liquid-filled tissue equivalent ionization chamber has been developed which has many applications.[197]

Instrumentation has always been a highly developed aspect of radiation protection, and maintenance is a continual need. In estimating the costs of the protection program, this maintenance factor must not be overlooked. The detection and measurement of radiation lends itself so well to amplification, energy discrimination, alarm systems, and all forms of automation that there is a real temptation to overdo the use of these devices in the interests of "saving manpower." The result is often having trained men waiting for equipment repairs or doing it themselves. This can be very costly.

CONTROL METHODS

In contrast to other branches of industrial hygiene, the literature dealing with radiation protection contains relatively little on control measures and equipment. Design of shielding, glove boxes, hot cells, ventilation, remote handling equipment, etc., generally is considered the responsibility of other professions. In large measure, this is because of the complexity involved. The field of ionization chambers, Geiger counters, spectrometers, scintillometers, and similar electronic equipment is intricate enough and far removed from remote manipulators, exhaust blowers, and periscopes. Shielding is often designed by specialists in this aspect of the radiation protection field. Many health physicists actually do considerable work in shielding design using penetration tables from various sources, but such work is not usually reported in the literature since it seems relatively simple. Occasionally, the existing tables are more complex than is desirable for shielding to serve in simple installation and then measurements are made and reported on common materials of construction.[198] Shielding is a serious problem around all types of high energy accelerators and the complexity of the calculations involved is well illustrated in one of the very few articles on this subject in *Health Physics*.[199]

A common method of working with γ-emitting isotopes is behind a shielding wall with an open top. This is an economical design, but consideration must be given of possible exposure from radiation scattered by air or other materials above the cell. The necessary calculations to predict this scatter are given in an article by Birchall who, significantly, is from a department of mechanical engineering.[200] The sole article on ventilation was an interesting description of a system used to permit repair of a reactor vessel without the uses of bulky protective equipment.[201] The International Atomic Energy Agency has published a "Manual on Safety Aspects of the Design and Equipment of Hot Laboratories," which contains descriptions of many important features of such equipment.[202]

RADIATION UNITS, STANDARDS, REGULATIONS, AND GUIDES

For purposes of radiation protection control, the unit of dose equivalence (H) is called the rem and is defined by ICRU as the product of the absorbed dose (D) in rads, the quality factor (Q), and other dose-modifying factors (N). As a practical matter, Q is defined soley in terms of the linear energy transfer, as follows:

$keV/\mu m$	Q
3.5 or less	1
7	2
23	5
53	10
175	20

In tissues, most β- and γ-radiation have $Q = 1$ and α-radiation $Q = 10$. For bone-seeking α-emitting radionuclides other than radium, N is conventionally taken as 5 to take into account the potential increased toxicity from less uniform distribution than radium.

It is improper to use the rem as a unit to express radiobiologic effect since it has a reasonably rigorous definition. Unfortunately, this distinction is not always observed, as was the case for the recent National Academy of Sciences BEIR report. The choice of Q and N is guided, however, by the results of biologic experiments so that there is an approximate adjustment made to weigh radiation doses to more nearly reflect their relative biologic importances. Still, for radiobiologic work the radiobiologic effectiveness of two types of radiation depend on the dose, sometimes dose rate, species under study, and biologic endpoint under consideration.

The question of the adequacy of the occupational dose limits has been addressed in recent years by ICRP. The commission observed that the major risk was that of a potentially increased probability of the development of malignancy late in life. Sowby has calculated that this is equivalent to a 0.6% risk of malignancy from a 40-year occupational exposure to 1 rem/year (about 20% of annual ICRP and NCRP occupational dose limit). The present risk of death from malignancy as compared to all other causes is roughly 1 in 6 in the United States, although the chance of experiencing a malignancy is higher. That occupational exposure regimen would then lead to an increase of less than 4% in the probability of developing a malignancy. At the dose limits this would be less than 20%. The latter figure may not sound very reassuring, but it should be borne in mind that a great deal of conservatism is built into the risk estimates, which are mostly based on considerations of exposures to much higher doses delivered very rapidly.

One of the recommendations of ICRP and NCRP has been, in addition to dose limits, that exposures be kept as low as practicable. This recommendation has been the source of much controversy and confusion in the United States, especially with regard to exposure of the public. Most of this controversy has not directly involved the industrial hygienist since it has focused on exposure of the public rather than the worker. Nevertheless, the industrial hygienist is interested and affected, since this concept is now being applied to occupational exposure. It should be recognized that the establishment of a permissible level for exposure of the public or worker is not solely a scientific procedure. This does not mean that it is unscientific, but only that value judgments enter which are correctly based on more concerns than scientific. The scientists can supply information on the effects or risks of various levels of radiation exposure, at least where such information is obtainable. Scientists and economists may estimate the values of the benefits from the use of radiation requiring various levels of exposure. Ultimately only the public can decide where the risks are commensurate with the gains. For this, education and debate are necessary. Fortunately, the ICRP has recently published an explanation of its recommendations that radiation exposure be kept as low as readily achievable along with suggestions about the manner in which to make assessments of costs and benefits.[202a] Another example of the serious problems of benefit versus risk is given by Morgan in a discussion of medical use of radiation.[203]

It is appropriate to list here the various standards-making agencies and organizations and their functions. A more extensive treatment is available elsewhere.

The International Commission on Radiological Protection has been the world's principal scientific standards-setting group in the field of radiation protection. It operates through subcommittees that include about 50 of the world's leaders in their fields and the Commission adopts and publishes its recommendations. Although their recommendations have no legal status, they have served as the basis for radiation protection legislation and standards throughout the world. Their publications salient to occupational protection are: Publication No. 2, "Permissible Dose for Internal Radiation"; No. 5, "The Handling and Disposal of Radioactive Materials in Hospitals and Medical Research Establishments"; No. 8, "The Evaluation of Risks from Radiation"; No. 9, "Recommendations of the ICRP" (adopted September 17, 1965); No. 10, "Evaluation of Radiation Doses to Body Tissues from Internal Contamination Due to Occupational Exposure"; No. 10a, "The Assessment of Internal Contamination Resulting from Recurrent or Prolonged Uptake"; No. 11, "A Review of the Radiosensitivity of the Tissues in Bone"; No. 12, "General Principles of Monitoring for Radiation Protection of Workers"; No. 14, "Radiosensitivity and Spatial Distribution of Dose"; No. 15, "Protection Against Ionizing Radiation from External Sources"; No. 18, "The RBE for High LET-Radiations with Respect to Mutagenesis"; No. 19, "The Metabolism of Compounds of Plutonium and other Actinides"; No. 20, "Alkaline Earth Metabolism in Adult Man"; No. 21, "Data for Protection Against Ionizing Radiation from External Sources; Supplement to ICRP Publication No. 15"; No. 22, "Implications of Commission Recommendations that Doses Be Kept As Low As Readily Achievable."

The National Council of Radiation Protection and Measurement is the United States analogue of ICRP, but exists under Congressional charter. Its recommendations are generally consistent with (although independent of) those of ICRP and generally serve as the basis for regulations adopted by official organizations in this country. Its basic dose limit recommendations and philosophy of radiation protection are embodied in NCRP Report 39, entitled "Basic Radiation Protection Criteria."[204] Their dose-limiting recommendations are summarized in Table III.

The Federal Radiation Council (FRC), whose functions have been absorbed into the Environmental Protection Agency, was organized to establish "guidance for all Federal agencies in the formulation of radiation standards. . . ." Their series of reports dealt primarily with environmental exposure. However, they did adopt essentially the NCRP limits for occupational exposure. Only one FRC report (No. 8) deals solely with occupational exposure. (See earlier section on uranium mining.)

The Atomic Energy Commission is not basically a standard-setting agency, although it has the responsibility for ensuring the safe development of the atomic industry. The Commission's radiation protection regulations are issued in the Code of Federal Regulations (10CFR20) and are based on NCRP, FRC, and EPA guidance. These go beyond the numerical limits to prescribe the technical and administrative means to determine whether standards are being met.

The American National Standards Institute (ANSI) develops consensus standards in radiation protection through its N-13 Committee. Members represent organizations that are industrial, private, or governmental. These

TABLE III

Dose-Limiting Recommendations

Maximum permissible dose equivalent for occupational exposure	
Combined whole body occupational exposure	
Prospective annual limit	5 rems in any one year
Retrospective annual limit	10–15 rems in any one year
Long-term accumulation to age N years	$(N - 18)$ ×5 rems
Skin	15 rems in any one year
Hands	75 rems in any one year (25/qtr)
Forearms	30 rems in any one year (10/qtr)
Other organs, tissues and organ systems	15 rems in any one year (5/qtr)
Fertile women (with respect to fetus)	0.5 rem in gestation period
Dose limits for the public, or occasionally exposed individuals	
Individual or occasional	0.5 rem in any one year
Students	0.1 rem in any one year
Population dose limits	
Genetic	0.17 rem average per year
Somatic	0.17 rem average per year
Emergency dose limits—life saving	
Individual (older than 45 years if possible)	100 rems
Hands and forearms	200 rems, additional (300 rems, total)
Emergency dose limits—less urgent	
Individual	25 rems
Hands and forearms	100 rems, total
Family of radioactive patients	
Individual (under age 45)	0.5 rem in any one year
Individual (over age 45)	5 rems in any one year

standards rely on numerical and policy guidance from NCRP and ICRP and serve the function of interfacing the application of their basic recommendation to the practical circumstances of engineering design and radiation protection practice.

The Department of Health, Education, and Welfare still has some responsibilities in radiation protection. The Radiation Control for Health and Safety Act of 1968 is designed to protect the public from unnecessary exposure to harmful radiation from "electronic products." This is consumer protection legislation and affects the industrial hygienist only if he also is concerned with product liability or as a member of the public. The law covers all forms of both ionizing and nonionizing radiation, including sound, and has had the effect of stimulating interest in developing standards for nonionizing radiation.

Activity in the field of ionizing radiation of interest to the industrial hygienist is too great to summarize in any single review or even a single book. It is hoped that this review will stimulate interest in further reading, and that the references may be a helpful introduction. To end, several additional general texts are recommended to the reader.[205-208,11]

REFERENCES

1. Schulte, H. F., Ionizing radiation. *In* "Industrial Hygiene Highlights" (L. V. Cralley, L. J. Cralley, and G. D. Clayton, eds.), p. 118. Industrial Hygiene Foundation of America, Pittsburgh, Pennsylvania, 1968.
2. Constitution of the International Radiation Protection Association (IRPA). *Health Phys. 14,* 59 (1968).
3. Snyder, W. S., Abee, H. H., Burton, L. K., Manshart, R., Benco, A., Duhamel, F., and Wheatley, B. M., eds., "Proceedings of the First International Congress of Radiation Protection, Rome 1966," Vols. 1 and 2. Pergamon, Oxford, 1968.
4. Second International Congress of the International Radiation Protection Association, Abstracts of Papers. *Health Phys. 19,* 67 (1970).
5. Letavet, A. A., and Kurlyandskaya, E. B., eds., "The Toxicology of Radioactive Substances." Pergamon, Oxford, 1970.
6. "Understanding the Atom" Series. Div. Tech. Inform., U.S. At. Energy Comm., Washington, D.C. [A single copy of any one booklet may be obtained from USAEC, Oak Ridge, Tennessee.]
7. Reports of the United Nations Scientific Committee on the Effects of Atomic Radiation, New York, 1958, 1962, 1964, 1966, 1969, 1973.
8. "Radioecological Concentration Processes," Proc. Int. Symp., 1966. Oxford Univ. Press, London and New York, 1967.
9. "Symposium on Radioecology," Proc. 2nd Nat. Symp., 1967, U.S. At. Energy Comm., CONF-670503, 1969.
10. "Radioecology," Proc. 3rd Nat. Symp., 1971. 1973.
11. Eisenbud, M., "Environmental Radioactivity," 2nd. ed. Academic Press, New York, 1973.
12. Clemente, G. F., Direct methods used at the Casaccia Nuclear Centre to assess body burdens. *In* "Assessment of Radioactive Contamination in Man," IAEA Symp., STI/PUB/290, p. 337. IAEA, Vienna, 1972.
13. U.S. Department of Health, Education and Welfare, "Survey of the Use of Radionuclides in Medicine," BRH/DMRE 70–1. USDHEW, Washington, D.C., 1970.
14. Nelson, N., Some biological effects of radiation in relation to other environmental agents. *AEC Symp. Ser. 16* (1969).
15. National Council on Radiation Protection and Measurements, "Basic Radiation Protection Criteria," Rep. No. 39. NCRP, Washington, D.C., 1971.
16. U.S. Atomic Energy Commission, "USAEC News Release," Vol. 5, No. 16. USAEC, Washington, D.C., 1974.
17. U.S. Atomic Energy Commission, "Annual Report to Congress, 1973," Vol. 2. USAEC, Washington, D.C., 1973.
18. International Atomic Energy Agency, Safe handling of plutonium, STI/PUB/358. *Saf. Ser., Int. At. Energy Ag. 39* (1974).

19. Hodge, H. C., Stannard, J. N., and Hursh, J. B., eds., "Handbuch der experimentellen Pharmakologie," Vol. 36. Springer-Verlag, Berlin and New York, 1973.

19a. Ross, D. M., *In* "A Statistical Summary of USAEC Contractors Exposure Experience 1955–67" in Diagnosis and Treatment of Deposited Radionuclides (H. A. Kornberg and W. D. Norwood, eds.). Excerpta Med. Found., Amsterdam, Netherlands, pp. 427–434 (1968).

19b. Ross, D. M., personal communication.

20. "Peaceful Uses of Nuclear Energy," Speeches by Glenn T. Seaborg. U.S. At. Energy Comm., Washington, D.C., 1970. [Available from Div. Tech. Inform. Extension, USAEC, Oak Ridge, Tennessee, 1970.]

21. Special Issue of Health Physics Dedicated to Duncan Holaday. *Health Phys. 16,* 545 (1969).

22. Holaday, D. A., History of the exposure of miners to radon. *Health Phys. 16,* 547 (1969).

23. Behounek, F., History of the exposure of miners to radon. *Health Phys. 19,* 56 (1970).

24. Evans, R. D., Engineers guide to the elementary behavior of radon daughters. *Health Phys. 17,* 229 (1969).

25. Morken, D. A., The relation of lung dose rate to working level. *Health Phys. 16,* 796 (1969).

26. Tompkins, P. C., Problems involved in setting basic guidance for radiological protection. *Amer. J. Pub. Health 59,* 305 (1969).

27. Federal Radiation Council, "Guidance for the Control of Radiation Hazards in Uranium Mining" (Staff Report of FRC). Rep. No. 8, revised. FRC, Washington, D.C., 1967.

28. Archer, V. E., Wagoner, J. K., and Lundin, F. E., Jr., Lung cancer among uranium miners in the United States. *Health Phys. 25,* 351–371 (1973).

29. Lundin, F. E., Jr., Wagoner, J. K., and Archer, V. E., "Radon Daughter Exposure and Respiratory Cancer: Quantitative and Temporal Aspects," NIEHS–NIOSH Joint Monogr. No. 1. Public Health Service, U.S. Dept. of Health, Education and Welfare, Washington, D.C., 1971.

30. Lundin, F. E., Jr., Lloyd, J. W., Smith, E. M., Archer, V. E., and Holaday, D. A., Mortality of uranium miners in relation to radiation exposure, hard rock mining and cigarette smoking, 1950 through Sept. 1967. *Health Phys. 16,* 571 (1969).

31. Wrenn, M. E., Cohen, N., Rosen, J. C., Eisenbud, M., and Blanchard, R. L., *In vivo* measurement of lead-210 in man. *In* "Assessment of Radioactive Contamination in Men," IAEA Symp. STI/PUB/290, 145ff. IAEA, Vienna, 1972.

32. Saccomonno, G., "Uranium Miners Health in Radiation Standards for Uranium Mining," Hearings before the subcommittee on Research, Development and Radiation of the JCAE Congress at U.S., 1969, Part I, pp. 301–315.

33. Bair, W. T., Inhalation of radionuclides and carcinogenesis. *Symp. Ser., Int. At. Energy Ag. 18* (1970).

34. Boyd, J. T., Doll, R., Faulds, J. S., and Leiper, J. Cancer of the lung in iron ore (haematite) miners. *Brit. J. Ind. Med. 27,* 97 (1970).

35. Duggan, M. J., Soilleux, P. J., Strong, J. C., and Howell, D. M., The exposure of United Kingdom miners to radon. *Brit. J. Ind. Med. 27,* 106 (1970).

36. Altshuler, B., Nelson, N., and Kuschner, M., Estimation of the lung tissue dose from inhalation of radon and daughters. *Health Phys. 10,* 1137 (1964).

37. Jacobi, W., The dose to the human respiratory tract by inhalation of short lived radon-22 decay products. *Health Phys. 10,* 1196 (1964).

37a. Haque, A. K. M., and Collinson, A. J. L., Radiation dose to the respiratory system due to radon and its daughter products. *Health Phys. 13,* 431–443 (1967).

37b. National Academy of Sciences–National Research Council, "The Effects on Populations of Exposure to Low Levels of Ionizing Radiation" (Report of the Advisory Committee on the Biological Effects of Ionizing Radiation). NAS–NRC, Washington, D.C., 1972.

37c. Parker, H. M., The dilemma of lung dosimetry. *Health Phys. 16,* 553 (1969).

38. Raabe, O. G., The adsorption of radon daughters to some polydisperse submicron polystyrene aerosols. *Health Phys. 14,* 397 (1968).

39. Raabe, O. G., Concerning the interaction that occur between radon decay products and aerosols. *Health Phys. 17,* 177 (1969).

40. Holleman, D. F., Martz, D. E., and Schiager, K. J., Total respiratory deposition of radon daughters from inhalation of uranium mine atmospheres. *Health Phys. 17,* 187 (1969).

41. George, A., and Breslin, A., Deposition of radon daughters in humans exposed to uranium mine atmospheres. *Health Phys. 17,* 115 (1969).

42. U.S. Public Health Service. Control of radon daughters in uranium mines and calculations on biologic effects. *U.S., Pub. Health Serv., Publ. 494* (1957).

43. Loysen, P., Errors in measurement of working level. *Health Phys. 16,* 629 (1969).

44. Harley, N. H., and Pasternack, B. S., The rapid estimation of radon daughter working levels when daughter equilibrium is unknown. *Health Phys. 17,* 109 (1969).

45. Martz, D. E., Holleman, D. F., McCurdy, D. E., and Schiager, K. J., Analysis of atmospheric concentrations of RaA, RaB and RaC by alpha spectroscopy. *Health Phys. 17,* 131 (1969).

46. Raabe, O. G., and Wrenn, M. E., Analysis of the activity of radon daughter samples by weighted least squares. *Health Phys. 17,* 593 (1969).

47. Thomas, J. W., Modification of the Tsivoglou method for radon daughters in air. *Health Phys. 19,* 691 (1970).

48. Rolle, R., Improved radon daughter monitoring procedure. *Amer. Ind. Hyg. Ass., J. 30,* 153 (1969).

49. Waters, J. R., and Howard, B. Y., Calibration of instrument for measurement of radon concentrations in mine atmospheres. *Health Phys. 16,* 657 (1969).

50. Costa-Ribeiro, C., Thomas, J., Drew, R. T., Wrenn, M. E., and Eisenbud, M., A radon detector suitable for personnel or area monitoring. *Health Phys. 17,* 193 (1969).

51. Thomas, J. W., and LeClare, P. C., A study of the two filter method for radon-222. *Health Phys. 18,* 113 (1970).

51a. Budnitz, R. J., Radon-222 and its daughters Rad-Nuc. *In* "Instrumentation for Environmental Monitoring." Lawrence Livermore Laboratory, U.S. At. Energy Comm., 1973.

52. Rock, R. L., Lovett, D. B., and Nelson, S. C., Radon-daughter exposure measurement with track etch films. *Health Phys. 16,* 617 (1969).

53. Lovett, D. B., Track etch detectors for alpha exposure estimation. *Health Phys. 16,* 623 (1969).

54. McCurdy, D. E., Schiager, K. J., and Flack, E. D., Thermoluminescent dosimetry for personal monitoring of uranium miners. *Health Phys. 17,* 415 (1969).

55. White, O., An evaluation of six radon dosimeters. *U.S. At. Energy Comm., Health Saf. Lab. Rep. 69-23A* (1969).

56. Duggan, M. J., and Howell, D. M., The measurement of the unattached fraction of airborne RaA. *Health Phys. 17,* 423 (1969).

57. Fusamura, N., Kurosawa, R., and Maruyama, M., Determination of f-value in uranium mine air. *In* "Assessment of Airborne Radioactivity," p. 213. IAEA, Vienna, 1967.

58. Black, S. C., Archer, V. E., Dixon, W. C., and Saccomanno, G., Correlation of radiation exposure and lead-210 in uranium miners. *Health Phys. 14,* 81 (1968).

59. Blanchard, R. L., Archer, V. E., and Saccomanno, G., Blood and skeletal levels of lead-210–polonium-210 as a measure of exposure to inhaled radon daughter products. *Health Phys. 16,* 585 (1969).

60. Fisher, H. L., A model for estimating the inhalation exposure to radon-222 and daughter products from the accumulated lead-210 body burden. *Health Phys. 16,* 597 (1969).

61. Holtzman, R. B., Sources of lead-210 in uranium miners. *Health Phys. 18,* 105 (1970).

62. Raabe, O. G., Concerning the relationship of lead-210 and inhalation exposure to radon-222. *Health Phys. 18,* 733 (1970).

63. Fisher, H. L., Relationship of lead-210 and short-lived radon-222 daughter products. *Health Phys. 19,* 697 (1970).

64. Blanchard, R. L., Radon-222 daughter concentrations in uranium mine atmospheres. *Nature (London) 223,* 287 (1969).

65. Cohen, N., and Kneip, T. J., A method for the analysis of lead-210 in the urine of uranium miners. *Health Phys. 17,* 125 (1969).

66. Gotchy, R. L., and Schiager, K. J., Bioassay methods for estimating current exposures to short-lived radon progeny. *Health Phys. 17,* 199 (1969).

67. Eisenbud, M., Laurer, G. R., Rosen, J. C., Cohen, N., Thomas, J., and Hazle, A. J., *In vivo* measurement of lead-210 as an indicator of cumulative radon daughter exposure in uranium miners. *Health Phys. 16,* 637 (1969).

68. Pohl-Rüling, J., and Pohl, E., The radon-222 concentration in the atmospheres of mines as a function of the barometric pressure. *Health Phys. 16,* 579 (1969).

69. Wrenn, M. E., Rosen, J. C., and Van Pelt, W. R., Steady state solutions for the diffusion equations of radon-222 daughters. *Health Phys. 16,* 647 (1969).

70. Wrenn, M. E., Eisenbud, M., Costa-Ribeiro, C., Hazle, A. J., and Siek, R. D., Reduction of radon daughter concentrations in mines by rapid mixing without makeup air. *Health Phys. 17,* 405 (1969).

71. Rock, R. L., and Walker, D. K., "Controlling Employee Exposure to Alpha Radiation in Underground Uranium Mines," Vol. 1. U.S. Bureau of Mines, Washington, D.C., 1970.

72. Martz, D. E., and Schiager, K. J., Protection against radon progeny inhalation using filter type respirators. *Health Phys. 17,* 219 (1969).

73. U.S. Bureau of Mines, Filter-type dust, fume, and mist respirators: requirements for investigation, testing, and certification. *Fed. Regist. 34,* 9617 (1969).

74. Burgess, W. A., and Shapiro, J., Protection from the daughter products of radon through the use of a powered air-purifying respirator. *Health Phys. 15,* 115 (1968).

75. Sill, C. W., An integrating air sampler for the determination of radon-222. *Health Phys. 16,* 371 (1969).

76. Shearer, S. D., and Sill, C. W., Evaluation of atmospheric radon in the vicinity of uranium mill tailings. *Health Phys. 17,* 77 (1969).

77. Ziemer, P. L., Personal radiation dosimetry. *Health Phys. 14,* 1 (1968).

78. Tochilin, E., Goldstein, N., and Miller, W. G., Beryllium oxide as a thermoluminescent dosimeter. *Health Phys. 16,* 1 (1969).

79. Jones, J. L., and Martin, J. A., Strontium fluoride as a thermoluminescent dosimeter. *Health Phys. 16,* 790 (1969).

80. McDougall, R. S., and Rudin, S., Thermoluminescent dosimetry of aluminum oxide. *Health Phys. 19,* 281 (1970).

81. Berstein, I. A., Bjarngard, B. E., and Jones, D., On the use of phosphor-Teflon thermoluminescent dosimeters in health physics. *Health Phys. 14,* 33 (1968).

82. Lin, F. M., and Cameron, J. R., A bibliography of thermoluminescent dosimetry (letter). *Health Phys. 14,* 495 (1968).
83. Spurny, I., Additional bibliography of thermoluminescent dosimetry. *Health Phys. 17,* 349 (1969).
84. Becker, K., Radiophotoluminescence dosimetry. Bibliography II. *Health Phys. 17,* 631 (1969).
85. Becker, K., Radiophotoluminescence dosimetry. Bibliography *Health Phys. 12,* 1367 (1966).
86. Goldstein, N., Tochilin, E., and Miller, W. G., Millirad and magarad dosimetry with LiF (letter). *Health Phys. 14,* 159 (1968).
87. Ehrlich, M., and Placious, R. C., Thermoluminescence response of CaF_2 : Mn in polytetrafluoroethylene to electrons. *Health Phys. 15,* 341 (1968).
88. Korba, A., and Hay, J. E., A thermoluminescent personnel neutron dosimeter. *Health Phys. 18,* 581 (1970).
89. Cusimano, J. P., and Cipperley, F. V., Personnel dosimetry using thermoluminescent dosimeters. *Health Phys. 14,* 339 (1968).
90. Kocher, L. F., Kathren, R. L., and Endres, G. W. R., Thermoluminescence personnel dosimetry at Hanford. *Health Phys. 18,* 311 (1970).
91. Endres, G. W. R., Kathren, R. L., and Kocher, L. F., Thermoluminescence personnel dosimetry at Hanford. II. *Health Phys. 18,* 665 (1970).
92. Hine, G. J., and Brownell, G., "Radiation Dosimetry," 1st ed. Academic Press, New York, 1956.
93. Attix, F. H., "Radiation Dosimetry," 2nd ed., Vol. 2. Academic Press, New York, 1966.
94. Price, W. J., "Nuclear Radiation Detection," 2nd ed. McGraw-Hill, New York, 1964.
95. International Commission on Radiological Protection, "Radiation Protection Instrumentation and its Application," Rep. No. 20. ICRU, Washington, D.C., 1971.
96. Rhyner, C. R., and Miller, W. G., Radiation dosimetry by optically stimulated luminescence of BeO. *Health Phys. 18,* 681 (1970).
97. Becker, K., and Robinson, E. M., Integrating dosimetry by thermally stimulated exoelectron (after) emission. *Health Phys. 15,* 463 (1968).
98. Becker, K., Thermally-stimulated exoelectron emission (TSEE) as a method for dose measurements using lithium fluoride. *Health Phys. 16,* 527 (1969).
99. Robinson, E. M., and Oberhofer, M., A sensitive ceramic BeO-TSEE dosimeter. *Health Phys. 18,* 434 (1970).
100. Becker, K., Cheka, J. S., and Oberhofer, M., Thermally-stimulated exoelectron emission, thermoluminescence, and impurities in LiF and BeO. *Health Phys. 19,* 391 (1970).
101. Becker, K., Principles of TSEE dosimetry. *At. Energy Rev. 8,* 173 (1970).
102. Duffy, T. L., and Kasper, R. B., Studies of gamma dosimetry systems used for nuclear accident dosimetry. *Health Phys. 14,* 45 (1968).
103. Brady, J. M., Aarestad, N. O., and Swartz, H. M., *In vivo* dosimetry by electron spin resonance spectroscopy. *Health Phys. 15,* 43 (1968).
104. Hankins, D. E., Direct counting of hair samples for phosphorous-32 activation. *Health Phys. 17,* 740 (1970).
105. National Council on Radiation Protection and Measurement, "Protection Against Neutron Radiation," Rep. No. 38. NCRP, Washington, D.C., 1971.
106. International Commission on Radiation Protection, Report of Committee II on permissible dose for internal radiation. *Health Phys. 3,* 1 (1960).
107. International Commission on Radiation Protection, "Evaluation of Radiation Doses to Body Tissues from Internal Contamination due to Occupational Exposure." ICRP

Publ. No. 10. Pergamon, Oxford, 1968, "The Assessment of Internal Contamination resulting from Recurrent or Prolonged Uptakes," ICRP Publ. No. 10a. Pergamon, Oxford, 1969.

108. Laurer, G. R., and Eisenbud, M., *In vivo* measurements of nuclides emitting soft penetrating radiations. *In* "Diagnosis and Treatment of Deposited Radionuclides" (H. Kornberg and W. Norwood, eds.), p. 189. Excerpta Med. Found., Amsterdam, 1968.

109. Dean, P. N., Ide, H. M., and Langham, W. H., External measurement of plutonium lung burdens. Paper presented at the Health Physics Society Meeting. 1970.

110. Newton, D., Fry, F. A., Taylor, B. T., and Eagle, M. C., Factors affecting the assessment of Pu-239 *in vivo* by external counting methods. *In* "Assessment of Radioactive Contamination in Man," IAEA Symp., STI/PUB/290, p. 83ff. IAEA, Vienna, 1972.

111. Wrenn, M. E., Rosen, J. C., and Cohen, N., *In vivo* measurement of Am-241 in man. *In* "Assessment of Radioactive Contamination in Man," IAEA Symp., STI/PUB/290, p. 595ff. IAEA, Vienna, 1972.

112. Ramsden, D., The measurement of plutonium-239 *in vivo*. *Health Phys. 16*, 145 (1969).

113. Taylor, B. T., A proportional counter for low level measurement of plutonium-239 in lungs. *Health Phys. 17*, 59 (1969).

114. Tomitani, T., and Tanaka, E., Large area proportional counter for assessment of plutonium lung burden. *Health Phys. 18*, 195 (1970).

115. Johnson, L. J., Watters, R. L., Lagerquist, C. R., and Hammond, S. E., Relative distribution of plutonium and americium following experimental PuO_2 implants. *Health Phys. 19*, 743 (1970).

116. Dudley, R. A., and Ben Haim, A., Assay of skeletally-deposited strontium-90 in humans by measurement of bremsstrahlung. *Health Phys. 14*, 499 (1968).

117. Chabra, A. S., A whole body counter for routine monitoring. *Health Phys. 16*, 719 (1969).

118. Masse, F. X., and Bolton, M. M., Experience with a low-cost chair-type detector system for the determination of radioactive body burdens of M.I.T. radiation workers. *Health Phys. 19*, 27 (1970).

119. Anderson, J. I., Parker, D., and Olson, D. G., A whole body counter with rotating detectors. *Health Phys. 16*, 709 (1969).

120. Dyson, E. D., and Beach, S. A., The movement of inhaled material from the respiratory tract to blood. *Health Phys. 15*, 385 (1968).

121. Nelson, I. C., Urinary excretion of plutonium deposited in the lung. *Health Phys. 17*, 514 (1969).

122. International Commission on Radiological Protection, "Report of Committee IV on Evaluation of Radiation Doses to Body Tissues from Internal Contamination Due to Occupational Exposure." ICRP Publ. No. 10. Pergamon, Oxford, 1968.

123. West, C. M., and Scott, L. M., Uranium cases showing long chest burden retention—an updating. *Health Phys. 17*, 781 (1969).

124. Ramsden, D., Bains, M. E. D., and Fraser, D. C., *In vivo* and bioassay results from two contrasting cases of plutonium-239 inhalation. *Health Phys. 19*, 9 (1970).

125. Lagerquist, C. R., Bokowski, D. L., Hammond, S. E., and Hylton, D. B., Plutonium content of several internal organs following occupational exposure. *Amer. Ind. Hyg. Ass., J. 30*, 417 (1969).

126. Hammond, S. E., Lagerquist, C. R., and Mann, J. R., Americium and plutonium urine excretion following acute inhalation exposures to high-fired oxides. *Amer. Ind. Hyg. Ass., J. 29*, 169 (1968).

127. Bains, M. E. D., and Rowbury, P. W. J., The biological excretion pattern from a person

involved in the inhalation of a mixture of enriched uranium oxide and lead metal powders. *Health Phys. 16*, 449 (1969).

128. Moss, W. D., Campbell, E. E., Schulte, H. F., and Tietjen, G. L., A study of the variations found in plutonium urinary data. *Health Phys. 17*, 571 (1969).

129. Lafuma, J., Nenot, J. C., and Movin, M., Problèmes posé par L'utilization des donnés d'excrétion urinaire pour l'evaluation de la charge corporelle. *In* "Assessment of Radioactive Contamination in Man," IAEA Symp., STI/PUB/290, p. 235ff. IAEA, Vienna, 1972.

130. Newton, C. E., Larson, H. V., Heid, K. R., Nelson, I. C., Fuqua, P. A., Norwood, W. D., Marks, S., and Mahony, T. D., Tissue analysis for plutonium at autopsy. *In* "Diagnosis and Treatment of Deposited Radionuclides" (H. Kornberg and W. Norwood, eds.), p. 460. Excerpta Med. Found., Amsterdam, 1968.

131. Bruner, H. D., A plutonium registry. *In* "Diagnosis and Treatment of Deposited Radionuclides" (H. Kornberg and W. Norwood, eds.), p. 661. Excerpta Med. Found., Amsterdam, 1968.

132. Pusch, W. M., Determination of effective half-life of ruthenium-103 in man after inhalation. *Health Phys. 15*, 515 (1968).

132a. Stradling, G. N., Design and implementation of biological monitoring program for tritium. *In* "Assessment of Radioactive Contamination in Man," IAEA Symp., STI/PUB/290, p. 385ff. IAEA, Vienna, 1972.

133. Evans, A. G., New dose estimates from chronic tritium exposures. *Health Phys. 16*, 57 (1969).

134. Moyer, R. A., Savannah River experience with transplutonium elements. *Health Phys. 15*, 133 (1968).

135. Denham, D. H., Health physics considerations in processing transplutonium elements. *Health Phys. 16*, 475 (1969).

136. Wright, C. N., Radiation protection for safe handling of californium-252 sources. *Health Phys. 15*, 466 (1968).

137. Lindell, B., Occupational hazards in x-ray analytical work. *Health Phys. 15*, 481 (1968).

138. Lubenau, J. O., Davis, J. S., McDonald, D. J., and Gerusky, T. M., Analytical x-ray hazards: A continuing problem. *Health Phys. 16*, 739 (1969).

139. Matthews, J. D., Accidental extremity exposures from analytical x-ray beams. *Health Phys. 18*, 75 (1970).

140. Paschal, L., Flash x-ray machines. *Amer. Ind. Hyg. Ass., J. 31*, 109 (1970).

141. Matthews, J. D., Radiation emission from a television projection system. *Health Phys. 18*, 451 (1970).

142. Neely, G. W., Thermal neutron activation of adhesive tapes. *Health Phys. 18*, 285 (1970).

143. Moghessi, A. A., Toerber, E. D., Regneir, J. E., Carter, M. W., and Posey, C. D., Health physics aspects of tritium luminous dial painting. *Health Phys. 18*, 255 (1970).

144. Howley, J. R., Robbins, C., and Brown, J. M., Health physics considerations in the use of radioactive foils for gas chromatography detectors. *Health Phys. 18*, 76 (1970).

145. Morris, J. O., Menker, D. F., and Dauer, M., A comparison of leak test procedures for sealed radium sources. *Amer. Ind. Hyg. Ass., J. 29*, 279 (1968).

146. International Commission on Radiological Protection, "General Principles of Monitoring for Radiation Protection of Workers," ICRP Publ. No. 12. Pergamon, Oxford, 1969.

147. U.S. Air Force, *Nuc. Saf. 65*, Part 2, Spec. ed. (1970).

148. Stevens, D. C., Churchill, W. L., Fox, D., and Large, N. R., A data processing system for radioactivity measurements on air samples. *Ann. Occup. Hyg. 13*, 177 (1970).

149. Sanders, M., *in* "Assessment of Airborne Radioactivity," p. 297. IAEA, Vienna, 1967.
150. Lister, B. A. J., *in* "Assessment of Airborne Radioactivity," p. 37. IAEA, Vienna, 1967, Brunskill, R. T., and Holt, F. B., *in* "Assessment of Airborne Radioactivity," p. 463. IAEA, Vienna, 1967.
151. Holliday, B., Dolphin, G. W., and Dunster, H. J., Radiological protection of workers exposed to airborne plutonium particulate. *Health Phys. 18,* 529 (1970).
152. Sherwood, R. J., and Stevens, D. C., A phosphor-film technique to determine the activity of individual particles on air sample filters. *Ann. Occup. Hyg. 11,* 7 (1968).
153. Stevens, D. C., The particle size and mean concentration of radioactive aerosols measured by personal and static air samples. *Ann. Occup. Hyg. 12,* 33 (1969).
154. Langmead, W. A., and O'Connor, D. T., The personal centripeter—a particle size-selective personal air sampler. *Ann. Occup. Hyg. 12,* 185 (1969).
155. Tanaka, E., Iwadate, S., and Miwa, H., A high-sensitivity continuous plutonium air monitor. *Health Phys. 14,* 473 (1968).
155a. Albert, R. E., "Thorium: Its Industrial Hygiene Aspects." Academic Press, New York, 1966.
156. Bradshaw, R. L., Empson, F. M., McClain, W. C., and Houser, B. L., Results of a demonstration and other studies on the disposal of high level solidified, radioactive wastes in a salt mine. *Health Phys. 18,* 63 (1970).
157. International Atomic Energy Agency, "Treatment of Airborne Radioactive Wastes." IAEA, Vienna, 1968.
158. "Proceedings of the Eleventh AEC Air Cleaning Conference," CONF-70016. Clearinghouse for Federal Scientific and Technical Information, National Bureau of Standards, Springfield, Virginia, 1970.
159. Burchsted, C. A., and Fuller, A. B., "Design, Construction and Testing of High Efficiency Air Filtration Systems for Nuclear Application," ORNL-NSIC-65. Clearinghouse for Federal Scientific and Technical Information, National Bureau of Standards, Springfield, Virginia, 1970.
160. Craig, D. K., Adrian, H. W. W., and Bouwer, D. J. J. C., Effect of iodine concentration on the efficiency of activated charcoal adsorbers. *Health Phys. 19,* 223 (1970).
161. International Atomic Energy Agency, Management of radioactive wastes at nuclear power plants. *Saf. Ser., Int. At. Energy Ag. 28* (1968).
162. Stannard, J. N., Toxicology of radionuclides. *Annu. Rev. Pharmacol. 13,* 325–357 (1973).
163. International Commission on Radiation Protection, "The Metabolism of Compounds of Plutonium and Other Actinides," ICRP Publ. 19. Pergamon, Oxford, 1972
163a. Stover, B. J., and Jee, S. S., eds., "Radiobiology of Plutonium." J. W. Press, University of Utah, Salt Lake City, 1972.
164. Evans, R. D., Keane, A. T., Kolenhow, R. J., Neal, R. W., and Shanahan, M. M., Radiogenic tumors in the radium and mesothorium case studies at MIT. *In* "Delayed Effects of Bone Seeking Radionuclides" (C. W. Mays, W. S. S. Jee, and R. D. Lloyd, eds.), pp. 157–194. Univ. of Utah Press, Salt Lake City, 1969.
165. Argonne National Laboratory, "Radiological Physics Division Annual Report," ANL-7760 Part II. Center for Human Radiobiology, 1969–1970, Argonne National Laboratory, "Radiological and Environmental Research Division," ANL-7960 Part II. Center for Human Radiobiology, 1971–1972.
166. Sanders, C. L., Busch, R. H., Ballou, J. E., and Mahlum, D. D., eds., "Radionuclide Carcinogenesis," AEC Symp. Ser. 29, U.S. At. Energy Comm., CONF-920505. 1973.
167. Van Cleave, C. D., "Late Somatic Effects of Ionizing Radiation," TID-24310. Div. Tech. Inform., U.S. At. Energy Comm., Washington, D.C., 1968.
168. Berke, H. L., The metabolism of rare earths. I. *Health Phys. 15,* 301 (1968).

169. Morgan, A., Morgan, D. J., and Block, A., A study of the deposition, translocation and excretion of radioiodine inhaled as iodine vapor. *Health Phys. 15,* 313 (1968).

170. Furchner, J. E., Richmond, C. R., and Drake, G. A., Comparative metabolism of radionuclides in mammals. IV. Retention of silver 110-m in the mouse, rat, monkey and dog. *Health Phys. 15,* 505 (1968).

171. Thomas, R. G., Thomas, R. L., and Wright, S. R., Retention of cesium-137 and strontium-90 administered in lethal doses to rats. *Amer. Ind. Hyg. Ass., J. 29,* 593 (1968).

172. Fletcher, C. R., The radiological hazards of zirconium-95 and niobium-95. *Health Phys. 16,* 209 (1969).

173. Palmer, H. E., Nelson, I. C., and Crook, G. H., The uptake, distribution and excretion of promethium in humans and the effect of DTPA on these parameters. *Health Phys. 18,* 53 (1970).

174. Morgan, B. N., Thomas, R. G., and McClellan, R. O., Influence of chemical state of cerium-144 on its metabolism following inhalation by mice. *Amer. Ind. Hyg. Ass., J. 31,* 479 (1970).

175. Wenzel, W. J., Thomas, R. G., and McClellan, R. O., Effect of stable yttrium concentration on the distribution and excretion of inhaled radioyttrium in the rat. *Amer. Ind. Hyg. Ass., J. 30,* 630 (1969).

176. Phillips, R., and Cember, H., The influence of body burden of radiomercury on radiation dose. *J. Occup. Med. 11,* 170 (1969).

177. Quastel, M. R., Taniguichi, H., Overton, T. R., and Abbatt, J. D., Excretion and retention by humans of chronically inhaled uranium dioxide. *Health Phys. 18,* 233 (1970).

178. Leach, L. J., Maynard, E. A., Hodge, H. C., Scott, J. K., Yuile, C. L., Sylvester, G. E., and Wilson, H. B., A five-year inhalation study with natural uranium dioxide (UO_2) dust. I. Retention and biological effect in the monkey, dog and rat. *Health Phys. 18,* 599 (1970).

179. Hursh, J. B., Neuman, W. R., Toribara, T., Wilson, H., and Waterhouse, C., Oral ingestion of uranium by man. *Health Phys. 17,* 619 (1969).

180. Thomas, R. G., Transport of relatively insoluble materials from lung to lymph nodes. *Health Phys. 14,* 11 (1968).

181. Johnson, L. J., Bull, E. H., Lebel, J. L., and Watters, R. L., Kinetics of lymph node activity accumulation from subcutaneous PuO_2 implants. *Health Phys. 18,* 416 (1970).

182. Sanders, C. L., Maintenance of phagocytic functions following $^{239}PuO_2$ particle administration. *Health Phys. 18,* 82 (1970).

183. Sanders, C. L., The distribution of inhaled plutonium-239 dioxide within pulmonary macrophages. *Arch. Environ. Health 18,* 904 (1969).

184. Richmond, C. R., Langham, J., and Stone, R. S., Biological response to small discrete highly radioactive sources. *Health Phys. 18,* 401 (1970).

185. Dean, P. N., and Langham, W. H., Tumorigenicity of small highly radioactive particles. *Health Phys. 16,* 79 (1969).

186. Letavet, A. A., and Kurlyandskaya, E. B., eds., "The Toxicology of Radioactive Substances," Vol. 4. Pergamon, Oxford, 1970.

187. Bender, M. A., Somatic chromosomal aberrations: Use in the evaluation of human radiation exposures. *Arch. Environ. Health 16,* 556 (1968).

188. Franco, S. C., A medical program for nuclear power stations. *J. Occup. Med. 11,* 16 (1969).

189. Tabershaw, I. R., Control of radiation hazards; role of the physician. *J. Occup. Med. 11,* 26 (1969).

190. Joint Publication of the World Health Organization, the International Labor Office and the International Atomic Energy Agency, Medical supervision of radiation workers. *Saf. Ser., Int. At. Energy Ag., 25* (1968).

191. Trombropoulos, E. G., Bair, W. J., and Park, J. F., Removal of inhaled ^{144}Ce–^{144}Pr oxide by diethylenetriaminepentaacetic acid (DTPA) treatment. I. *Health Phys. 16,* 333 (1969).

192. Sanders, C. L., and Bair, W. J., The effect of DTPA and calcium on the translocation of interperitoneally administered ^{239}PuO$_2$ particles. *Health Phys. 18,* 169 (1970).

193. Johnson, L. J., Watters, R. L., Lebel, J. L., Lagerquist, C. R., and Hammond, S. E., The distribution of plutonium and americium: Subcutaneous administration of PuO$_2$ and the effect of chelation therapy. *In* "Radiobiology of Plutonium" (B. J. Stover and W. S. S. Jee, eds.), p. 213. Univ. of Utah Press, Salt Lake City, 1972.

194. Pfleger, R. C., Wilson, A. J., and McCellan, R. O., Pulmonary lavage as a therapeutic measure for removing inhaled "insoluble" materials from the lung. *Health Phys. 16,* 758 (1969).

195. Sagan, L. A., Radiobiological problems associated with adjudication of workmen's compensation claims. *J. Occup. Med. 11,* 335 (1969).

196. Jones, A. R., A portable area monitor for gamma rays. *Health Phys. 18,* 333 (1970).

197. Blanc, D., Mathieu, J., Bouet, J., and Prigent, R., A portable electronic system equipped with an ionization chamber filled with a liquid equivalent to the biological tissue. *Health Phys. 18,* 432 (1970).

198. O'Riordan, M. C., and Cott, B. R., Low energy x-ray shielding with common materials. *Health Phys. 17,* 516 (1969).

199. Jenkins, T. M., and Nelson, W. R., The effect of target scattering on the shielding of high energy electron beams. *Health Phys. 17,* 305 (1969).

200. Birchall, I., Gamma scatter from open-top cells. *Health Phys. 16,* 47 (1969).

201. Caldwell, R. D., and Cooley, R. C., Ventilation for control of tritium air contamination during reactor vessel repair. *Health Phys. 18,* 167 (1970).

202. International Atomic Energy Agency, "Manual on Safety Aspects of the Design and Equipment of Hot Laboratories." IAEA, Vienna, 1969.

202a. International Commission on Radiological Protection, "Implications of Commission Recommendations that Doses Be Kept As Low As Readily Achievable," No. 22, Pergamon, Oxford, 1973.

203. Morgan, K. Z., Ionizing radiation: Benefits versus risks. *Health Phys. 17,* 539 (1969).

204. National Council on Radiation Protection and Measurements, "Basic Radiation Protection Criteria," Rep. No. 39. NCRP, Washington, D.C., 1971.

205. Spiers, F. W., "Radioisotopes in the Human Body: Physical and Biological Aspects." Academic Press, New York, 1968.

206. Morgan, K. Z., and Turner, J. E., eds., "Principles of Radiation Protection: A Textbook of Health Physics." Wiley, New York, 1967.

207. Cember, H., Introduction to health physics. *Int. Ser. Monogr. Nucl. Energy 105* (1969).

208. Hendee, W. R., "Medical Radiation Physics." Yearbook Publ., Chicago, Illinois, 1970.

Work in Hot Environments:
Threshold Limit Values and Proposed Standards

BRUCE A. HERTIG

Professor Harwood S. Belding* reviewed the physiologic factors, environmental factors, and techniques for evaluation of heat stress and resultant strain in the industrial setting in two previous volumes concerned with industrial environment.[1,2] In the intervening three years, attention has been sharply focused on industrial heat stress through activities at the federal level to draft and promulgate a standard for work in hot environments.

It is the purpose here to trace the historic and conceptual development of the proposed standard and to examine critically the implications of such a standard for the hot industries.

HEAT AS AN INDUSTRIAL HAZARD

Heat has long been recognized as an acute hazard around processes involving molten metals, glass, and other intense radiant sources. In the early days of industrialization, heat deaths were accepted as inevitable, as part, along with the other hazards, of the cost to human health and safety of producing goods. Fortunately, industrial heat deaths are now essentially a matter of history; the hot processes have in fact evolved around the capacities of man to deal effectively with the stress—usually. It is the exceptions that set the stage for overt heat illnesses: the unusually hot days or an individual's personal debilitating condition, such as respiratory infection.

In spite of the successes of mechanization and work practices in reducing industrial heat overstrain to an occasional occurrence, the ubiquity of heat stress

* Deceased August 1973.

219

makes it an important concern of industrial hygienists and medical personnel. The multiplicity of independent environmental and physiologic factors makes evaluation of heat hazards difficult, requiring considerable specific training in the area. Short courses and presentations of papers on heat stress at scientific meetings are always well attended. Attempts to simplify the analysis of heat stress fill volumes, and many integrative indices have been proposed over the years.[1] With this sustained interest, it is logical to expect that criteria should be established for upper limits of exposure to work in hot environments.

THRESHOLD LIMIT VALUES (TLV)

In June 1971, the Physical Agents Committee of the American Conference of Governmental Industrial Hygienists (ACGIH) introduced its proposed Threshold Limit Values for heat stress to the industrial and scientific community at a Hot Job Workshop sponsored jointly by the Industrial Health Foundation (IHF), the University of Pittsburgh, and the National Institute for Occupational Safety and Health (NIOSH).[3] Later, in 1973, the ACGIH published a "Notice of Intent to Establish Threshold Limit Values: Heat Stress."[4] As proposed standards for work in hot environments are based on these TLV's, and the ACGIH will most likely adopt the TLV's in 1974, it is pertinent here to review the essential features of these TLV's for heat stress.

Wet Bulb–Globe Temperature Index

The Wet Bulb–Globe Temperature (WBGT) was chosen as the index of choice by the ACGIH for assessment of heat stress as "... the simplest and most suitable technique to measure the environmental factors." The WBGT is determined as follows:

1. Outdoors with solar load:
   $$WBGT = 0.7WB + 0.2GT + 0.1DB$$
2. Indoors or outdoors with no solar load:
   $$WBGT = 0.7WB + 0.3GT$$

where WB is the natural wet-bulb temperature, DB, the dry-bulb temperature, and GT is the globe thermometer temperature.

Specific instructions for instrumentation are contained in the TLV[4] and NIOSH's Criteria Document, described below.

Permissible Heat Exposure Threshold Limit Values

The ACGIH's recommended TLV's for heat are given in Table I. This table emphasizes the importance of work load on the one hand, and the percentage of time spent working, on the other.

TABLE I
Permissible Heat Exposure Threshold Limit Values[a, b]

	Work load		
Work-rest regimen	Light	Moderate	Heavy
Continuous work	30.0 (86.0)	26.7 (80.1)	25.0 (77.0)
75% Work–25% rest, each hr	30.6 (87.1)	28.0 (82.4)	25.9 (78.6)
50% Work–50% rest, each hr	31.4 (88.5)	29.4 (84.9)	27.9 (82.2)
25% Work–75% rest, each hr	32.2 (90.0)	31.1 (88.0)	30.0 (86.0)

[a] From Reference 4; used with permission of the American Conference of Governmental Industrial Hygienists.

[b] Values are given in °C (°F) WBGT.

The specific WBGT limit values in each of the cells of Table I were determined from data in the literature which correlated environmental conditions with deep body temperatures not exceeding 38°C (100.4°F) at the various work loads. Selection of this level of 38°C as a safe upper limit for deep body temperature was based on the consensus of an international panel of experts.[5] Deep body temperatures (t_r) may reach this level under conditions of hard work alone without superimposed environmental heat load. The rationale in establishing this as the upper limit of work in the heat is certainly reasonable: when environmental conditions impose a heat load and/or impede rejection of metabolic heat to the environment such that heat is stored in the body $(t_r = 38°C)$, heat overstrain may occur quickly.[6] The margin for safety in effect becomes small, requiring close supervision of the worker. However, the level of WBGT at which deep body tends to exceed this safe limit, or even whether WBGT is in fact a valid index of heat stress, remain controversial.

The data contained in Table I may be presented graphically as a continuum (Fig. 1). From this it can be seen that "heavy work" corresponds to about 500 kcal/hr (2000 Btu/hr), "moderate work" 325 kcal/hr (1300 Btu/hr), and "light work" about 200 kcal/hr (800 Btu/hr). Few industrial jobs require 500 kcal/hr on a sustained basis; this is equivalent to running up a 5° grade at 3 mph, or heavy pick and shovel work.

In the months that followed the introduction of the TLV concept and the ensuing discussions at the Hot Job Workshop of 1971, the hot industries initiated field studies to test the validity of the TLV's on the job. The results of these studies were reported at a second workshop held in January 1972. Data presented there revealed that many jobs within these industries required work in environments that substantially exceeded the TLV WBGT's. Special selection of personnel for these jobs was one explanation of this nonconformity of the field experience with the TLV's. Another explanation was that the WBGT was not a

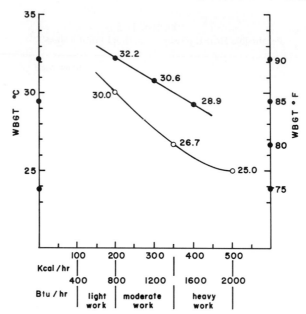

Fig. 1. Permissible heat exposure threshold limit value. (–○–), Continuous work, low air velocity (<300 fpm); (–●–), continuous work, high air velocity (>300 fpm). Adapted from Ref. 4.

valid index for the industrial setting, as it was validated originally for environmental conditions at military camps. In any event, the need for additional field data was apparent. As a result, it was agreed at the second workshop that during the summer of 1972 extensive efforts in industry would be mounted further to determine environmental stress–physiologic strain relationships.

NIOSH CRITERIA DOCUMENT: CRITERIA FOR A RECOMMENDED STANDARD ... OCCUPATIONAL EXPOSURE TO HOT ENVIRONMENTS

In March 1972, NIOSH personnel were directed to produce a criteria document on heat stress; it was drafted, reviewed, and revised during the spring and published in July 1972.[7]

The Criteria Document differed from the ACGIH TLV in certain fundamental respects. Continuous heavy work (at about 400 kcal/hr) was assumed. From the appropriate work curve in Fig. 1, the corresponding WBGT was selected as 26.1°C (79.0°F). It is important to note that work in hot environments at levels above these WBGT's was not proscribed, but rather that "any one or combination of the following work practices shall be initiated to ensure that the employee's body core temperature does not exceed 38.0° C (100.4° F).

Work Practices

The work practices specified included:

(i) Acclimatization

(1) Unacclimatized employees shall be acclimatized over a period of 6 days. The acclimatization schedule shall begin with 50% of the anticipated total work load and time exposure on the first day, followed by daily 10% increments building up to 100% total exposure on the sixth day.

(2) Regular acclimatized employees who return from nine or more consecutive calendar days of leave, shall undergo a four day acclimatization period. The acclimatization schedule shall begin with 50% of the anticipated total exposure on the first day, followed by daily 20% increments building up to 100% total exposure on the fourth day.

(3) Regular acclimatized employees who return from four consecutive days of illness should have medical permission to return to the job, and should undergo a four day re-acclimatization period as defined in (2) above.

(ii) A work and rest regimen shall be implemented to reduce the peaks of physiological strain and to improve recovery during rest periods.

(iii) The total work load shall be evenly distributed over the entire work day when possible.

(iv) When possible hot jobs shall be scheduled for the coolest part of the work shift.

(v) Regular breaks, consisting as a minimum of one every hour, shall be prescribed for employees to get water and replacement salt. The employer shall provide a minimum of 8 quarts of cool potable 0.1% salted drinking water or a minimum of 8 quarts of cool potable water and salt tablets per shift. The water supply shall be located as near as possible to the position where the employee is regularly engaged in work, but never further than 200 feet (except where a variance had been granted) therefrom.

(vi) Appropriate protective clothing and equipment shall be provided and used.

(vii) Engineering controls to reduce the environmental heat load shall be utilized.

In addition to the above specific work practices, the Criteria Document outlined other requirements for management of personnel exposed to WBGT's in excess of 79°F (or 76°F, for women). Medical examination, with particular emphasis on capacity to deal with hot environments, was required prior to assignment to a hot job with reexamination at 2-year intervals (1 year for employees over 45 years of age).

WBGT profiles for each work place were required, these profiles serving as guides for determining when the work practices should be implemented. The document also outlined in detail the recordkeeping required to comply with the proposed standard. Perhaps these latter two provisions—determining the WBGT profiles and the recordkeeping—elicited the most negative response from the hot industries. In the southern tier of states, WBGT's in excess of 79°F exist out-of-doors every day for several months of the year; in effect, every work station or stations for every employee would have to have a profile established, a truly formidable task!

Needless to say, the Criteria Document stimulated discussion and concern among the industries affected. A 2-day symposium sponsored by NIOSH and organized jointly by the IHF and the University of Pittsburgh in February 1973 was attended by several hundred representatives of industry, labor, government, and academia.[8] Results of studies during the preceding two summers in aluminum, steel, chemical, and other hot industries were presented. One salient finding was that substantial numbers of workers suffered no demonstrable effects detrimental to health from exposures to heat in environments considerably in excess of the 79°F WBGT limit specified in the Document. The implication was that the WBGT is not a universally valid index when applied to certain industrial environments. Non-equivalence physiologically of environments with various combinations of humidities and globe temperatures, but with equal WBGT levels, has been demonstrated by Ramanathan and Belding in their laboratory studies.[9]

STANDARDS ADVISORY COMMITTEE ON HEAT STRESS

In spring of 1973, the Secretary of Labor empaneled an advisory committee to attempt to resolve some of the apparent discrepancies between heat stress limits in the Criteria Document and industrial experience. Professor Belding was selected to chair this committee, which included representatives of industry, labor, military, and the public sector. Upon his death he was succeeded by Professor Jerry Ramsey of Texas Tech University. Deliberations of the Committee throughout the balance of 1973 resulted in a "Recommended Standard for Work in Hot Environments," which was transmitted to the Secretary of Labor on January 9, 1974.[10]

Many features of the NIOSH Criteria were discussed at length and modified to reflect input from recent industrial data:

1. An attempt was made better to fit the WBGT index to industrial situations.

2. The importance of workload in the heat balance equation was recognized in setting threshold WBGT values.

3. Work practices were revised and reworded to be more satisfactory to management and labor groups, although full agreement among the committee

members was not achieved. The full text of the Committee's Recommended Standard, including alternative wordings, is contained in Reference 10.

Standards Advisory Committee Recommendations

The WBGT was retained as the index by the Committee because of its inherent ease of application. The importance of air motion in promoting evaporation of sweat from man and the inadequacy of the WBGT properly to weight this factor suggested that separate WBGT threshold values be given for air speeds below 300 ft/min and for above 300 ft/min (1.5 meter/sec).

Workloads were separated into four levels:

Workload—The metabolic energy which is expended in performing physical work.

(i) Level 1. Resting is the condition with no workload and involves metabolic energy expenditure of 100 kcal/hr (kilocalories) or less per hour or 400 Btu (British thermal units) per hour.

(ii) Level 2. Light work involves metabolic energy expenditure greater than 100 kcal (400 Btu) per hour, up to 200 kcal (800 Btu) per hour.

(iii) Level 3. Moderate work involves metabolic energy expenditure greater than 200 kcal (800 Btu) per hour, up to 300 kcal (1200 Btu) per hour.

(iv) Level 4. Heavy work involves metabolic energy expenditure greater than 300 kcal (1200 Btu) per hour.

WBGT Threshold Values. In contrast to the Criteria Document, which specified the single 79° WBGT as the threshold for initiation of work practices, the Advisory Committee recommended threshold values of WBGT depending on air speed and workload. Table II lists this matrix of WBGT values.

TABLE II
Threshold Wet Bulb Globe Temperature Index Values for Work in Hot Environments[a]

	Threshold WBGT values degrees °C (°F)	
Work load	*Low air velocity* *(Up to 300 fpm)*	*High air velocity* *(300 fpm or above)*
Light (level 2) (200 kcal/hr or below)	30 (86)	32.2 (90)
Moderate (level 3) (201 to 300 kcal/hr)	27.8 (82)	30.6 (87)
Heavy (level 4) (above 300 kcal/hr)	26.1 (79)	28.9 (84)

[a] After Table I of Ref. 10.

These **WBGT** threshold values, while not applicable to all situations, nevertheless provide conservative guidelines for implementation of work practices in hot environments. The low air speed values are, in fact, points on the continuous work curve of the ACGIH TLV (Fig. 1, lower curve). For comparison, the points for high air speed, continuous work, have been plotted on the original TLV axes. (In Fig. 1, the other curves included in the ACGIH TLV representing 75, 50, and 25% work have been deleted for simplicity.) Note that "Level 2" workload corresponds to "Light" workload in the ACGIH TLV, but that "Level 3" and "Level 4" are not as high as "Moderate" and "Heavy," as evidenced by the correspondingly higher threshold WBGT's (Table II) than in the ACGIH TLV's (Table I).

Work Practices. Work practices proposed by the Advisory Committee follow, in general, those in the Criteria Document quoted above. However, they are more detailed and, in contrast to the more general guidelines of the Criteria Document, the Advisory Committee outlines mandatory work practices, special work practices for special conditions, and work practices for extreme heat exposures.

There was considerable discussion about each of the work practices during the deliberations of the Committee. Of interest is the distribution of votes on the work practices over which there was major disagreement. These votes are given in parentheses following the work practice where 13 (86%) or more of the members cast a vote. The order represents votes "for," "against," and "abstain," respectively.

Work practices:

(1) During any two-hour period of the work day [refer to Paragraph (d)], workers shall not be exposed to hot environmental conditions and workload stresses in excess of the levels shown in Table II without the following work practices being initiated.

(i) An adequate supply of potable water shall be made available near the work site, and workers shall be informed that working in hot environments requires frequent water intake. One quart of water per worker per hour approximates the water loss from man working at a maximum sweat rate.

(ii) Newly assigned employees or those recently returning from serious illness or vacations in excess of two weeks who are normally assigned to moderate or heavy workload tasks shall not be required to perform at full normal pace until they have had an opportunity to become acclimatized.

(iii) The importance of acclimatization for the well-being of workers shall be recognized by the formulation of a written statement of employer's policy which shall meet the conditions existing at workplaces for which he is responsible. This policy shall be explained and made available to all employees exposed to hot environments. This policy statement shall also be kept on file and be available for inspection by an authorized representative of the Secretary of Labor; and shall be consistent with the guidelines established and issued by OSHA.

(iv) Persons trained to render first aid shall be given training in recognition and first aid treatment of heat-related disorders and be available to those workplaces where heat strain may occur. The names and location of persons so qualified shall be made known to all workers exposed to hot environmental conditions.

(v) Fitness of employees for heavy workload (Level 4) at hot environmental conditions shall be determined on the basis of the preplacement medical evaluation as specified in Paragraph (f) (1). (Vote: 8–6–1).

(2) Special work practices.

In addition to those work practices specified in Paragraphs (2) (i)–(v) above, one or more of the following work practices shall be applied where necessary to comply with the purposes of this standard.

(i) The employer shall adopt engineering controls which are appropriate for reducing and controlling the level of heat exposure.

(ii) The duration of the work period, the frequency and length of rest pauses, and pace and tempo of work shall be adjusted to avoid heat strain.

(iii) Because cases of heat illness in hot industries often occur at the sudden onset of increases in climatic temperature or humidity, the rate of heavy work and frequency of rest pauses shall be adjusted to allow for acclimatization at such times.

(iv) When feasible, heavy work shall be scheduled during the cooler parts of the work shift.

(v) Appropriate protective clothing or equipment shall be provided.

(vi) Workers in a hot environment shall be allowed to interrupt their work when necessary due to extreme discomfort. (Vote: 10–3–2).

(3) Work practices required for extreme heat exposure.

In addition to those work practices specified in Paragraphs (1) (i)–(v) and (2) (i)–(vi) above, the following work practices are required for conditions of extreme heat exposure.

(i) Duration of any extreme heat exposure is to be determined by experienced and/or professional judgment based on similar work under similar conditions. Nevertheless, in extreme heat exposure, each worker shall have the option of terminating any particular exposure because of heat disorder. (Vote: 8–5–2).

(ii) Fitness of all employees for work in extreme heat exposures shall be determined on the basis of preplacement and periodic medical evaluation as specified in Paragraphs (f) (1) and (f) (2).

(iii) Workers shall be under observation of a trained supervisor or fellow worker who can note any early signs of heat effects.

(iv) Appropriate protective clothing or equipment shall be provided for reducing the intensity of extreme exposure.

These work practices provide excellent guidelines for the regulation of exposure of workers in hot environments. In effect, they are outlines of work practices that have been found virtually to eliminate serious heat strain in industry.

Other sections of the Recommended Standard deal with required medical examinations, training of employees, monitoring of the environment, and keeping of records; space does not permit the reproduction of the Recommended Standard in its entirety here.

Despite the devoted effort expended by the members of the Committee, a document satisfactory to all did not emerge. There was substantial support for the thesis that a heat stress standard is inappropriate at this point in time.

The vote within the Committee was 10 to 5 that the final draft be the basis of a proposed rule to be published by the Secretary of Labor. Thus the Recommended Standard was not a "consensus document." Consequently, the Secretary judged that more study is in fact needed before a hot jobs standard should be promulgated, and in late March 1974 the recommendations of the Committee were transmitted to the National Institute for Occupational Safety and Health for further evaluation and reassessment of appropriate criteria.

WBGT VERSUS HSI

In the previous volume of this series, Belding cites an example of actual industrial data,[2] calculating heat stress by means of the Belding and Hatch Heat Stress Index (HSI) and interpreting the results in terms of predicted physiologic strain. It is of interest to compare the conclusions based on HSI with those calculated using the WBGT for the same set of data.

Example: "Warm day," outside air temperature = $82°F*$:

	At the job site (50% of time)	At the rest site (50% of time)
Globe temp. (t_g)	$113°F$	$88°F$
Air temp. (t_a)	$91°F$	$84°F$
Wet bulb temp. (t_{wb})	$70°F$	$70°F$
Air motion (V)	300 ft/min	60 ft/min
Determination of HSI:		
Metabolic workload (M)	1300 Btu/hr	400 Btu/hr
E_{req}	2240	270
E_{max}	2130	810
	av E_{req} = 1260	
	av E_{max} = 1470	
	HSI = 86	

Belding's Interpretation. "Heat balance should be maintainable by a fit acclimatized 'standard man' (154 pounds) without undue strain . . . heat stress estimates on this day indicating only a marginal safety allowance."

DETERMINATION OF WBGT

Assume "natural wet bulb" temperature

$$t_{nwb} = t_{wb} \quad \text{at} \quad V = 300 \text{ ft/min, } 70°\text{F}$$
$$t_{nwb} = t_{wb} + 2° \quad \text{at} \quad V = 60 \text{ ft/min, } 72°\text{F}$$

$$WBGT_{work} = 0.7 \times 70 + 0.3 \times 113 = 82.9°\text{F}$$
$$WBGT_{rest} = 0.7 \times 72 + 0.3 \times \quad 88 = 76.8°\text{F}$$
$$\text{av WBGT* } = 79.9°\text{F}$$

$$\text{av Workload} \dagger = \frac{1300 + 400}{2} = 850 \text{ Btu/hr}$$

INTERPRETATION OF WBGT

Workload = 850 Btu/hr   moderate (level 3)
V = 300 ft/min   high air speed

From Table II, threshold **WBGT** for work practices = 87. Av **WBGT** of example = 79.9; no work practices need be initiated.

Comment. The HSI method indicates that the safety allowance is only *marginal.* The average WBGT is well below threshold, providing no quantitative indication of how close the exposure is to the limit of tolerance.

Example "Hottest weather," outside temperature = 89° F.

DETERMINATION OF HSI[2]

Metabolic workload (M)	1300 Btu/hr	400 Btu/hr
E_{req}	2380	320
E_{max}	1610	620
	av E_{req} = 1350	
	av E_{max} = 1120	
	HSI = 120	

* From Reference 2, pages 272–273; see for complete description of example.

† For this example of 50% work, 50% rest, av WBGT and av WL are straightforward numerical averages. For more complex situations, the av WBGT is calculated by 2-hr weighted time and workload formulae[10]:

$$\text{av (WBGT} = \frac{(WBGT_1)\,(t_1) + (WBGT_2)\,(t_2) + \cdots + (WBGT_n)\,(t_n)}{120 \text{ min}}$$

$$\text{av workload (WL)} = \frac{(WL_1)\,(t_1) + (WL_2)\,(t_2) + \cdots + (WL_n)\,(t_n)}{120 \text{ min}}$$

Belding's Interpretation. Well above the recommended upper limit such "... that the overall physiologic cost would be high and risk of heat injury would be real."

DETERMINATION OF WBGT*

At the work site

$$t_g = 126°F \quad t_{nwb} = 79°F$$
$$WBGT_{work} = 0.7 \times 79 + 0.3 \times 126 = 93.1°F$$

At the rest site

$$t_g = 91.5°F \quad t_{nwb} = 78°F$$
$$WBGT_{rest} = 0.7 \times 78 + 0.3 \times 91.5 = 82°F$$

$$av \ WBGT = 87.6°F$$
$$av \ workload = 850 \ Btu/hr$$

From Table II, threshold WBGT = 87° F.

Interpretation. Exposure slightly above threshold, work practices should be initiated, particularly since air speed falls on the border between "low" and "high."

These illustrations support several important observations that emerged during the deliberations of the Standards Advisory Committee. (1) There are insufficient industrial data upon which to base a heat stress standard applicable to the many types of hot jobs encountered. To this end, members of the Committee have urged the Secretary of Labor to initiate epidemiologic studies. (2) The WBGT has serious limitations as a universal heat stress index in industry. Before it may be accepted with confidence, it needs to be validated in many more places. Perhaps separate WBGT threshold values will need to be established for specific types of hot jobs or classes of industries, e.g., mining, farming, hot metal pouring. (3) Instrumentation to assess accurately and quickly the imposed environmental heat stress is as yet not available, although several WBGT meters have been introduced in recent years.† In addition, one of the most difficult tasks in estimating heat load occurs when the worker is moving from work place to work place frequently, perhaps in no set sequential pattern. The best of the instruments available take several minutes to equilibrate with the environment; within this time the worker may have been exposed to several additional totally different environments.

---

* t_g and t_{nwb} calculated "backwards" from values of radiation (R) and convection (C) given by Belding in his example, Reference 2, page 275.

† Some of them are the YSI Heat Stress Instrument (Yellow Springs Instrument Co., Yellow Springs, Ohio); Reuter Stokes RSS–211 Heat Stress Monitor (Reuter–Stokes Canada Ltd., Ontario); ENVIREC and WBGT Index Instrument (Bendix Corp., Baltimore, Maryland).

Briefly, to summarize, although a heat standard has not yet been promulgated, industrial hygienists who are concerned about potential heat hazards in their plants may find portions of each of the several documents reviewed here—the ACGIH TLV's, NIOSH Criteria Document, and Standards Advisory Committee's Recommended Standard—useful for assessing the degree of heat hazard and implementing preventive measures.

REFERENCES

1. Belding, H. S., Work in hot environments. *In* "Industrial Hygiene Highlights" (L. V. Cralley, L. J. Cralley, and G. D. Clayton, eds.), p. 214. Ind. Hyg. Found. Amer., Pittsburgh, Pennsylvania, 1968.
2. Belding, H. S., Engineering approach to analysis and control of heat exposures. *In* "Industrial Environmental Health" (L. V. Cralley, ed.), Vol. 1, p. 271. Academic Press, New York, 1972.
3. "Assessment of Heat Stress and Strains," Bull. 8–71. Industrial Health Foundation, Pittsburgh, Pennsylvania, 1971.
4. "Threshold Limit Values for Chemical Substances and Physical Agents in the Workroom Environment with Intended Changes for 1973." Amer. Conf. Govt. Ind. Hyg., Cincinnati, Ohio, 1973.
5. Health factors involved in working under conditions of heat stress. *World Health Organ., Tech. Rep. Ser. 412* (1969).
6. Lind, A. R., A physiological criterion for setting thermal environmental limits for everyday work. *J. Appl. Physiol. 18,* 51–56 (1963).
7. "Criteria for a Recommended Standard ... Occupational Exposure to Hot Environments," Cat. No. HSM 72–10269. U.S. Department of Health, Education and Welfare, National Institute for Occupational Safety and Health, US Govt. Printing Office, Washington, D.C., 1972.
8. "Symposium on Standards for Occupational Exposures to Hot Environments," sponsored by the National Institute for Occupational Safety and Health, Pittsburgh, Pennsylvania, 1973 (unpublished).
9. Ramanathan, N. L., and Belding, H. S., Physiological evaluation of the WBGT index for occupational heat stress. *Amer. Ind. Hyg. Ass., J. 34,* 375 (1973).
10. "Recommendations for a Standard for Work in Hot Environments," Draft No. 5, Standards Advisory Committee on Heat Stress, Department of Labor, Washington, D.C., 1974. (Full text may be found in Bureau of National Affairs' Occupational Safety and Health Reporter, Vol. 3, No. 33, p. 1055, January 17, 1974.)

Evaluation of
Chemical Hazards in the Environment

ROBERT G. KEENAN AND RICHARD R. KEENAN

This chapter presents a review of the more significant developments in sampling and analytic methods for inorganic and organic substances in air, water, and biologic materials during the 1971–1973 period. The methods have been selected upon due consideration of the substantiating data provided by the original authors, as has been our practice during the compilation of the corresponding chapter in the previous edition of this work. As the sophistication of our methodology continues to increase, so does our treatment of this subject. The reader, however, will note that we have attempted to maintain a sensible balance between the fundamental types of analytic methods represented in our treatment of the subject.

STANDARDIZATION

At the time of publication of the previous edition of this work, the Intersociety Committee on Methods for Ambient Air Sampling and Analysis had published 63 tentative methods of analysis for substances of concern on air pollution studies. This collection of methods, selected by the expert subcommittees of the Intersociety Committee, has proved to be very helpful to engineers and chemists engaged in the evaluation of workroom and community environments. Since that time 35 additional methods have been published by the Intersociety Committee in *Health Laboratory Science,* including the April 1974 issue. Copies of these methods may be purchased from the American Public Health Association, Washington, D.C.

The important work of Project Threshold of the American Society for Testing and Materials, in its critial evaluation of methods of sampling and analysis for specific substances in the atmosphere and in stack gases, has continued through Phases I and II since early 1971. This important approach to the collaborative sampling of contaminants under field conditions is unique, and is providing valuable data on the actual performance of these methods of test under the exacting environmental conditions of the real world. Continuation of Project Threshold's Phase III, which is concerned with manual methods of sampling and analysis of ambient atmospheres, is being planned at present.

METHODS FOR INORGANIC SUBSTANCES

Ammonia

The ammonia ion selective electrode has been evaluated as a tool for the determination of ammonia in water and wastes.[1] Accurate and precise results with recoveries greater than 90% have been obtained when adequate controls are imposed on the procedure. The ammonia electrode has been shown to give results comparable to those obtained with the indophenol blue method at comparable concentrations.

A new sensitive method for the determination of ammonia and aliphatic amines in air has been reported.[2] The ammonia and amines are collected in dioxane containing o-(benzenesulfonamido)-p-benzoquinone. The absorbance at 480 nm is subsequently determined. Aromatic amines react slowly and require heating to produce coloration. The dye formed is extremely stable, fading only slightly over a 2-hr period. In the range of 1.7×10^{-5} to 6.0×10^{-5} moles/liter of solution, a linear calibration curve is obtained. This method was found to be three to four times more sensitive than nesslerization. However, its use may be limited as a result of the reaction of the reagent with primary, secondary, and tertiary amines.

Antimony

A fluorometric procedure for the determination of antimony in air, water, soil, and biologic materials has been reported.[3] This method, which uses 3,4',7-trihydroxyflavone, has a detection limit of 0.04 μg of antimony and a precision of approximately 2% at the 5 μg level. The sample is decomposed by pyrosulfate fusion, and the antimony is extracted from the sulfuric acid solution as the triiodide into methyl isobutyl ketone (MIBK). The 3,4',7-trihydroxy-flavone solution is added to the extract. After 30 min, the intensity of the fluorescence is measured. Tin and aluminum most seriously interfere in this determination. The extraction step, however, removes greater than 95% of these interferences. Substances that form insoluble sulfates or phosphates will interfere. Such interferences are readily eliminated by filtration.

Arsenic

A method for the determination of arsenic at the submicrogram level by the evolution and subsequent measurement of arsine by flameless atomic absorption spectrophotometry has been developed.[4] The reduction of arsenic by zinc to arsine is followed by passing the generated arsine gas through the reaction cell and into an electrically heated absorption tube. The arsine absorbance increases as the temperature of the absorption cell is raised. Replicate determinations on 0.4 μg arsenic standards gave a relative standard deviation of 0.36%. Recoveries of 94.7 and 92.6% were obtained from 0.1 μg and 0.2 μg arsenic levels, respectively.

Beryllium

Ross and Sievers have described a routine method for the determination of ultratrace concentrations of beryllium in water and in airborne particulate matter collected on glass fiber filters.[5] The particulate matter is ashed, the residue digested with acid and the resulting solution buffered to the optimum pH for solvent extraction. Interfering metals are effectively masked with EDTA. Trifluoroacetylacetone (TFA) is reacted with the beryllium to form the volatile chelate $Be(TFA)_2$. The organic extract is subsequently analyzed by gas chromatography utilizing electron capture detection. The authors claim this procedure is more sensitive and reproducible than any other method now being used for the determination of beryllium in environmental samples. They have determined the limit of detection to be approximately 4×10^{-14} gm of beryllium.

A procedure for the analysis of beryllium in spiked blood containing as little as 0.02 μg of Be/ml of whole blood has been reported.[6] Whole blood containing Na_2 EDTA as an anticoagulant was analyzed with preliminary acid digestion. The procedure involves placing 50 μl of whole blood into an ampoule followed by the addition of 0.5 ml of the appropriate chelating solution containing trifluoroacetylacetone and 1,1,2,2-tetrabromoethane (TBE). After cooling, the tube is flame sealed, shaken for 20 sec, and heated at 115°C in an oven for 15 min. The ampoule is opened and 50 μl of 28% ammonium hydroxide is added. The ampoule is corked, shaken for 10 sec, centrifuged, and a 1 μl aliquot of the benzene layer is injected into a gas chromatograph equipped with an electron capture detector. The average recovery of beryllium from blood was approximately 97% with a relative standard deviation of approximately 7.7%.

Boron

Bailey and Lo have presented a procedure for the flame photometric determination of boron which has increased the sensitivities and detection limits by two orders of magnitude over previous experiments in which the hotter oxyacetylene flame was used.[7] Aqueous solutions containing boron are diluted four- to sixfold with methanol resulting in an enhanced signal due to reduced surface tension, which increases the rate of aspiration and results in the formation of smaller droplets. The investigators proposed that the chemiluminescence of the trimethyl borate species is at least partially responsible for greatly increased emission of the borates when diluted with methanol and the high sensitivity observed when the relatively cool air/hydrogen flame is used. The emission intensity is measured at 546 nm. A number of cations cause interference due to emission of radiation in the vicinity of the band head emission of the boron species at 546 nm—Ba, Ca, Co, Cr, Cu, Na, Ni, and K. Some of the interferences could be eliminated by measuring the emission intensity at 518 or 492 nm. Other interferences had to be removed by ion exchange.

Free Chlorine

A procedure for the determination of free chlorine (hypochlorous acid, hypochlorite ion) in water without interference from chloramines has been reported by Bauer and Rupe.[8] Syringaldazine, the chromophoric agent employed, is insensitive to bound chlorine. Only o-tolidine has been widely accepted as a convenient field test for free chlorine even though it reacts with various chloramines.[9] The use of o-tolidine may lead to serious error when water containing ammonia and other contaminants is analyzed. The proposed method produces a straight-line calibration curve at low concentration levels of chlorine, exhibits a high degree of reproducibility, and shows excellent agreement with the o-tolidine procedure in the absence of chloramines. In the presence of chloramines, significant discrepancies exist. Whereas o-tolidine reacts with free and bound chlorine, syringaldazine reacts only with the free chlorine, as indicated by its agreement with the amperometric determination of free chlorine present.

Chromium

Booth and Darby have presented a gas chromatographic procedure for the determination of chromium in complex biologic tissues.[10] The tissues are wet digested, and analyzed by gas–liquid chromatography with electron capture detection. A chromium concentration of 20 ng/gm of tissue is detectable. The average recovery of chromium from liver was 95%.

The determination of chromium in blood and plasma by gas chromatography has also been reported.[11] The sample is heated at 175°C for 30 min in a sealed tube with a hexane solution of trifluoroacetylacetone. The hexane extract is then analyzed by gas–liquid chromatography with an average recovery of 90% for spiked blood and plasma samples. The limit of detection was stated to be 5 ng/ml of blood.

The analysis of blood, hair, and urine for trace quantities of chromium by emission spectroscopy has been reported.[12] These determinations were made possible by an increased stability of the direct current arc and the use of a static argon atmosphere.[13-15] With these improvements, excellent reproducibility is obtained along with increased signal : noise ratios. The limit of detection for chromium is 1 ng. The reported mean relative standard deviation in the 1–7 ng range was 6% for triplicate analyses.

Cyanide

The rapid reaction of cyanide ion with nickel ion forms a stable anion complex, tetracyanonickelate(II), which has a characteristic ultraviolet spectrum and is the basis of an analytic method for the determination of cyanide in water.[16] Hydrogen cyanide is distilled into ammoniacal nickel chloride, and without further treatment to the absorbing solution, the absorbance due to the anionic complex $Ni(CN)_4^{2-}$ is measured at 267 nm. Beer's law is followed over the range of 5–200 μg of cyanide ion per 10 ml of ammoniacal nickel chloride solution. The limit of detection is 0.1 mg cyanide/liter of sample solution.

Frant and co-workers have reported a procedure for the determination of low levels of cyanide using a silver ion selective electrode.[17] The known addition method[18] using a Gran's plot[19] is used. The lower limit of detection is approximately 0.025 mg/liter whereas the limit of detection of the cyanide ion electrode is 0.3 mg/liter.

Ryan and Holzbecher have presented two methods for the fluorometric determination of cyanide in aqueous solution.[20] With copper present, leuco-fluorescein permits the determination of 0–100 parts per billion (ppb) cyanide. The fluorescence intensity is a linear function of concentration in the low concentration range (0–5 ppb) with a relative standard deviation of approximately 10%. Sulfide and strongly oxidizing and reducing anions must be absent.

The copper–calcein metallofluorescent indicator permitted the determination of 10–250 ppb cyanide. The relative standard deviation was 6.5% at the 26 ppb level. Sulfide does not interfere.

Fluoride

A sensitive method for the determination of fluoride was reported by Har and West,[21] who have designed an intensified fluorescent method with a sensitivity of 2 ppb (10^{-7} M). The procedure involves the formation of a ternary complex between zirconium, calcein blue, and fluoride. Fluoride enhances the intensity of the fluorescence of the zirconium—calcein blue complex. The method is rapid, reproducible, and shows a precision of ±3%. Phosphate was found to seriously interfere at fivefold excess.

Hydrogen Sulfide

Natusch and co-workers have reported a method for the measurement of trace levels of atmospheric hydrogen sulfide as low as 5 parts per trillion (ppt, 10^{-12}).[22] Hydrogen sulfide is extracted from the air by reacting with a silver nitrate-impregnated filter. The silver sulfide formed is dissolved with sodium cyanide solution and analyzed fluorometrically using fluorescein mercuric acetate.[23] The procedure provides efficient collection of hydrogen sulfide, results in the formation of a stable sulfide, and the analytic method is both sensitive and specific. The limit of detection is 5 ppt, and only mercaptans and high ozone levels interfere.

A fluorometric procedure for the determination of hydrogen sulfide in natural waters at the microgram per liter level has been suggested.[24] Average recoveries greater than 95% have been demonstrated for hydrogen sulfide concentrations of 0.1–200 μg/liter. The procedure involves the extraction of hydrogen sulfide as triethyllead sulfide followed by the fluorometric titration with mercurated fluorescein. As an alternative, the titration can be performed with o-hydroxymercuribenzoic acid in the presence of dithizone. Common ions do not interfere. Thiols, cyanide, xanthate, and dithiocarbamate do not change the fluorometric endpoint.

Lead

A method for the determination of organic and total lead in the atmosphere by atomic absorption spectrophotometry was recently reported[25] and involves the collection of particulate lead on a membrane filter backed by an iodine monochloride solution for collecting organic lead compounds. The particulate lead is determined by atomic absorption spectrophotometric analysis of the acid extracts of the membrane filter. The lead in the iodine monochloride solution is complexed with ammonium pyrrolidine dithiocarbamate (APDC) in methyl isobutyl ketone (MIBK) followed by AAS analysis. Organic lead concentrations in air of 0.1–>4.0 $\mu g/m^3$ can be determined. No detectable organic lead was found in the second impinger at flow rates of 1.89 liters/min.

A method that eliminates the need for double absorption measurements through the use of automatic background correction and frequent standardization techniques has been presented for the determination of lead in 25 μl of a 1 : 10 water-diluted whole blood sample.[26] An Instrumentation Laboratory Model No. 355 Atomization Chamber is used in place of the regular burner head. The blood is dried, ashed, and atomized directly from a tantalum ribbon in the chamber. Highly acceptable agreement with the lead levels in a series of reference blood samples obtained from Baltimore City Hospital was reported.

An extraction procedure for the determination of lead in biologic tissues and fluids has been developed.[27] Lead is chelated with APDC at pH 8.5, extracted into MIBK, and analyzed by atomic absorption spectrophotometry. Only bismuth and cadmium are not masked by cyanide when APDC is used for chelation purposes. This method has been used with confidence for the analysis of samples containing up to 100 μg of lead. Average recoveries from blood and urine specimens were 100.2 and 98.7%, respectively. Preliminary ashing of the sample is required.

Mercury

A procedure for the determination of mercury in urine, blood, water, and air has been reported.[28] This procedure is simple and fast, and requires no prior sample digestion. The apparatus used is composed of a reaction vessel, a water scrubber, a filter, and an absorption cell. The mercury vapor is generated in the reaction vessel by reduction with stannous chloride. A linear calibration curve is obtained in the 0–0.06 μg region. The limit of detection for mercury in water and urine is at least 0.003 μg. Recoveries range from 90 to 110%, and is 104% at the 0.50 μg level in urine. Concentrations of mercury less than 1 ppb in a liquid sample can be detected accurately by increasing the aliquot of sample.

Using the analytic procedure of Krause and co-workers,[28] Nelson et al. have modified the sample preparation to permit the analysis of industrial effluents and wastewaters for mercury.[29] They developed a wet digestion procedure that removes all organics and eliminates the foaming problems that interfere in this method. The use of antifoam agents was shown to have an adverse effect on the analytic data. Typically, analytic signals are reduced by 50% when antifoam agents are used. Nelson et al. obtained increased sensitivity and reproducibility by using a heated gas line. As direct analysis of these aqueous solutions is not possible due to the high organic content, a preliminary digestion with sulfuric and nitric acids is required. Recovery of ionic mercury was reportedly 100% at the 5 and 10 ppb levels, and 117% at the 1 ppb level. Recovery of mercury from organomercurial compounds averaged 108%.

The recovery of mercury from wastewater was 101% at the 1 ppb level. The investigators stated that the limit of detection was at least 0.9 ppb.

The determination of mercury in water has been performed in a reduction aeration system similar to the one just described. In order to eliminate interferences, a silver amalgamator is used to selectively remove mercury prior to the final measurement, which is accomplished by atomic fluorescence.[30] The digestion of samples that required such treatment was performed overnight with sulfuric acid, nitric acid, potassium permanganate, and potassium peroxy-disulfate. As little as 0.6 ng of mercury can be determined.

The combination of electroreduction of mercury, followed by analysis by atomic absorption spectrophotometry, has been employed successfully for the determination of trace quantities of mercury in environmental water samples.[31] Mercury is reduced on a copper coil cathode at −3.0 volts for 90 min. This time period has been found to be sufficient to quantitatively reduce up to 50 ng of mercury. The mercury isolated on the coil is subsequently determined by atomic absorption using the method of Brandenberger.[32] The recovery of mercury is quantitative within the precision of the instrumentation used. A mercury concentration of 0.1 ppb in a 50 ml sample is easily measured. The precision and accuracy are estimated to be ±10% in the range 0.1–10 ppb mercury.

A highly sensitive and selective procedure for the determination of mercury using a dc discharge spectral type detector[33] has been reported.[34] The membrane probe–spectral emisson type detection system for the determination of mercury has proved to be more selective with lower sample size limits of detection than any other method. The lower limit of detection is 4 ppt, and is 4×10^{-10} gm in a batchwise analysis modification of the technique. Following reduction with sodium borohydride, mercury diffuses through a latex membrane and is flushed with helium through the dc discharge cell. The limits of detection are 10–20 times lower than those of flameless atomic absorption methods. The method has been applied to the analysis of mercury in various materials including fresh water, sea water, and urine.

The concentration of mercury in air has been successfully determined in the nanogram per cubic meter range.[35,36] Mercury is amalgamated with either a thin gold film on ceramic powder[35] or silver wool.[36] Heating the sample liberates the mercury from the gold or silver. Both procedures utilize flameless atomic absorption to detect the amount of mercury present in the sample. The method of Scullman and Widmark[35] has a sensitivity of less than 1 ng/m^3 of air; the percent relative standard deviation ranges from 1.9 to 7%. Long and co-workers,[36] whose method involves the collection of mercury on silver wool, claim the procedure permits the determination of mercury in air in the range of 15 ng/m^3 –10 $\mu g/m^3$ for 24-hr sampling periods. The limit of detection was 0.3 ng of mercury vapor. Precision was 11% at 0.5 ng and ±3% relative standard deviation beyond 6 ng. Ambient levels of dimethyl mercury, sulfur dioxide, hydrogen sulfide, and nitrogen dioxide did not seriously interfere. The investigators conclude that the use of the silver collection medium gives a simple, inexpensive, high capacity, and selective medium for the collection of elemental mercury.

Oxides of Nitrogen

A modification of the Saltzman method for the determination of low concentrations of oxides of nitrogen has been suggested.[37] The modification involves the use of ozone as an oxidizing agent for the conversion of nitric oxide to nitrogen dioxide. When ozone is used, this conversion is almost instantaneous, gives reproducible absorbance values, and provides a straight line calibration curve that passes through the origin. Interference from ammonia has been shown to be eliminated with boric acid added to the Saltzman reagent. The precision and accuracy of the method is acceptable using these modifications when compared to the chemiluminescence method of Niki.[38] The use of oxygen to convert nitric oxide to nitrogen dioxide by the Saltzman method requires 24 hr.[39]

A procedure describing a modification of the phenol–disulfonic acid (PDS) method, which eliminates the time-consuming evaporation step, has been presented.[40] Gas samples were collected in evacuated air sample bottles containing 4.00 ml of absorbent. Oxidation of nitric oxide to nitrate was judged to be complete after the samples were rotated for 1 hr. Total absorption was also obtained when samples were allowed to stand for 24 hr. Excess peroxide is destroyed in the gas collection bottle, and 0.50–2.00 ml aliquots are added to 2 ml of PDS reagent in a 25 ml volumetric flask that is cooled under cold running water. After the sample is heated on a steam bath, cooled, and diluted to the mark with 1 : 1 ammonium hydroxide, the absorbance at 410 nm is measured. The authors reported obtaining excellent agreement between the modified method and the currently used PDS method, as indicated by the correlation coefficient of 0.98. The sensitivities of the two methods are comparable.

Martens et al.[41] have improved the currently used PDS method for the determination of nitrogen oxides when chloride, turbidity, and carbon dioxide evolution are present. They have shown the effect of chloride ion, turbidity filtration, and carbon dioxide on the absorbance of the nitrochromogen, and how the nitrogen oxides concentration may be determined in the presence of these interferences.

A chemiluminescent method for the analysis of nitrogen compounds in mobile source emissions has been reported.[42] The method depends on the thermal dissociation of nitrogen dioxide to nitric oxide, the oxidation of ammonia to nitric oxide, and the reaction of nitric oxide with ozone to give detectable light emission. Levels of nitric oxide as low as 0.02 ppm can be detected, and response is linear into the percentage range.

Phosgene

Noweir and Pfitzer have tested a new reagent for the spectrophotometric determination of phosgene in air.[43] The reagent consists of 0.25% 4-p-nitrobenzylpyridine and 0.5% N-benzylaniline in diethylphthalate, and was found to be highly sensitive and rather specific for phosgene. The procedure allows for the reliable determination of less than 0.1 ppm concentrations of phosgene in air; substances generally encountered under industrial conditions do not interfere. The chromogenic reagent is stable and results in the formation of a reasonably stable color that is only slightly affected by humidity.

Phosphorus

A simplified wet ashing procedure for the analysis of total phosphorus of organophosphonates in biologic samples has been reported.[44] The digestion mixture is composed of sulfuric, nitric, perchloric acids, and water. The open digestion tube containing 1.5 ml of the digestion mixture, 40 mg of organic material, 1–50 nmoles of phosphorus, and less than 0.6 mEq of cations was placed in a heating block for 1.5 hr at $225°C$. After the heating period, the tube contained approximately 0.1 ml of clear, colorless digestion residue and 3 mEq of concentrated sulfuric acid. The residue was subsequently analyzed by the ammonium molybdate–aminonaphthol sulfonic acid method.[45] Recovery of phosphorus ranged from 95 to 101% with a relative standard deviation for replicates of 1.7%.

Phosphate

Kirkbright and co-workers[46] have optimized the conditions for the formation and extraction of molybdophosphate resulting in a highly selective and sensitive spectrofluorometric method for the determination of phosphate. A 0.04–0.6 μg quantity of phosphorus can be determined by way of the formation of the ion-association complex of molybdophosphate with Rhodamine B. The intensity of the fluorescence is measured at 575 nm with excitation at 350 nm. The procedure has a coefficient of variation of ±3.9%. Average recovery of phosphate from synthetic mixtures was 100.1% and ranged from 98 to 105%.

Selenium

Osburn and co-workers[47] have developed a new method for the determination of selenium at the ppb level in water and air samples. The method is based on the reaction of selenous acid (H_2SeO_3) with hydroxylamine to form nitrous acid, and the subsequent reaction of NO_2^- with sulfanilamide to form a diazonium salt, which in turn couples with N-(1-naphthyl)-ethylenediamine dihydrochloride to form intensely colored dyes. This represents an attempt to develop a sensitive, selective method for selenium. The range of determinations extended from 10 to 200 μg of selenium(IV) per liter of aqueous solution. The method is simple, sensitive, and reproducible. The relative error at the 50 μg/liter level is 4.8%. No common interferences exist which cannot be easily eliminated. Average recovery, based on comparison with the catalytic method of West,[48] was 92%.

Baird et al.[49] have proposed a method for the flameless atomic absorption determination of selenium using a carbon rod attachment. The advantage of this technique is low lamp intensity and the absence of the usual high levels of flame background normally responsible for the decreased sensitivity. The small sample volume required, plus the increased residence time spent by the selenium vapor in the analyzed volume of gas, results in an absolute detection limit of 72 pg of selenium.[50] Wastewaters were digested with nitric and perchloric acids to oxidize organic material prior to injection into the carbon rod. Following this procedure, Baird experimentally realized a detection limit of 33 pg of selenium in wastewater samples. The relative standard deviation was 3.5% at the 5×10^{-10} gm level. An average recovery of 88% was realized for samples containing 1 μg/ml.

A fluorometric procedure for the determination of selenium in lake sediments,[51] effluent streams,[52] and water[53] has been presented. The procedure developed by Wiersma and Lee[51] involves the digestion of lake bottom sediments in nitric and perchloric acids. Selenium is reduced and coprecipitated with arsenic and hypophosphorous acid. The precipitate is dissolved in nitric acid, allowed to react with 2,3-diaminonaphthalene, and extracted with cyclohexane. The fluorescence (λ_{ex} = 366 nm, λ_{em} = 522 nm) is measured for the complex in the extract. Submicrogram amounts of selenium are detectable in 1-g samples. Selenious acid reacts with 2,3-diaminonaphthalene in acid solution to form the strongly fluorescent naphtho-[2,3-d]-2-selena-1,3-diazole.[52] This method is specific for elemental selenium and selenium(IV). Standards and spiked effluent samples exhibit a straight line plot of fluorescence intensity versus concentration in the 0.005–0.2 μg selenium(IV) region; the method appears to be practically free of reagent interference.

Rankin[53] applied the fluorometric method of Wiersma and Lee[51] to the analysis of clean water for selenium. Selenium metal is oxidized with hydrogen peroxide to selenate [Se(VI)] followed by hydrogen chloride reduction to selenite [Se(IV)]. Selenite is reacted with 2,3-diaminonaphthalene to form the organic extractable piazselenol which is determined fluorometrically. This method is free of common interferences and capable of detecting selenium at the 1 ppb level. A plot of the fluorescence intensity versus concentration is linear over the region of 0.02–1.0 μg per 50 ml of water. Above that range, the relationship deviates from Beer's law. The average recovery from spiked potable water samples was 101.9% with a standard deviation of 5.9. The analysis of spiked effluents and streams gave an average recovery of 101.7% with a standard deviation of 4.6.

Oxides of Sulfur

A new spectrophotometric method for the determination of sulfur dioxide in air having definite advantages over the method of West and Gaeke has been proposed.[54] The procedure involves the collection of sulfur dioxide in sodium tetrachloromercurate solution. At pH 1.3 the ethanol–dye–formaldehyde complex displays a red color [due to the 4-(4-aminophenylazo)-1-naphthylamine dye]. In the presence of sulfur dioxide, the color is blue, having a maximum absorbance between 600 and 640 nm. The color development is instantaneous but starts fading within 15 min. When 0.1% o-toluidine is used to mask the nitrogen dioxide interference, color development reaches a maximum intensity after 30 min and is stable for more than 90 minutes. The use of o-toluidine reduces the sensitivity of the method by about a factor of two. However, a longer path-length cell may be used. Also, the range is extended by a factor of two when o-toluidine is employed. The working range for the method without o-toluidine is 0.07–2.4 μg SO_2/ml of absorbing solution.

Young and co-workers[55] have reported a method for the determination of sulfur dioxide in flue gases. The gas is collected as H_2SO_4 in aqueous hydrogen peroxide. The procedure involves the potentiometric titration of sulfate with 0.01 M lead perchlorate. The lead concentration is monitored with a lead ion selective electrode. A comparison of the potentiometric results with those obtained by the barium ion–thorin indicator and the barium chloranilate methods shows good agreement between the three methods.

Carlson and Black[56] have described a method for the determination of sulfur dioxide using lead candles. The method is based upon the fact that lead sulfate is significantly more soluble than lead dioxide in 30% ammonium acetate solution. Hence, the concentration of lead taken in solution is considered to be due to the lead sulfate dissolved from the candle. Average recovery of lead sulfate in simulated lead dioxide candles was 97.9%. Excellent agreement between the method of Carlson and Black and the gravimetric procedure was obtained. Substances that will reduce lead to a lower valence state would interfere and appear as sulfate. However, the results from the comparison with the gravimetric results show that these interferences are not normally present in a significant concentration to cause any measurable interference. The procedure is rapid and economical. It should be applicable to other types of lead dioxide samplers such as sulfation plates.

A coated piezoelectric crystal for the detection and measurement of sulfur dioxide in air has been designed and evaluated.[57] The detector response is linear with respect to the concentration of SO_2. The use of a "static" sampling system permits much greater sensitivity to be achieved than a dynamic gas system. The limit of detection is approximately 0.1 ppm. Nitrogen dioxide produces serious detector fatigue by deactivating the amine coating. Moisture may cause considerable interference by bringing about an increase in the weight of the crystal. Sulfur dioxide may then dissolve in the water, forming sulfurous acid, which will attack the amine coating and result in the formation of a salt.

Sulfur Compounds

A number of gas chromatographic procedures for the analysis of air samples for sulfur compounds have been reported.[58-62] Stevens *et al.* have described a procedure for the automated gas chromatographic analysis of sulfur dioxide, hydrogen sulfide, methyl mercaptan, and dimethyl sulfide using flame photometric detection.[58] Ambient air concentrations of these reactive sulfur gases down to 0.002 ppm can be determined. The column used was a 1% polyphenyl ether and 1% H_3PO_4 on Haloport–F (Teflon powder). The four compounds were typically eluted within 8 min.

Kremer and Spicer analyzed mixtures of sulfur compounds with a single-pass system consisting of two 30% tritolyl phosphate on Chromosorb P columns, one being 10 ft, the other 20 ft long.[59] They were able to adequately separate COS, H_2S, SCl_2, CH_3SH, SO_2, C_2H_5SH, CS_2, CH_2SCH_2, Cl_3CSCl, and thiophene. Recovery of the sulfur-containing components was excellent.

Bruner and co-workers have developed a procedure for the gas chromatographic determination of sulfur compounds at the ppb level in air (SO_2, H_2S, CH_3SH, and CH_3SCH_3).[60] Graphitized carbon black treated with 0.5% H_3PO_4 and 0.3% Dexsil in a Teflon column was used as the column packing. A flame photometric detector provided the necessary sensitivity.

The portable gas chromatographic analysis of SO_2, H_2S, and CH_3SH using a bromine titration cell for detection of the eluted sulfur compounds has been reported.[61] Limits of detection for SO_2, H_2S, and CH_3SH are 1.0 ppm, 0.2 ppm, and 0.1 ppm, respectively.

The response of the flame photometric detector has been shown to be predictably nonlinear due to self-absorption.[62] The maximum detector sensitivity occurs in the 0–60 ng range ($<10\%$ self-absorption).

METHODS FOR MINERAL SUBSTANCES

Asbestos

Improved techniques for the identification and determination of airborne asbestos have been reported.[63] Modifications include a longer plenum section for sample collection to provide a much more uniform distribution of particles over the filter surface, and the use of a liquid of a specific refractive index to separate asbestos particles from other airborne particulates. A liquid of refractive index 1.546 is used for the examination of airborne particulate for chrysotile. The liquid has the effect of making all asbestos particles invisible and permits the operator to determine the number of nonasbestos particles in the sample. The sample must first be ashed in a low-temperature asher to remove the membrane filter.

Rickards has reported the detection of as little as 10 μg of chrysotile asbestos on membrane filters using x ray diffraction.[64] To attain this sensitivity, a pulse height discriminator, step-scanning facilities with digital printout, and a rotating sample holder were used. In the presence of interferences, 50–100 μg of asbestos can be detected. This x ray diffraction method may be applied whenever airborne particulate samples are collected on membrane filters. The external standard procedure has a limit of detection of 10 μg with a relative standard deviation of 10%. At the 100 μg level the relative standard deviation is 2%.

In order to determine lower concentrations of asbestos in environmental samples, an electron microscopic procedure was developed.[65] The procedure is based on the morphology and electron diffraction patterns of the small asbestos fibers. Quantitative estimates are made recording the dimensions of the fibers and using the theoretical density of chrysotile to calculate the mass of chrysotile in the sample. The limit of detection was 0.1 ng/m^3. Filter samples were ashed at 450°C. Wetting of the filter with dibutylphthalate before ignition prevented loss of chrysotile which may occur during explosive combustion of the membrane.

Quartz

A procedure for the determination of quartz in coal dust by infrared spectroscopy has been reported.[66] Airborne coal dust is collected on 37 mm cellulose ester membrane filters, ashed in a low temperature asher, and the ash incorporated into a potassium bromide pellet for examination by infrared spectrophotometry. The infrared spectrum is recorded in the 900–700 cm^{-1} region. The absorbance at 800 cm^{-1} is calculated and the weight of quartz is determined from a calibration curve. This method is applicable to 10–100 μg of quartz. The limit of detection is 5–10 μg of quartz. Some polyvinyl chloride filter ashes interfere severely.

The determination of quartz in respirable coal mine dust has been reported.[67] The samples are ashed for 30 min at 800°C in a muffle furnace. The ash is thoroughly mixed with 360 mg of potassium bromide, pressed into a pellet, and analyzed by infrared spectrophotometry. The absorbance at 795 cm^{-1} is calculated using the baseline technique. The limit of detection is 4 μg of quartz.

A procedure for the determination of α-quartz in respirable airborne particulate matter by x ray diffraction has been reported.[68] The particulate matter is redeposited on a silver membrane filter that was shown to have a much lower background than the organic filters commonly used as collection media. In order to obtain reliable results when an uneven distribution of particulate exists on the filter, a flat sample spinner is used. The method is accurate to approximately ±30% of the quartz present. As little as 5 μg of quartz can be detected under carefully controlled conditions. Crystals having diffraction lines at 0.335 and 0.317 nm can interfere. Interferences include muscovite, mica (biotite), sillimanite, graphite, and aragonite.

METHODS FOR ORGANIC SUBSTANCES

Carcinogens

The combination of thin-layer chromatography (TLC) and mass spectrometry (MS) is effective in confirming the presence or absence of aflatoxins in agricultural commodities.[69] The use of TLC-fluorescence can lead to incorrect conclusions if fluorescing artifacts or nonfluorescing materials of coincident R_f values are present. The TLC–MS combination applies to all aflatoxins, appears to have approximately equal sensitivity for them, and allows for their positive identification in many cases with 50 ng or less of aflatoxin. Mass spectrometry extends the lower limit of reliable detection at least two orders of magnitude below existing chemical confirmatory tests for these compounds. TLC analysis for aflatoxins was done on silica gel (G–HR, Brinkmann Instrument Company). The plates were developed with 10% acetone in chloroform. Distilled water is required to dislodge the aflatoxins from the active sites of the silica gel.

A method for the determination of bis(chloromethyl)ether at the ppb level in air has been developed.[70] The method involves the collection of organics on $1\frac{1}{2}$ inches of 80/100 mesh Chromosorb 101 supported in a $\frac{1}{4}$ × 2 inch stainless steel tube with subsequent analysis by gas chromatography–mass spectrometry. Positive identification is made by the retention time, the mass of the base peak, and the chlorine isotope ratio. This procedure is highly specific for bis(chloromethyl)ether (bis-CME) and provides a limit of detection of 2.1 ppb in a 1-liter air sample within 10% accuracy.

Previously, Collier had analyzed air for the presence of bis-CME at the ppb level by mass spectrometry with a limit of detection of 0.1 ppb.[71] He concentrated airborne organics on Porapak Q. Adsorbed compounds were thermally eluted into the reservoir of a high-resolution mass spectrometer. The preliminary separation of bis-CME by gas chromatography prior to mass spectrometric analysis would greatly simplify the observed mass spectrum. Increased specificity would result as the analyst would also have a chromatographic retention time for the material.

A method for the determination of fluorenes in cigarette smoke has been reported.[72] The procedure involves the partitioning of the nonvolatile particulate matter of cigarette smoke between three solvent pairs, chromatographing on alumina, and analyzing by gas chromatography. Analysis of each of the individual methylfluorene isomers is possible on either an OV–17 or an OV–1 column.

The separation of polynuclear aromatic hydrocarbons (PNA) can be accomplished by gas chromatography on a 1% OV–7 column,[73] high-pressure liquid chromatography on 2,4,7-trinitrofluorenone-impregnated Corasil I,[74] high-pressure liquid chromatography on cellulose acetate,[75] and gel permeation chromatography followed by identification by fluorescence spectrometry.[76] Qualitative identification is most easily performed by fluorescence spectrometry.

Lane and co-workers have reported the use of a single gas chromatographic column, 1% OV–7, for the analysis of PNA's, some heterocyclics, and aliphatics.[73] Complete separation is reported for benzo[k]fluoranthene [B(k)F], benzo[a]pyrene [B(a)P], and perylene, and for B(k)F, benzo[e]pyrene [B(e)P], and perylene. B(a)P and B(e)P overlap. However, distinct peaks are evident. This column can also produce a separation of a number of alkanes making it well suited to the analysis of the organic fraction of atmospheric particulate matter. The retention time of 7H-dibenzo[c,g] carbazole was 86 min.

Karger et al. separated PNA's on a 3-meter U-shaped liquid–solid chromatography column with 2,4,7-trinitrofluorenone-impregnated Corasil I as the stationary phase, dry n-heptane as the mobile phase, and an ultraviolet detector.[74] Separation of a large number of PNA's was possible with this setup. Retention times were reasonable for these materials (36 min for 1,2,3,4-dibenzpyrene). The inlet head pressure was 185 atm. The use of a spectrofluorometer should increase the sensitivity of the method.

Klimisch separated PNA's by high-pressure liquid chromatography on cellulose acetate column with spectral photometric detection.[75]

McKay and Latham isolated PNA's by gel permeation chromatography and subsequently identified seven of them by fluorescence spectrophotometry.[76] The GPC fractions each contained three or more PNA's. Each fraction was subsequently separated by TLC on a 2 : 1 mixture of aluminum oxide type E and 20% acetylated cellulose, developed in two directions with ethyl ether–toluene–cyclohexane (2 : 1 : 7). Several fluorescence emission spectra are given.

A gas phase fluorescence detector has been developed for the analysis of PNA's by gas chromatography.[77] Use of a nondestructive fluorescence detector has the advantages of being more sensitive and specific than electron capture detection. A number of PNA pairs cannot be separated on any presently known column packing. The use of the gas phase fluorescence detector overcomes this problem. The inherent specificity of the fluorometric detector results from the fact that each PNA has its own characteristic excitation and emission maxima. This requires a change in the excitation and emission monochromators. However, this inconvenience can be readily overcome by automation.

Bhatia reports the analysis of high-boiling PNA mixtures by using gas chromatographic columns packed with OV–7-coated glass beads and using temperature programming.[78] The author believes that this method can be adapted to the analysis of airborne particulates and distillates containing PNA's.

Pesticides and Herbicides

Ali and Wheelock have investigated the extraction of chlorinated pesticides followed by their subsequent analysis by thin-layer and gas chromatographic procedures.[79] Hexane and petroleum ether were found to be the most satisfying solvents for extraction of the pesticides while benzene and chloroform were less so. The best separation of chlorinated compounds found in river water by TLC was achieved with hexane : acetone (90 : 10) on Silica Gel G. The silver nitrate/bromphenol blue chromogenic reagent of Bates[80] was satisfactory for all the pesticides investigated and gave distinct spots with the river water samples. The silver nitrate chromogenic reagent of Morley and Chiba[81] gave sharply defined spots with all the standard organochlorine pesticides except the BHC isomers. Spots became visible after exposure to ultraviolet light for 20 min. A QF–1 column was found to be more versatile for separating pesticides than SE–30 due to less overlap of neighboring peaks.

Frei and Mallet have developed a method for the quantitative analysis of organothiophosphorus pesticides in natural water samples by *in situ* fluorometry after separation on Silica Gel N layers.[82] They describe the application of fluorescence measurements to the quantitative analysis of sulfur-containing organophosphorus compounds directly on thin-layer chromatograms by means of a spectrofluorometer. After development of the chromatogram, the plate was dried for 5 min at 105°C, brominated for 10 sec while still hot, and after cooling was sprayed with a mixture of manganese(II) and salicyl-2-aldehyde-2-quinolylhydrazone (SAQH). The limit of detection ranges from 0.02 to 0.08 μg

per spot; a relative standard deviation of 2.4% is observed for 1 μg samples. Recoveries of 80–92% for Guthion from natural water samples were obtained. *In situ* fluorometry results agreed well with the gas chromatographic data.

Identification of organochlorine pesticides is possible by the gas chromatographic (GC) examination of the parent pesticide followed by GC analysis of the ultraviolet photolysis products on the same column.[83] Leavitt and co-workers have analyzed mixtures of organochlorine pesticides in the presence of polychlorinated biphenyls following photolysis with ultraviolet irradiation.[84] The lower limits of practical quantitation are 0.5 ppm for the PCB's and 0.05 ppm for the individual chlorinated pesticides in hexane solution. However, the determination of pesticide concentrations in the presence of 20- to 40-fold excess of PCB's was difficult.

Gabica *et al.*[85] have described the advantages of flame photometric detection for the gas chromatographic analysis of methyl parathion in rat whole blood and brain tissue. Flame photometric detection results in a more constant base line, a much reduced solvent peak, and greatly reduced background. This detector also gives an increased degree of specificity needed for the reliable authoritative determination of organophosphates.

An accurate and precise procedure for the analysis of whole blood for chlorinated hydrocarbon pesticide residues has been developed.[86] The method involves extraction of the pesticides from blood (acidified with sulfuric acid) with 10% acetone in hexane. Following concentration of the extract, addition of silica gel, mixing, and centrifugation, the sample is analyzed by gas chromatography with electron capture detection. Heparin, EDTA, and sodium citrate were each used as anticoagulants and found not to interfere in the recovery. Recoveries in excess of 88% were observed for all the pesticides examined with a relative standard deviation of ±3%. Comparison of this method with other methods indicates that this procedure represents an improvement in the accuracy, precision, and analysis time required.

A sampling and analytic system for the measurement of atmospheric levels of pesticides has been developed.[87] The sampling train consists of an unimpregnated glass cloth filter followed by a Greenburg–Smith impinger containing 100 ml of hexylene glycol, and subsequently followed by an adsorption tube filled with alumina. The pesticides are extracted from the filter, alumina, and hexylene glycol, passed through a Florisil cleanup column which effects a separation of the chlorinated and organophosphate pesticides. The pesticides were subsequently analyzed by gas chromatography. Correction factors for losses, incurred during extraction and cleanup, ranged from 1.00 for o,p'-DDT to 2.82 for malathion.   Atrazine and linuron residues can be simultaneously detected in water, soil, plant, and animal tissue samples by thin-layer chromatography.[88] Excellent separation of the two herbicides from each other and other materials is achieved on both silica gel and aluminum oxide GF using several different solvent systems, including methylene chloride and chloroform. Visualization on the silica gel layer was effected with tertbutyl hypochlorite-iodide-starch with the ureas giving yellowish bleached spots and the triazines producing blue spots. On the alumina layer, gray spots were visible on a white background following addition of 0.05 N silver nitrate and ultraviolet irradiation.

Shafik *et al.* have developed a gas chromatographic method for the determination of trace quantities of 2,4-dichlorophenoxyacetic acid (2,4-D), 2,4,5-trichlorophenoxyacetic acid (2,4,5-T), 2,4-dichlorophenol (2,4-DCP), and 2,4,5-trichlorophenol (2,4,5-TCP) in human and rat urine.[89] The average recoveries of the phenols and acids from spiked rat urine ranged from 90 to 98%. The limits of detection for 2,4-D, 2,4,5-T, DCP, and TCP were 0.05, 0.01, 0.10, and 0.01 ppm, respectively. This method involves the acid hydrolysis of the conjugated phenols, followed by the benzene extraction of the herbicides. The phenols and acids are ethylated with diazoethane reagent,[90] cleaned up on a silica gel chromatography column, and analyzed by gas chromatography on 20% OV-101 at 175°–195°C with electron capture detection.

Dichloroacetylene

A procedure for the gas chromatographic analysis of dichloroacetylene at the ppb level has been developed.[91] The chromatographic separation is performed on a 15% polyethylene glycol 400 column. Following separation, the eluent is pyrolyzed and titrated coulometrically with silver ion. The precision of the method is ±5% above 10 ppm and decreases to ±50% at the 10 ppb level.

Fluorocarbons

A gas chromatographic procedure for the determination of several common fluorocarbon propellants in blood was evaluated by Terrill.[92] The fluorocarbons are extracted from the blood with hexane and analyzed by gas chromatography on a Porapak Q column utilizing electron capture detection. This procedure was found to be satisfactory for the analysis of Fluorocarbon-11, Fluorocarbon-12, and Fluorocarbon-114. Five milliliters of hexane were injected into a 1 ml Vacutainer and cooled in an ice bath. Two milliliters of blood were obtained from the animal and immediately injected in the Vacutainer containing the hexane. The tube was shaken for 1 min and placed in a −20°C freezer for 30 min. The frozen blood remains on the bottom of the tube facilitating sampling of the liquid hexane layer.

Recoveries of F-11 and F-12 were generally better than 90%. A slightly lower recovery (85%) was observed for F-114 and could not be readily explained. Gas chromatographic separation of F-11, F-12, F-114, and F-115 was performed on a Porapak Q column. While there was no significant loss of the fluorocarbons upon storage for 1–7 days, the results do tend to be low (5–10%) due to nonquantitative extraction with hexane. The limits of detection for F-11 and F-12 were 0.005 μg/ml and 0.15 μg/ml, respectively.

Formaldehyde

Bailey and Rankin have proposed a spectrophotometric method for the determination of formaldehyde based on the catalytic effect of formaldehyde on the hydrogen peroxide oxidation of p-phenylenediamine to form bis(2′,5′-diaminophenyl)-benzoquinone diimine (Bandrowski's base).[93] The investigators believe this procedure to be applicable to the quantitative determination of formaldehyde at low concentrations in air with a relatively high degree of selectivity. Nitrogen dioxide and hydrogen sulfide do not interfere. Sulfur dioxide does interfere but this interference can be eliminated by its prior oxidation with dilute hydrogen peroxide. The calibration curves demonstrate agreement with Beer's law in the concentration range of 0.05–2.5 μg HCHO/ml of solution.

Methylene-bis-*ortho*-chloroaniline

Linch *et al.* have evaluated the hazards of methylene-bis-*ortho*-chloroaniline (MOCA) and discussed means for control of its exposure.[94] The investigators report that MOCA would be classified as mildly cyanogenic in comparison with p-chloroaniline. The analysis of urine and air for MOCA by paper, thin-layer, and gas chromatographic procedures is described. The limits of detection for MOCA in urine by paper, thin-layer, and gas chromatography are 1.5, 0.2, and 0.04 mg/liter. The limit of detection for the analysis of MOCA in air by gas chromatography is 0.01 mg/m^3. Visualization of MOCA on alumina is done under ultraviolet irradiation. The spot is cut from the plate, extracted into acetone–hydrochloric acid, and analyzed by an acid coupling procedure.

Methylene Chloride

The analysis of breath, blood, and urine for relatively low concentrations of methylene chloride can be performed by gas chromatography by means of a 20% Carbowax 20M column and using a gas sampling valve.[95] The head space technique was used as it offers convenience, speed, and sensitivity, and avoids column contamination and cumbersome sample preparation. The method has a sensitivity of at least 0.2 ± 0.1 ppm in breath and 0.022 mg/liter of whole blood.

Phenol

The use of liquid chromatography for the determination of trace quantities of phenol in aqueous solution and industrial waste ($<$mg/liter) has been described.[96] Increased sensitivity can be realized with an ultraviolet detector set at 270 nm. The authors have shown that most other phenols do not interfere. Aqueous solutions are chromatographed on Corasil/C-18 and strong anion exchange material (1% quaternary ammonium substituted methacrylate polymer on 45 μm "Zipax" particles). An inlet pressure of 1000 psi was used.

Polychlorinated Biphenyls

The quantitative estimation of the amount of total polychlorinated biphenyls (PCB's) present in environmental samples has been simplified by the exhaustive chlorination procedure suggested by Hutzinger et al.[97] Problems generally associated with the analysis of PCB's include the interference by 1,1-dichloro-2,2-bis(p-chlorophenyl)ethylene [DDE], the major metabolite of 1,1,1-trichloro-2,2-bis(p-chlorophenyl)ethane (DDT). The proposed procedure eliminates this gas chromatographic interference and permits the separate determination of PCB's, DDT and DDE. The suggested approach greatly simplifies the analytic problem by reducing all the various polychlorinated biphenyls to decachlorobiphenyl and lowers the limit of detection by greatly increasing the halogen content. Two perchlorinating reagents are suggested: (1) the BMC reagent[98] (sulfuryl chloride, sulfur monochloride, and anhydrous aluminum chloride) and (2) antimony pentachloride–iodine. Both reagents can be used in the quantitative conversion of the PCB isomers to decachlorobiphenyl. Extending this procedure to the analysis of the chlorinated dibenzo-dioxins, dibenzofurans, and naphthalenes is accomplished only with the BMC reagent as the antimony pentachloride–iodine reagent results in extensive decomposition, especially at high temperature.

Toluene Diisocyanate

A gas chromatographic procedure for the determination of toluene diisocyanate (TDI) in mixtures of TDI–diphenylmethane diisocyanate (MDI) and polymethylene polyphenyl isocyanate (PAPI) has been developed.[99] MDI and PAPI are not volatile and a pyrolyzer accessory fitted with an aluminum boat was used to keep the pyrolyzer clean. The investigators have not reported the results of its application to environmental samples. However, in view of the difficulties experienced by others with the chemical methods for these determinations, this approach may prove to be rewarding.

Trichloroacetic Acid

The rapid gas chromatographic analysis of trichloroacetic acid (TCA), the major metabolite of trichloroethylene, in urine has been developed by Ehrner–Samuel et al.[100] TCA was extracted from the diluted acidified urine with toluene, esterified with boron trifluoride–methanol reagent, and subsequently analyzed by gas chromatography on 5% QF-1. It has been shown that trichloroethylene does not interfere with the analysis of the methyl ester of TCA. The limit of detection reported for this procedure is 3 μg/ml.

REFERENCES

1. Thomas, R. F., and Booth, R. L., Selective electrode measurement of ammonia in water and wastes. *Environ. Sci. Technol. 7*, 523 (1973).
2. Kramer, D. N., and Sech., J. M., New sensitive method for quantitative assay of ammonia in air. *Anal. Chem. 44*, 395 (1972).
3. Filer, T. D., Fluorometric determination of submicrogram quantities of antimony. *Anal. Chem. 43*, 725 (1971).
4. Chu, R. C., Barron, G. P., and Baumgarner, P. A. W., Arsenic determination at sub-microgram levels by arsine evolution and flameless atomic absorption spectro-photometric technique. *Anal. Chem. 44*, 1476 (1972).
5. Ross, W. D., and Sievers, R. E., Environmental air analysis for ultratrace concentrations of beryllium by gas chromatography. *Environ. Sci. Technol. 6*, 155 (1972).
6. Taylor, M. L., and Arnold, E. L., Ultratrace determination of metals in biological specimens. Quantitative determination of beryllium by gas chromatography. *Anal. Chem. 43*, 1328 (1971).
7. Bailey, B. W., and Lo, F. C., Flame photometric determination of submicrogram quantities of boron. *Int. J. Envir. Anal. Chem. 1*, 267 (1972).
8. Bauer, R., and Rupe, C. O., Use of syringaldazine in a photometric method for estimating "free" chlorine in water. *Anal. Chem. 43*, 421 (1971).
9. Sconce, J. S., ed., "Chlorine, its Manufacture, Properties and Uses," pp. 461–482. Van Nostrands, Reinhold, Princeton, New Jersey, 1962. , 10.
10. Booth, G. H., Jr., and Darby, W. J., Determination by gas-liquid chromatography of physiological levels of chromium in biological tissues. *Anal. Chem. 43*, 831 (1971).
11. Hansen, L. C., Scribner, W. G., Gilbert, T. W., and Sievers, R. E., Rapid analysis for sub-nanogram amounts of chromium in blood and plasma using electron capture gas chromatography. *Anal. Chem. 43*, 349 (1971).
12. Hambidge, K. M., Use of static argon atmosphere in emission spectrochemical determination of chromium in biological materials. *Anal. Chem. 43*, 103 (1971).
13. Gordon, W. A., Use of temperature buffered argon arc in spectrographic trace analysis. *NASA Tech. Note D-2598* (1965).
14. Gordon, W. A., Stabilization of dc arc in static argon atmospheres for use in spectrochemical analysis. *NASA Tech. Note D-4236* (1967).
15. Gordon, W. A., A servocontroller for programming sample vaporization in direct current arc spectrochemical analysis. *NASA Tech. Note D-4769* (1968).
16. Scoggins, M. W., Ultraviolet spectrophotometric determination of cyanide ion. *Anal. Chem. 44*, 1294 (1972).

17. Frant, M. S., Ross, J. W., Jr., and Riseman, J. H., Electrode indicator technique for measuring low levels of cyanide. *Anal. Chem. 44*, 2227 (1972).
18. Orion Research, Inc., *Newslett./Specific Ion Technol. 1*, 9 (1969); *2*, 5 (1970).
19. Gran, G., Determination of the equivalence point in potentiometric titrations. Part II. *Analyst 77*, 661 (1952).
20. Ryan, D. E., and Holzbecher, J., Fluorescence and anions determination. *Int. J. Environ. Anal. Chem. 1*, 159 (1971).
21. Har, T. L., and West, T. S., Spectrofluorimetric determination of traces of fluoride ion by ternary complex formation with zirconium and calcein blue. *Anal. Chem. 43*, 136 (1971).
22. Natusch, D. F. S., Klonis, H. B., Axelrod, H. D., Teck, R. J., and Lodge, J. P., Jr., Sensitive method for measurement of atmospheric hydrogen sulfide. *Anal. Chem. 44*, 2067 (1972).
23. Axelrod, H. D., Cary, J. H., Bonelli, J. E., and Lodge, J. P., Jr., Fluorescence determination of sub-parts per billion hydrogen sulfide in the atmosphere. *Anal. Chem. 41*, 1856 (1969).
24. Wroński, M., Thiomercurimetric determination of hydrogen sulfide in natural waters below and above microgram per liter level. *Anal. Chem. 43*, 606 (1971).
25. Purdue, L. J., Enrione, R. E., Thompson, R. J., and Bonfield, B. A., Determination of organic and total lead in the atmosphere by atomic absorption spectrometry. *Anal. Chem. 45*, 527 (1973).
26. Hwang, J. Y., Ullucci, P. A., and Mokeler, C. J., Direct flameless atomic absorption determination of lead in blood. *Anal. Chem. 45*, 795 (1973).
27. Yeager, D. W., Cholak, J., and Henderson, E. W., Determination of lead in biological and related material by atomic absorption spectrophotometry. *Environ. Sci. Technol. 5*, 1021 (1971).
28. Krause, L. A., Henderson, R., Shotwell, H. P., and Culp, D. A., The analysis of mercury in urine, blood, water, and air. *Amer. Ind. Hyg. Ass., J. 32*, 331 (1971).
29. Nelson, K. H., Brown, W. D., and Staruch, S. J., Determination of trace levels of mercury in effluents and wastewaters. *Int. J. Environ. Anal. Chem. 2*, 45 (1972).
30. Muscat, V. I., Vickers, T. J., and Andren, A., Simple and versatile atomic fluorescence system for determination of nanogram quantities of mercury. *Anal. Chem. 44*, 218 (1972).
31. Doherty, P. E., and Dorsett, R. S., Determination of trace concentrations of mercury in environmental water samples. *Anal. Chem. 43*, 1887 (1971).
32. Brandenberger, H., and Bader, H., The determination of nanogram levels of mercury in solution by a flameless atomic absorption technique. *At. Absorption Newslett. 6*, 101 (1967).
33. Braman, R. S., and Dynako, A., Direct current discharge spectral emission-type detector. *Anal. Chem. 40*, 95 (1968).
34. Braman, R. S., Membrane probe-spectral emission type detection system for mercury in water. *Anal. Chem. 43*, 1462 (1971).
35. Scullman, J., and Widmark, G., Collection and determination of mercury in air. *Int. J. Environ. Anal. Chem. 2*, 29 (1972).
36. Long, S. J., Scott, D. R., and Thompson, R. J., Atomic absorption determination of elemental mercury collected from ambient air on silver wool. *Anal. Chem. 45*, 2227 (1973).
37. Fisher, G. E., and Becknell, D. E., Saltzman method for determination of low concentrations of oxides of nitrogen in automotive exhaust. *Anal. Chem. 44*, 863 (1972).

38. Niki, H., Warnick, A., and Lord, R. R., An ozone–NO chemiluminescence method for NO analysis in piston and turbine engines. *SAE Transactions* No. 710072 (1971).

39. Fine, D. H., Critical evaluation of Saltzman technique for NO_x analysis in the 0-100 ppm range. *Environ. Sci. Technol. 6,* 348 (1972).

40. Coulehan, B. A., and Lang, H. W., Rapid determination of nitrogen oxides with use of phenoldisulfonic acid. *Environ. Sci. Technol. 5,* 163 (1971).

41. Martens, H. H., Dee, L. A., and Nakamura, J. T., Improved phenoldisulfonic acid method for determination of NO_x from stationary sources. *Environ. Sci. Technol. 7,* 1152 (1973).

42. Sigsby, J. E., Jr., Black, F. M., Bellar, T. A., and Klosterman, D. L., Chemiluminescent method for analysis of nitrogen compounds in mobile source emissions (NO, NO_2 and NH_3). *Environ. Sci. Technol. 7,* 51 (1973).

43. Noweir, M. H., and Pfitzer, E. A., An improved method for determination of phosgene in air. *Amer. Ind. Hyg. Ass., J. 32,* 163 (1971).

44. Kirkpatrick, D. S., and Bishop, S. H., Simplified wet ash procedure for total phosphorus analysis of organophosphonates in biological samples. *Anal. Chem. 43,* 1707 (1971).

45. Bartlett, G. R., Phosphorus assay in column chromatography. *J. Biol. Chem. 234,* 466 (1959).

46. Kirkbright, G. F., Narayanaswamy, R., and West, T. S., Spectrofluorimetric determination of orthophosphate as Rhodamine B molybdophosphate. *Anal. Chem. 43,* 1434 (1971).

47. Osburn, R. L., Shendrikar, A. D., and West, P. W., New spectrophotometric method for determination of submicrogram quantities of selenium. *Anal. Chem. 43,* 594 (1971).

48. West, P. W., and Ramakrishna, T. V., A catalytic method for determining traces of selenium. *Anal. Chem. 40,* 966 (1968).

49. Baird, R. B., Pourian, S., and Gabrielian, S. M., Determination of trace amounts of selenium in wastewaters by carbon rod atomization. *Anal. Chem. 44,* 1887 (1972).

50. Matousek, J. P., A carbon rod atomizer for AAS. *Amer. Lab. 3,* 45 (1971).

51. Wiersma, J. H., and Lee, G. F., Selenium in lake sediments–analytical procedure and preliminary results. *Environ. Sci. Technol. 5,* 1203 (1971).

52. Raihle, J. A., Fluorometric determination of selenium in effluent streams with 2,3-diaminonaphthalene. *Environ. Sci. Technol. 6,* 621 (1972).

53. Rankin, J. M., Fluorometric determination of selenium in water with 2,3-diaminonaphthalene. *Environ. Sci. Technol. 7,* 823 (1973).

54. Baiulescu, G. E., Marcuta, P. C., and Marinescu, D. M., Spectrophotometric determination of atmospheric sulfur dioxide with 4(4-aminophenylazo)-1-naphthylamine. *Int. J. Environ. Anal. Chem. 2,* 203 (1973).

55. Young, M., Driscoll, J. N., and Mahoney, K. Potentiometric determination of sulfur dioxide in flue gases with an ion selective lead electrode. *Anal. Chem. 45,* 2283 (1973).

56. Carlson, G. D., and Black, W. E., Rapid method for estimation of mean sulfur dioxide pollution using lead candles and atomic absorption spectrophotometry. *Environ. Sci. Technol. 7,* 1040 (1973).

57. Frechette, M. W., and Fasching, J. L., Simple piezoelectric probe for detection and measurement of SO_2. *Environ. Sci. Technol. 7,* 1135 (1973).

58. Stevens, R. K., Mulik, J. D., O'Keefe, A. E., and Krost, K. J., Gas chromatography of reactive sulfur gases in air at the parts-per-billion level. *Anal. Chem. 43,* 827 (1971).

59. Kremer, L., and Spicer, L. D., Gas chromatographic separation of hydrogen sulfide,

carbonyl sulfide, and higher sulfur compounds with a single pass system. *Anal. Chem. 45*, 1963 (1973).

60. Bruner, F., Liberti, A., Possanzini, M., and Allegrini, I., Improved gas chromatographic method for the determination of sulfur compounds at the ppb level in air. *Anal. Chem. 44*, 2070 (1972).

61. Robertus, R. J., and Schaer, M. J., Portable continuous chromatographic coulometric sulfur emission analyzer. *Environ. Sci. Technol. 7*, 849 (1973).

62. Greer, D. G., and Bydalek, T. J., Response characterization of the melpar flame photometric detector for hydrogen sulfide and sulfur dioxide. *Environ. Sci. Technol. 7*, 153 (1973).

63. Bartosiewicz, L., Improved techniques of identification and determination of airborne asbestos. *Amer. Ind. Hyg. Ass., J. 34*, 252 (1973).

64. Rickards, A. L., Estimation of trace amounts of chrysotile asbestos by x ray diffraction. *Anal. Chem. 44*, 1872 (1972).

65. Rickards, A. L., Estimation of submicrogram quantities of chrysotile asbestos by electron microscopy. *Anal. Chem. 45*, 809 (1973).

66. Larsen, D. J., von Doenhoff, L. J., and Crable, J. V., The quantitative determination of quartz in coal dust by infrared spectroscopy. *Amer. Ind. Hyg. Ass., J. 33*, 367 (1972).

67. Goldberg, S. A., Raymond, L. D., and Taylor, C. D., Bureau of mines procedure for analysis of respirable dust from coal mines. *Amer. Ind. Hyg. Ass., J. 34*, 200 (1973).

68. Bumsted, H. E., Determination of alpha-quartz in the respirable portion of airborne particulates by x ray diffraction. *Amer. Ind. Hyg. Ass., J. 34*, 150 (1973).

69. Haddon, W. F., Wiley, M., and Waiss, A. C., Jr., Aflatoxin detection by thin-layer chromatography—mass spectrometry. *Anal. Chem. 43*, 268 (1971).

70. Shadoff, L. A., Kallos, G. J., and Woods, J. S., Determination of bis(chloromethyl)ether in air by gas chromatography—mass spectrometry. *Anal. Chem. 45*, 2341 (1973).

71. Collier, L., Determination of bis-chloromethyl ether at the ppb level in air samples by high-resolution mass spectroscopy. *Environ. Sci. Technol. 6*, 930 (1972).

72. Hoffmann, D., and Rathkamp, G., Quantitative determination of fluorenes in cigarette smoke and their formation by pyrosynthesis. *Anal. Chem. 44*, 899 (1972).

73. Lane, D. A., Moe, H. K., and Katz, M. Analysis of polynuclear aromatic hydrocarbons, some heterocyclics, and aliphatics with a single gas chromatograph column. *Anal. Chem. 45*, 1776 (1973).

74. Karger, B. L., Martin, M., Loheac, J., and Guiochon, G., Separation of polyaromatic hydrocarbons by liquid-solid chromatography using 2,4,7-trinitrofluorenone impregnated Corasil I columns. *Anal. Chem. 45*, 496 (1973).

75. Klimisch, H.-J., Determination of polycyclic aromatic hydrocarbons. Separation of benzpyrene isomers by high-pressure liquid chromatography on cellulose acetate columns. *Anal. Chem. 45*, 1960 (1973).

76. McKay, J. F., and Latham, D. R., Polyaromatic hydrocarbons in high-boiling petroleum distillates. Isolation by gel permeation chromatography and identification by fluorescence spectrometry. *Anal. Chem. 45*, 1050 (1973).

77. Burchfield, H. P., Wheeler, R. J., and Bernos, J. B., Fluorescence detector for analysis of polynuclear arenes by gas chromatography. *Anal. Chem. 43*, 1976 (1971).

78. Bhatia, K., Gas Chromatographic determination of polycyclic aromatic hydrocarbons. *Anal. Chem. 43*, 609 (1971).

79. Ali, K. H., and Wheelock, J. V., Pesticides in effluents and polluted river water. *Int. J. Environ. Anal. Chem. 2*, 261 (1973).

258   Robert G. Keenan and Richard R. Keenan

80. Bates, J. A. R., The general method for the determination of organophosphorus pesticide residues in foodstuffs. *Analyst (London) 90*, 453 (1965).
81. Morley, H. V., and Chiba, M., Thin-layer chromatography for chlorinated pesticide residue analysis without cleanup. *J. Ass. Offic. Agr. Chem. 47*, 306 (1964).
82. Frei, R. W., and Mallet, V., Quantitative thin-layer chromatography of organothiophosphorus pesticides by *in situ* fluorimetry. *Int. J. Environ. Anal. Chem. 1*, 99 (1971).
83. Glotfelty, D. E., Identification of organochlorine pesticide residues by ultraviolet solid-phase photolysis. *Anal. Chem. 44*, 1250 (1972).
84. Leavitt, R. A., Su, G. C. C., and Zabik, M. J., Analytical methodology for bioactive compounds. Photochemically assisted analysis of chlorinated hydrocarbon pesticides in the presence of polychlorinated biphenyls. *Anal. Chem. 45*, 2130 (1973).
85. Gabica, J., Wyllie, J., Watson, M., and Benson, W. W., Example of flame photometric analysis for methyl parathion in rat whole blood and brain tissue. *Anal. Chem. 43*, 1102 (1971).
86. Henderson, S. J., DeBoer, J. G., and Stahr, H. M., Improved method for determination of chlorinated hydrocarbon pesticide residues in whole blood. *Anal. Chem. 43*, 445 (1971).
87. Stanley, C. W., Barney, J. E., II, Helton, M. R., and Yobs, A. R., Measurement of atmospheric levels of pesticides. *Environ. Sci. Technol. 5*, 430 (1971).
88. Purkayastha, R., Simultaneous detection of the residues of atrazine and linuron in water, soil, plant, and animal samples by thin-layer chromatography. *Int. J. Environ. Anal. Chem. 1*, 147 (1971).
89. Shafik, M. T., Sullivan, H. C., and Enos, H. F., A method for determination of low levels of exposure to 2,4-D and 2,4,5-T. *Int. J. Environ. Anal. Chem. 1*, 23 (1971).
90. Stanley, C. W., Derivatization of pesticide-related acids and phenols for gas chromatographic determination. *J. Agr. Food Chem. 14*, 321 (1966).
91. Williams, F. W., Determination of dichloroacetylene in complex atmospheres. *Anal. Chem. 44*, 1317 (1972).
92. Terrill, J. B., Determination of fluorocarbon propellants in blood and animal tissue. *Amer. Ind. Hyg. Ass., J. 33*, 736 (1972).
93. Bailey, B. W., and Rankin, J. M., New spectrophotometric method for determination of formaldehyde. *Anal. Chem. 43*, 782 (1971).
94. Linch, A. L., O'Connor, G. B., Barnes, J. R., Killian, A. S., Jr., and Neeld, W. E., Jr., Methylene-bis-*ortho*-chloroaniline (MOCA): evaluation of hazards and exposure control. *Amer. Ind. Hyg. Ass., J. 32*, 802 (1971).
95. DiVincenzo, G. D., Yanno, F. J., and Astill, B. D., The gas chromatographic analysis of methylene chloride in breath, blood and urine. *Amer. Ind. Hyg. Ass., J. 32*, 387 (1971).
96. Bhatia, K., Determination of trace phenol in aqueous solution by aqueous liquid chromatography. *Anal. Chem. 45*, 1344 (1973).
97. Hutzinger, O., Safe, S., and Zitko, V., Analysis of chlorinated aromatic hydrocarbons by exhaustive chlorination: Qualitative and structural aspects of the perchloroderivatives of biphenyl, naphthalene, terphenyl, dibenzofuran, dibenzodioxin and DDE. *Int. J. Environ. Anal. Chem. 2*, 95 (1972).
98. Ballester, M., Molinet, C., and Castañer, J., Preparation of highly strained aromatic chlorocarbons(I) a powerful nuclear chlorinating agent—relevant reactivity phenomena traceable to molecular strain. *J. Amer. Chem. Soc. 82*, 4254 (1960).
99. Bovee, H. H., Monteith, L. E., and Breysse, P. A., Analysis of TDI–MDI–PAPI mixtures by gas chromatography. *Amer. Ind. Hyg. Ass., J. 32*, 256 (1971).
100. Ehrner-Samuel, H., Balmér, K., and Thorsell, W., Determination of trichloroacetic acid in urine by a gas chromatographic method. *Amer. Ind. Hyg. Ass., J. 34*, 93 (1973).

Hazard Evaluation and Control

ROBERT D. SOULE

INTRODUCTION

The period of time represented by the literature pertaining to developments in hazard evaluation and control reviewed in this chapter coincides with the first years of federal activity associated with implementation of the Occupational Safety and Health Act of 1970. Understandably enough, therefore, the literature of this period indicates an increase in interest in, and concern for, development of more relevant methodology for evaluation and control of the industrial environment.

Much of the recent literature pertaining to evaluation and control of physical stresses and analysis of chemical stresses is reviewed in other chapters of this text. The material reviewed in this chapter will be limited to pertinent developments in evaluation and control concepts per se. Obviously, "pertinent" concepts need not necessarily be innovative in nature. In fact, more often than not they are merely new applications of basic principles of industrial hygiene control. Traditionally, these have included replacement of a hazardous material with one of less hazard, modification of a process or work practices associated with the process, isolation, enclosure, and either or both local and general exhaust ventilation.

Specific control problems that arise in various industrial operations are never so unique and insurmountable that application of some types of hazard evaluation and control concepts is impossible, although there is a tremendous range of complex individual problems encountered. Necessary and relevant information is usually available from one of many sources: abstracting and indexing services; technical journals; publications of various universities, research organizations, and trade associations; rules, regulations, and guidelines published by various federal, state, and local agencies; publications of professional societies and results of studies conducted by private companies. As was the case with the previous edition of this book, the major portion of the material discussed in this chapter was published in the *American Industrial Hygiene Association Journal,* which traditionally has been the primary source of new information on hazard evaluation and control.

AIR SAMPLING INSTRUMENTATION

Correlation of Particle Number and Mass Concentration Techniques

In recent years there have been many attempts to determine relationships between various sampling techniques that have evolved in the industrial hygiene profession. One such investigation[1] consisted of collecting samples of airborne dust in several industrial plants including a flour mill, sand preparation plant, granite grinding facility, gray iron foundry, and a steel casting foundry. Particle number concentrations were determined by three different techniques: (1) use of the midget impinger with microscopic analysis at 100x magnification, (2) the membrane filter–optical microscope technique using Millipore type AA filters and analyses at both 100x and 1000x magnification, and (3) use of an optical counter (Bausch and Lomb Model No. 40–1A) to automatically obtain particle number–size distribution and concentration.

Mass concentrations were also determined using three different techniques: (1) a total filter system incorporating preweighed 47-mm diameter glass fiber filters with subsequent determination of weight gain on the filter, (2) a two-stage sampler employing a small cyclone to collect the larger particles and a 1-inch glass fiber filter used to collect the so-called "respirable" particles with subsequent gravimetric analysis of both fractions, and (3) a Lundgren impacter that was used to acquire data on both particle mass concentration and size distribution by separating the sampled particulate into five fractions.

The conclusions drawn by these investigators included the following observations. The optical counter yielded data that agreed well with direct microscopic examinations of non-light-absorbing particles; however, for highly absorbing particles the optical counter tended to underestimate the size of the particles. Assuming that the impinger technique produces data that can be interpreted as concentrations of particles larger than 1 μm, results obtained with this technique ranged between $\frac{1}{4}$ and 10 times those indicated by the light-scattering counter and optical microscope techniques. Total mass concentration data determined by the total filter, two-stage sampler, and Lundgren impacter[1] all agreed within a factor of approximately two for all test conditions.

Also, the "respirable" particle concentrations determined with the two-stage sampler and the Lundgren impacter agreed within a factor of three.

Piezoelectric–Electrostatic Mass Concentration Sampler

Olin *et al.*[2] describe an instrument that has been developed to measure particle mass concentration rather than light-scattering ability or soiling properties as was common with previous mass measuring instrumentation.

This instrument, the principle of operation of which is discussed in detail in the article, operates on the basis of using a point-to-plane electrostatic precipitator to deposit sampled particles onto a piezoelectric microbalance mass sensor since the natural vibrational frequency of a piezoelectric material can be shifted if a mass of particles can be made to adhere to it. The instrument described in this article uses a combination of airflow and electric field to carry sampled particles to the electrode surface of a piezoelectric crystal with a measurement of resulting change in frequency of vibration of the crystal. The authors point out that the instrument holds promise for application in the measurement of exhaust from automobile engines as well as in industrial hygiene particulate sampling, ambient air monitoring, and as an industrial process control device.

Instantaneous Mass Monitor

Lilienfeld and Dulchinos[3] describe a battery-operated mass sampler that was developed originally for use in evaluation of dust levels in coal mines based on measurement of β-radiation absorption by particles collected on a thin polyester film substrate by inertial impaction. The sampler can be operated with or without a cyclone precollector so as to obtain samples of either total or respirable mass.

Typically, the sampler is allowed to run for 1 min for each sample. During the initial and final periods of sampling, the β-pulse rate is measured. The ratio of logarithms of the initial to final pulse rates is proportional to the mass of material collected on the plate and is displayed in digital format on the instrument. The unit samples at a flow rate of nominally 2 liters/min and has a mass concentration measuring range of 1–50 mg/m^3.

Piezoelectric–Cascade Impactor

Another instrument utilizing the ability to observe a shift in vibrational frequency of piezoelectric quartz crystals as a result of deposition of particles onto them has been described.[4] This instrument utilizes a four-stage cascade impactor with a capability of installing piezoelectric mass sensors in any or all of the stages, thus permitting the quantitation of the mass of the various size fractions separated by the impactor. It is apparent that, with some minor modifications, primarily in the physical characteristics of the crystal, this type of instrument could have many applications in the field of particle sizing and mass concentration measurements.

Passive Monitor of Gaseous Contaminants

The development of a novel type of personal monitoring device for estimating exposure to airborne gases has been described by Palmes and Gunnison.[5] Briefly, the device consists of a cylinder approximately 1 cm in diameter and 3 cm long. An orifice, 0.32 cm in diameter and 0.5-4 cm in length, is inserted into the chamber. The chamber is filled with a material that will collect the material to be tested quantitatively and permit subsequent chemical or physical estimation. Since it is necessary for the concentration within the chamber to be essentially zero, it requires that a highly effective collecting medium be placed in the chamber. Determination of the quantity of gas transferred by diffusion from the atmosphere being tested through the orifice of known dimensions into a chamber maintained at essentially zero concentration by means of the collecting medium can be used as the basis for calculating average concentrations during the time the sampler is in the environment. Tests with water vapors and sulfur dioxide have indicated that this sampling principle is workable and theoretically applicable to any gaseous airborne contaminant.

Halogen Detector

A field instrument that can be used to continuously monitor concentrations of halogenated compounds has been developed, based on the enhancement of the nitrogen and NO molecular spectrum that occurs when halogenated substances are present in an ac spark.[6] Although the exact mechanism of this enhancement is not fully understood, the increase in brightness in the spectrum definitely is a function of the amount of halogenated material present and is predictable and reproducible in nature.

Briefly, the air sample is drawn into the instrument through a glass wool filter, which removes particulate matter and water droplets, then through a valve to an air pump, which forces the gas into the spark chamber. If halogens are present in the airstream the spark brightens and the intensity of the spectrum is monitored by a photocell that displays the reading on an ammeter. The instrument appears to be a definite refinement of and improvement upon the previously available spark-type halide detectors in that it is considerably lighter and smaller and requires no batteries.

Pyrolyzer–Microcoulomb Detector

A pyrolyzer and microcoulomb detector (Mast ozone meter) connected in series were evaluated as a direct-reading air sampling instrument.[7] This arrangement extended the usefulness of the microcoulomb detector to measurement of a variety of materials in concentrations well below 1 ppm with direct readout capabilities. In general, the combination system is more effective because the pyrolyzer decomposes certain compounds to substances that can be measured by the microcoulomb detector. It should be pointed out that this system is nonspecific in nature and therefore normally has application only in situations where the contaminants are known and interferences are not present.

Developments in Respirable Mass Sampling

There has been a trend toward increased utilization of sampling instrumentation which, by one means or another, determines concentrations of "respirable" mass. To a great extent this has consisted of development and refinement of the 10-mm cyclone sampler for use in personal monitoring programs. The appropriateness and validity of gravimetric measurements obtained using the cyclone and filter assemblies have been discussed. Of particular concern were shortcomings of the overall system, documented in an article by Morse et al.,[8] when viewed in light of the legal requirements and standards relative to use of this method in coal mines. Although it is generally agreed that the gravimetric method is superior to the microscopic count method in many respects, there does not appear to be much information available relative to adverse health affects as a function of concentrations of respirable dust to which workers have been exposed.

Efficiency of the 10-mm Nylon Cyclone

For many years the 10-mm nylon cyclone has been used as a size-selective presampler to separate total particulate into respirable and nonrespirable fractions. Developmental work has demonstrated that the cyclone provides a good approximation of the deposition and retention curves for particles in the respiratory system.

In an attempt to ascertain the operating conditions that best enable the cyclone to approximate the theoretical deposition curve, a study was undertaken by the National Institute for Occupational Safety and Health with particular attention to the critical parameter of flow rate through the cyclone.[9] On the basis of a series of studies conducted with the cyclone, in which detailed attention was paid to the sphericity, optical size, aerodynamic size, and actual density of the particles being sampled, it was concluded that a flow rate of 1.7 liters/min was the critical flow at which the cyclone assembly best approximated the theoretical lung deposition curve. The authors pointed out that the recommended flow rate should be a constant, critically controlled flow rate and would not necessarily be the recommended flow rate for personal sampling units that incorporate pulsating pumps. Preliminary studies of small personal sampling units have indicated that pulsations created by diaphragms, valves, and/or pistons significantly alter the efficiency of the cyclone. The authors pointed out a need for more research before a recommended flow rate could be established for optimum operation of personal sampling units in general.

Pulsation Dampeners for Respirable Mass Sampling Units

Because of the recognized adverse effects that pulsating pumps have on the operating characteristics of the 10-mm cyclone used in conjunction with respirable mass sampling, considerable effort has been expended in recent years to develop optimum ways to minimize the effect of pulsation in these units. At essentially the same time, and apparently independently of each other, similar designs of four pulsation dampeners were published by Lamonica and Treaftis[10] and by LaViolette and Reist.[11] Incorporation of pulsation dampeners into sampling units used for respirable mass sampling has shown a reduction in the peak-to-peak amplitude of pulse flow to within 10% of that existing without dampeners in line.

The cyclone is supposed to pass those particles with aerodynamic diameters such that they could be inhaled and collect all other particulate material. The collection efficiency for the cyclone for a given size particle, however, is extremely sensitive to flow rate through the unit. For example, a 30% drop in flow rate, from 2.0 to 1.4 liters/min, resulted in a sixfold increase in the weight of the 4- to 5-μm diameter particles that penetrate the cyclone. This means that, at lower flow rates, larger particles that normally could not penetrate the cyclone are able to pass through it. Increasing the flow rate through the cyclone has the opposite effect. Pumps commercially available for use in respirable mass sampling programs are principally of either the diaphragm or piston type, and thus inherently produce a pulsed flow rather than a constant flow.

Evaluation of Performance of Detector Tubes

Because of obvious advantages of portability, low cost, rapid readout, and simplicity of operation, sampling devices using various indicating tubes have become commonplace within the industrial hygiene profession. To be sure, it has been recognized that many such tubes are useful more in a qualitative than a quantitative sense. The variability of response from tube to tube, problems with interfering substances, and general lack of accuracy and precision for many such tubes have long been recognized. On the other hand, with increasing demand for fast and accurate means of estimating concentrations of specific contaminants in the atmosphere, the desirability of such sampling devices has increased tremendously. Such devices would be of particular value to industrial hygienists having responsbilities for enforcement of occupational health standards.

Over the course of the past several years, the National Institute for Occupational Safety and Health and its predecessor agency has performed evaluations of detector tube systems for several specific substances. The results of these evaluations are presented below, not so much as representative of new information as to point out, with specific examples, the performance of detector tubes in general. It should be cautioned that the detector tube evaluation project undertaken by NIOSH and its predecessor agency was an approval program in which tubes from all manufacturers marketing such devices in the United States were tested provided that they were intended for use over the range from $\frac{1}{2}$ to 5 times the threshold limit value for specific compounds. This approval process should not be construed as a "certification" since the results were based strictly on one lot of tubes and the manufacturers' testing and quality control procedures necessary to ensure continued acceptable qualities were not reviewed.

For all chemicals discussed below, concentrations of the substance in air over the range of essentially $\frac{1}{2}$–5 times the threshold limit value were generated dynamically by means of either a double-dilution, vapor-pressure system or a permeation tube system. Confirmation of the actual concentrations generated by the systems at each of the test levels was made by sampling and analyzing the atmosphere within the mixing chamber by at least two independent methods for which the accuracy and reproducibility were known.

The criterion used to evaluate the performance of the detector tubes was that suggested by the ACGIH–AIHA joint committee in its report of August 9, 1965: "Each calibration point listed by the manufacturer shall be correct to within ±25% of the stated concentration over the working range of the tube". The results of the evaluations of commercially available tubes for six specific substances are presented below.

BENZENE

Of the commercially available tubes evaluated for accuracy of response to known concentrations of benzene in air, none met the ±25% criterion.[12] Therefore, an alternative performance level was set based on the documented performance of the test population of tubes as a whole. Those tubes that were consistently and significantly below the performance of the alternate criteria level were rejected statistically. Of detector tubes manufactured for use in the range from 20 to 160 ppm of benzene, the following were found to be ±50% accurate at the 95% confidence level.

Manufacturer	Type
Mine Safety Appliances	93074
Scott Draeger	Ch-248
Unico-Kitagawa	118-A

CARBON TETRACHLORIDE

Tubes supplied by various manufacturers claiming to have tubes that measured concentrations of carbon tetrachloride in air over the range of at least 10–50 ppm were evaluated.[13] None of the tubes submitted met the 25% criterion and, in fact, none was found to be satisfactory for use at even ±50% accuracy. Therefore, all tubes marketed for use in evaluating atmospheric levels of carbon tetrachloride were judged to be unsatisfactory for practical use. The authors point out that these tubes should be employed at best for no more than qualitative determinations since, with poor reproducibility, calibration of the tubes would be of little value.

CHLORINE

Chlorine tubes manufactured for use in a range including 0.5–5 ppm were evaluated.[14] Of the tubes tested, only those supplied by Mine Safety Appliances Company (type 82399) were found to meet the performance criteria of ±25% accuracy over the range of test concentrations. The Bacharach tubes (type 19–0239) performed acceptably at the highest three concentrations, but failed to meet the performance standard of ±35% at the lowest concentration tested, namely 0.5 ppm. In addition, the Draeger tube (type CH–243) and the Unico tube (type 109) were found to be acceptable at the alternate criterion level of ±50% accuracy.

HYDROGEN SULFIDE

Tubes manufactured for use in detecting concentrations of hydrogen sulfide in air in the range of 5–50 ppm were evaluated as part of these tests.[15] Of the tubes tested, only the Draeger tube (type CH–298 5/b) was found to meet the performance criteria at all concentrations tested. In addition, the Bacharach (type 19–0198) and the Unico (type 120 b) tubes were found to be acceptable by the alternative accuracy limit of ±50% over the range of test concentrations used.

SULFUR DIOXIDE

Detector tubes manufactured for use in the range including 2.5–25 ppm of sulfur dioxide in air were evaluated.[16] Of the tubes tested, the following were found to be ±25% accurate at the 95% confidence level at the higher concentrations. Apparently, none of the tubes performed within the desired performance criteria at the lowest concentration. Although the percentage errors were large at this concentration, they actually represented relatively small absolute deviations.

Manufacturer	Type
Mine Safety Appliances	92623
Scott-Draeger	CH-317
Unico-Kitagawa	103-C
Unico-Kitagawa	103-D

TETRACHLOROETHYLENE

Only tubes manufactured for use in the range including 50–500 ppm tetrachloroethylene (perchloroethylene) in air were evaluated.[17] Tubes from one batch only for each brand submitted were evaluated. Of the tubes submitted, and based on the particular batches tested, the following tubes were found to be ±25% accurate at the 95% confidence limit over the range of test concentrations used.

Manufacturer	Type
Unico-Kitagawa	134
Unico-Kitagawa	135
Scott-Draeger	CH-307

EVALUATIONS OF SPECIFIC HAZARDS

Asbestos

Concern for the occupational health hazard posed by exposure of workers to airborne asbestos during a variety of applications has continued in recent years.

Recommendations for a total control program for handling and use of asbestos-containing materials have been published in several forms.[18-20] These recommendations are based on the firm conviction that asbestos can be used safely in modern industrial applications provided that adequate precautions are taken to prevent exposures of persons, directly or indirectly affected by the operations, to excessive levels of asbestos. The basic elements of the control programs outlined in the several publications can be summarized as follows:

1. Appropriate engineering control procedures should be used to prevent dissemination of dust into the air wherever asbestos fibers can be generated. Such control measures are necessary not only to keep the exposure levels of workers involved in the asbestos handling operations at acceptable levels but, perhaps more importantly, to assure that atmospheres of adjacent areas do not become inadvertently contaminated.

2. Increased concern for the packaging and storage of asbestos-containing materials must be shown. Containers used to package asbestos should be leak-proof, resistant to breakage, and capable of being maintained in clean conditions during shipping, storage, and use. Containers should be clearly marked and provided with appropriate precautionary labels. Storage of asbestos should be done in such a way, and in such locations, that there is a minimum of container breakage. Spillage of asbestos-containing materials should be cleaned immediately, preferably by means of a vacuum system, in order to prevent dispersion of asbestos into the atmosphere.

3. All processing, handling, and dust control equipment should be maintained in good state of repair. Asbestos-containing wastes should be disposed of in a manner that prevents contamination of areas or subsequent redispersion of the fibers into the air. A rigid program of good housekeeping should be enforced in all areas in which asbestos-containing materials are used.

4. A policy of education of workers involved in handling and use of asbestos should become a part of the routine program. Workers should be made aware of the dangers of breathing asbestos dust and educated as to proper use of engineering controls and personal protective equipment, as well as good industrial hygiene work practices.

5. Approved respiratory protective equipment should be used whenever high exposures to asbestos are likely and where other means of controlling the exposures are not feasible. Whenever a respiratory protective equipment program is instituted, it must be accompanied by the establishment of a program for proper selection, fitting, inspection, and maintenance of the equipment.

6. Where excessive contamination of work clothing is a significant potential hazard, workers should wear special clothing that should be changed at the end of the work shift and handled in a manner that prevents exposure to asbestos of those laundering the clothes. Washroom facilities should be made available to

those workers exposed to excessive levels of airborne asbestos so as to prevent excessive contamination of the skin with asbestos fibers.

7. The air in work areas occupied by persons handling asbestos should be monitored routinely to assure that instituted control procedures are adequate and that airborne levels of asbestos are maintained within acceptable limits.

8. Workers exposed to asbestos should receive periodic medical examinations with particular emphasis on chest roentgenography and pulmonary function measurements.

A detailed discussion of the health hazards associated with exposure of workers to asbestos in the construction industry where asbestos-containing fireproofing material is applied to support structures of multi-storied buildings has been presented by Reitze et al.[21] This presentation indicated that over 40,000 tons of asbestos-containing insulation material was used in 1970 for this purpose. The classical method of applying this material was by spray techniques using one of two basic methods. In the "dry" method, dry insulation material is dumped into a large hopper where the material is agitated and subsequently blown into a 2- or 4-inch hose that conveys the material to a nozzle at the site of application. As the dry material leaves the nozzle, it passes through a ring of fine water jets. Mixing of the dry material and the water takes place at the focal point of these spray jets. The spraying mechanism is controlled by the operator who can adjust the air, dry material, and water mix with valves at the nozzle and determine the point of application for the resulting wet material. The "wet" method differs in that the material is premixed with water in the hopper and the resulting slurry is pumped to the nozzle and sprayed directly upon the surface to be coated, using a nozzle similar to that used to apply plaster.

The authors present the results of an evaluation of exposures of workers to asbestos during the spraying of asbestos-containing fire-proofing materials. The concentrations to which the operators were exposed ranged from approximately 30 to over 100 fibers/cm^3. Of as much concern as the operators were those nearby workers who were exposed indirectly as a result of the spraying operations. Concentrations of asbestos in air as high as 45 fibers/cm^3 were measured 75 ft away from the point of application. The article discusses in detail the various control measures and work practices that are necessary to adequately contain and reduce the concentrations of airborne asbestos resulting from such operations.

Hazards Encountered during Fire-Fighting Training

A discussion of the health hazards associated with fire-fighting training has been published by Hill et al.[22] Part of fire-fighting programs frequently include lessons and demonstrations in extinguishing oil fires in confined spaces. Since it was known that combustion of oil under such oxygen-deficient conditions could lead to formation of polycyclic aromatic hydrocarbons, a study was made of the chemicals contained in the smoke and soot resulting from such fires in an attempt to assess the potential hazards to which participants in such activities might be exposed.

Analysis of air samples obtained during a series of tests indicated the presence of over 45 specific compounds in either the atmosphere within the enclosure or in samples of settled soot. Of most interest and concern were the several polycyclic hydrocarbons identified in the samples. These included benzo(*a*)-pyrene, benzo(*a*)anthracene, benzofluoranthenes, dibenzo(*a,j*)anthracene, and others. The authors point out that until long-term studies have been conducted, the data presented support the belief that chronic exposure to the fine chemical-laden soots produced in these oil fires may constitute a severe potential health hazard.

Carbon Monoxide Personal Monitors

An article by Linch and Pfaff discusses the practicability of using length-of-stain detector tubes as devices for monitoring the exposures of workers to carbon monoxide.[23] The study was undertaken because fixed-station monitors in a large warehouse in which gasoline-powered lift-trucks were operated indicated peak concentrations of carbon monoxide above the threshold limit value of 50 ppm. In an attempt to determine whether workers assigned to this area were exposed to excessive concentrations, it was desirable to use personal monitoring devices if such could be developed.

Monitoring of the employees' exposures was accomplished by use of small battery-operated pumps that provided the airflow through length-of-stain indicator tubes connected to the pumps by means of plastic tubing. In order to provide a constant, low-volume airflow through the detector tubes, and yet allow the pump to operate in the 1 liter/min optimum range, a bypass mechanism was fitted to a tee that was inserted beneath the rotameter. Total airflow through the sampling tube then was maintained at approximately 8 ml/min.

Obviously, the effect of flow rate on development of stain in the tube was critical. However, the article presents data showing that, provided proper calibration of the sampling system is accomplished, the sampling technique could be used to determine the exposures of workers over a 4-hr sampling period. The authors point out that the range of analytic uncertainty could be reduced significantly by improving control of flow rates through the detector tube by either reduction of the pressure drop variability between detector tubes or introduction of a compensator within the air sampler.

Carbon Monoxide–Oxygen Personal Monitor

A self-contained personal monitoring sampling unit has been described in an article by Sidor *et al.*[24] The sampler was developed as a device for monitoring the exposures of fire fighters to both carbon monoxide and oxygen during actual fire-fighting activities. A nonspecific combustible gas indicator modified to be fairly specific for carbon monoxide in a concentration range of 200–100,000 ppm and a commercial membrane oxygen sensor system (without modification) were incorporated as basic components of the sampler. The data were recorded on a small cassette tape recorder by using a simple voltage-to-frequency circuit. Tests during actual fire-fighting activities indicated mean errors of 14 and 3.2% in the carbon monoxide and oxygen measurements, respectively, by comparison of results with standard sampling methods.

Use of these samplers permitted the collection of information, for the first time, on exposures of men during actual fire-fighting and permitted some definition of the term "overcome by smoke." It was the expressed hope of the authors that this method would allow specification of fire situations that presented acute previously unidentified hazards to fire fighters. Aside from that, the sampler also showed promise as a training device to assist fire fighters in recognizing hazards associated with their occupation.

Carbon Monoxide and Nitrogen Dioxide Exposures in Ice Arenas

Several episodes of illnesses among patrons of ice arenas, symptoms of which were typically headache and nausea among children and headache principally in adults, prompted the Minnesota Department of Health to investigate the situation.[25] The study revealed that concentrations of carbon monoxide and nitrogen dioxide from the exhaust of engines of vehicles used to resurface the ice could be built up to the point where they were capable of producing adverse affects in exposed persons. Apparently, more reports of adverse affects had not been received for many reasons: most patrons spend only limited amounts of time in the ice arenas; many arenas located in less densely populated areas resurface only five or six times each day; many arenas resurface frequently only under conditions of heavy use, such as hockey games, at which times the ventilation systems are operated to control heat and smoke generated by spectators; and most arenas do not have a summer ice program when ventilation would be minimal. The article presents guidelines for control of exhaust fumes by means of mechanical ventilation. Based on situations where (1) the resurfacing machine operates approximately 10 min/hr, (2) air distribution in the arena is "good," and (3) the engine of the resurfacing machine receives proper maintenance, these recommendations in essence are that

10,000–15,000 ft^3/min of outside air be supplied to the arena, the actual required air volumes being dependent upon the types of engines in use and the number of vehicles operated at any one time.

Carbon Monoxide Hazard in Aviation

An article by Howlett and Shephard outlines the significance of potential hazard associated with exposures to carbon monoxide of personnel assigned to air crews.[26] Reports of the sources of carbon monoxide were reviewed in detail with discussion of the quantitative significance of each source. These sources include ambient levels of carbon monoxide which are generated by local vehicular traffic from service vehicles associated with operations at the airports, other local ground services including test and repair facilities, ground level contamination by exhaust from aircraft, and exposure resulting from smoking. The article discusses and compares the susceptibility of aviation crew personnel to carbon monoxide intoxication with that of the general population. Taxi drivers and baggage handlers at airport operations may encounter relatively high concentrations of carbon monoxide. Although the personnel assigned to air crews are typically exposed to relatively low concentrations of carbon monoxide, the exposures present a greater risk because of synergistic stresses and the severe demands of their tasks. It was recommended that exposures of personnel in air crews not exceed 40 ppm for 1 hr or 15 ppm for 8 hr. A discussion of methods for modifying air crew operations to meet these recommended standards is presented.

Decomposition of Carbon Tetrachloride

In two articles by Noweir *et al.,* discussions of potential hazards associated with the thermal decomposition of carbon tetrachloride at its threshold limit value concentration (10 ppm) were presented and measurements of the levels of phosgene, chlorine, chlorine dioxide, and hydrogen chloride were discussed.[27,28] Data presented in the study showed that hazardous, and possibly lethal, concentrations of decomposition products can be produced, under various conditions, from the decomposition of a "safe level" (10 ppm) of carbon tetrachloride. Concentrations as high as 10 ppm of phosgene, 15 ppm of chlorine, 1 ppm of chlorine dioxide, and 35 ppm of hydrogen chloride were obtained under various conditions. Although the study was conducted as a controlled laboratory project, the application of findings to the evaluation of maximum hazard situations in the work environment can be made.

Decomposition of Chlorinated Hydrocarbons

A discussion of the hazards associated with decomposition of chlorinated hydrocarbons in the presence of various welding operations was presented by Rinzema and Silverstein.[29] This report discusses the results of air sampling within a glovebox enclosure during gas tungsten, gas metal, and shielded metal arc welding in the presence of several chlorinated hydrocarbons, including methyl chloride, methylene chloride, chloroform, carbon tetrachloride, ethylene dichloride, 1,1,1-trichloroethane, trichloroethylene, perchloroethylene, and o-dichlorobenzene. Air samples collected within the glovebox were analyzed qualitatively and quantitatively for decomposition products including phosgene, chlorine, hydrogen chloride, nitrogen oxides, carbon oxides, ozone, and chlorinated hydrocarbons.

Of the chlorinated hydrocarbons tested, only trichloroethylene and perchloroethylene, when present in the air near welding operations, were decomposed to dangerous levels of phosgene. With these two solvents, the levels of hydrogen chloride and chlorine, although substantial, may not provide adequate warning against presence of phosgene. The other solvents tested appeared to be rather stable in the presence of arc-welding energy. Phosgene, if formed at all, would be at concentrations below the threshold limit value, whereas chlorine and hydrogen chloride, formed simultaneously, would likely act as adequate warning that decomposition of the solvent was taking place. Ventilation requirements may have to be modified to eliminate the irritation caused by the decomposition products.

Noweir et al. presented an up-to-date review and criticism of previously published reports on the decomposition of the chlorinated hydrocarbons.[30] The following conclusions were reached based upon this review of the literature.

1. Chlorinated hydrocarbons decomposed under certain stated conditions to form phosgene, hydrogen chloride, chlorine, chlorine dioxide, and other products.

2. Carbon tetrachloride produced higher concentrations of phosgene than any of the other chlorinated hydrocarbons tested.

3. Metallic surfaces, metal oxides, and metal salts expedited, but were not essential for, the thermal decomposition of chlorinated hydrocarbons. Iron was the most active metal surface for the decomposition.

4. Humidity apparently influenced the decomposition of the phosgene formed, but the degree of hydrolysis due to water vapor was only slight at low concentrations of phosgene.

5. There were marked variances between results of studies on the effect of flame and studies on the extinguishment of fires. The literature review indicated that open flames did cause production of phosgene, but the reports indicated

great variance presumably due to the complexity and nature of contact of the chlorinated hydrocarbons with the flame, the extent of heating, and the nature of the surfaces contacted.

Spontaneous Formation of Bischloromethyl Ether

Much controversy and concern developed following reports that bischloro-methyl ether can be formed spontaneously in ordinary humid air whenever formaldehyde and hydrochloric acid are present together. Initial reports indicated that, at ordinary room temperatures and humidity (70°F and 30% relative humidity), a steady-state level of bischloromethyl ether is reached within a minute following rapid reaction of formaldehyde and hydrogen chloride.[31,32] In general, parts per million of formaldehyde and hydrochloric acid were stated as being capable of reacting to produce parts per billion of the bischloromethyl ether. However, based upon continuing laboratory studies, it was shown that the spontaneous combination of hydrogen chloride and formaldehyde, in concen-trations at or below the respective threshold limit values, does not result in production of detectable amounts of the bischloromethyl ether.[33] It was found that at relatively high concentrations of the reactants (500–3000 ppm) bischloromethyl ether was produced at a detectable level, the highest concen-tration being 38 ppb generated by the reaction of 3000 ppm of formaldehyde and 10,000 ppm of hydrogen chloride. The authors concluded that occupational health problems would not be expected from hydrogen chloride and formal-dehyde reacting to form bischloromethyl ether since the latter was not produced at reactant concentrations of 100 ppm each, levels that are intolerable to humans because of the inherent irritation properties of formaldehyde and hydrogen chloride.

Coal Tar Pitch Volatiles from Coke Ovens

Results of evaluations of exposures of workers to coal tar pitch volatiles during activities associated with operation of coke ovens has been reported by personnel from the Pennsylvania Division of Occupational Health.[34] A total of 319 personal breathing zone and 31 general area samples were obtained. On the basis of determination of the benzene-soluble fraction of these samples, which were collected on silver membrane filters by means of battery-operated personal monitoring pumps, it was concluded that essentially all job classifications in the coking facility were characterized by exposures to concentrations of coal tar pitch volatiles in excess of 0.2 mg/m^3 of air (8-hr time-weighted average exposures), the recognized threshold limit value (TLV).

Attempts were made to correlate the exposures of workers by job classifications. In this respect, there appeared to be a direct correlation between exposures and average general proximity to coke ovens, that is, the nearer the worker is to the oven, the greater the exposure to coal tar pitch volatiles. Preliminary attempts were made to compare results of sampling for respirable dust, using a cyclone elutriator, to those obtained for total dust. However, very slight correlation was found between the amounts of benzene extractable material obtained using the cyclone prefilter versus that found in samples without the prefilter. The article includes a review of proposals for the reduction of exposures of workers to coal tar pitch volatiles, emphasizing that the suggested changes were expensive and complicated in nature. It was recommended that, until control measurers have been proven effective, reasonable enforcement and supervision of operating practices, maintenance, and use of personal protective equipment must be implemented.

A detailed set of work practices for persons employed in operations that have associated with them potential exposures to emissions from coke ovens was published by the National Institute for Occupational Safety and Health and submitted to the U.S. Department of Labor as a recommended work practices standard.[35] This criteria document contained detailed recommendations for necessary work practices, but did not specify an environmental standard.

Cotton Dust in a Textile Plant

The results of a comprehensive survey of concentrations of airborne cotton dust at various process operations in a large textile plant were reported by Hammad and Corn.[36] The sampling methodology included use of a specially designed and constructed horizontal elutriator similar to the Hexhlet. Membrane filters were used to obtain both gravimetric and microscopic data. Air was drawn through the instrument at a constant rate of 0.75 ft^3/min maintained by a critical orifice. Fine and medium dust fractions were collected together on a filter behind a wire gauze, the main function of which was to separate the coarse fraction, or lint, which would not be expected to pass into the respiratory tract. The weight of the medium dust fraction was calculated by subtracting the weight of the fine dust fraction from combined weights of the medium and fine dust fractions collected in the sampler. Total dust concentrations were determined separately using an open-faced 50-mm diameter filter positioned downward in the workroom air. The weight of the coarse fraction was determined by subtracting the weights of the medium and fine fractions from the total dust weights. In addition to sampling the general workroom areas, isokinetic sampling was conducted within air-conditioning ducts in the plants.

Results of the sampling program confirmed those of previously published reports indicating that dust concentrations throughout the facility were generally in excess of the TLV for cotton dust. In addition, the authors point out that most of the "fine" respirable dust fraction was returned to the workrooms either through air-conditioning systems or fabric dust collectors installed inside the rooms. It was apparent that, according to current practice in modern air-conditioned mills in the United States, the use of nonrecirculating air systems is considered impractical. It was the opinion of the authors, however, in light of findings of epidemiologic studies of the incidence of byssinosis in this country, that the practice of recirculating air in the textile plants should cease. Additional concepts for improving the atmospheric environment within the textile plants were presented.

Respirable Dust Generated at Belt Conveyor Transfer Points

An experimental study was conducted by the U.S. Department of Interior, Bureau of Mines, in which the formation of airborne respirable dust by the dropping of broken bituminous coal from a belt conveyor was evaluated.[37] The experimental setup included an enclosed drop tester combined with a laboratory-size belt conveyor. Coal used in the test was obtained from a mine during a dry operation and placed in plastic bags to maintain its natural surface moisture of about 0.8%. Air samples were obtained by means of a high-volume air sampler as well as an Anderson cascade sampler equipped for isokinetic sampling in the test chamber. Processing variables that were investigated included the height of the drop of coal, the loading of the belt, and speed of the conveyor belt. The following conclusions were drawn on the basis of the test results.

1. The fraction of the void space in falling broken coal significantly affected the amount of airborne dust formed during the drop.

2. Approximately 10% of the respirable dust adhering to the coal became airborne by the impact of dropping.

3. Reduction of the height of the material dropped reduced the amount of respirable airborne dust generated.

4. For heavy belt loads, an increase in thickness of the coal bed reduced the specific formation of airborne respirable dust; for light belt loads, an increase in belt speed reduced the formation of dust.

5. Preliminary studies indicated that addition of water upstream of the drop point or the use of an inclined chute significantly reduced the generation of airborne respirable dust.

Exposures to Detergent Enzymes

Two pertinent articles considering the potential health hazards associated with production of synthetic household detergents incorporating enzymes have appeared recently, the first considering primarily the general scope of the problem posed by the need for control of enzymes during production steps,[38] and the second discussing the development of a method for determining the concentrations of proteolytic enzymes in air.[39]

There are two separate and distinct occupational health hazards associated with exposures to enzymes. The first is a primary irritant dermatitis resulting from excessive skin contact with concentrated enzymes, particularly in the presence of moisture and/or skin abrasions. The second condition is one of acute respiratory tract obstruction, due to inhalation of enzyme dust. It should be emphasized here that the consumer aspects of enzyme detergents has been confirmed and reported previously. The articles reviewed here point out control measures necessary to prevent the development of health problems in the manufacturing processes. These include strict adherence to programs of personal hygiene and use of protective clothing for maintaining control of the dermatitis problem and engineering controls to eliminate or, at least, minimize exposures of workers to airborne dusts so as to prevent respiratory sensitization. A continuing program of comprehensive industrial hygiene surveys, complimented by periodical medical evaluations and follow-ups, was deemed essential to assure safe long-term handling of enzymes in the manufacturing of detergents.

The sampling methodology recommended for evaluation of airborne levels of proteolytic enzymes consists of collecting samples on glass fiber filters using high-volume sampling techniques. The level of total dust in the air sample is analyzed subsequently by gravimetric techniques to determine the total dust level. The amount of proteolytic enzymes present in the sample is determined by means of colorimetric techniques, using dimethylated casein as the substrate and trinitrobenzene sulfonic acid as the color reagent. Detailed information describing the analytic accuracy, precision, and limits of detection is presented.

Results of sampling conducted in various production areas indicated a definite reduction in levels of both total dust and proteolytic enzyme as the result of a conscientious program of implementing appropriate engineering controls and a rigorous program of good industrial hygiene work practices and general housekeeping. In a quantitative sense, the results of the air sampling program, conducted over an interval of 18 months, demonstrated the following:

1. Concentrations of total dust and proteolytic enzymes in the enzyme complex handling operations were reduced from approximately 5 mg/m^3 and $25 \text{ }\mu\text{g/m}^3$, respectively, to approximately 1 mg/m^3 and slightly in excess of $1 \text{ }\mu\text{g/m}^3$ for the toal dust and enzymes, respectively.

2. In the enzyme bin floor operations, levels of total dust were reduced from approximately 5 mg/m^3 to about 0.8 mg/m^3. Over this same time period, the concentration of enzyme in this general operations area was reduced correspondingly from approximately $10 \text{ }\mu\text{g/m}^3$ to $0.25 \text{ }\mu\text{g/m}^3$.

3. The average total dust and enzyme concentrations in the enzyme packing

operations were reduced from approximately 5 mg/m^3 and 10 μg/m^3, respectively, to approximately 1 mg/m^3 and 0.26 μg/m^3 for the total dust and enzyme, respectively.

Exposure of Insulation Workers to Fibrous Glass

A study reported by Fowler et $al.$ summarized the results of an evaluation of exposures of workers to airborne fibrous glass during handling and use of prefabricated, and other fibrous glass, insulation materials.[40] Samples of airborne fibers were collected during various operations with over 100 products.

The report concluded that insulation workers, during the application of fibrous glass insulation products, were exposed to concentrations of airborne glass fibers ranging from 0.5 to 8 fibers/ml of air. The computed gravimetric concentrations of airborne glass fibers less than 7 μm in diameter were shown to be well below the tentative threshold limit value of 10 mg/m^3, during even peak periods of activity. Although it was not possible to develop time-weighted average exposure values, it was obvious that such exposures would be considerably less than the peak concentrations measured which were themselves below the acceptable limit for time-weighted average exposures. Although insulators work with fibrous glass-containing materials from less than 10 to essentially 100% of their time, depending on their employer and type of construction site, the authors conclude that it is doubtful that the concentrations of airborne fibrous glass reported in their study were of long term biologic significance.

In a somewhat related study, Balzer et $al.$ reported the results of air sampling within air transmission systems that contained fibrous glass linings.[41] In general, the study showed that there was a general decrease in concentrations of glass fibers in air as the air passed through the system, both in terms of number of glass fibers per unit volume of air and in relative proportion of total fibers identified as glass. Although the data did not preclude the occurrence of erosion of fibers from the lining materials, any that did occur apparently was more than offset by deposition and entrapment of fibers in filters or elsewhere within the transmission systems. Typically, the concentrations of total fibers in outside air ranged between 1.77 and 7.80 fibers per liter with the glass fiber portion of the total fibers ranging from 15 to 57%. Average concentrations of total fibers in the filtered outside air ranged between 0.029 and 0.33 fiber per liter; the glass fiber content of total fibers ranged from 16 to 34%. Within the duct the average concentrations of total fibers ranged between 0.18 and 2.65 fibers per liter with the amount of glass fiber in the total fibers ranging between 8 and 46%. Within occupied areas of the building, the average concentrations of total fibers ranged between 1.52 and 11.76 fibers per liter with the average amounts of glass fibers in the total fibers ranging from 10 to 31%. The authors concluded that concentrations of total fibers and glass fibers in the ambient air, in the air exiting from the air-supply systems and in the occupied spaces within the building, were extremely low and did not appear to be of biologic significance.

Comparison of Respirable Mass Sampling with Impinger Counting Techniques

Ayer *et al.* have reported the results of a study conducted in the granite sheds in Vermont which had, as its primary objective, an attempt to relate respirable mass measurements to conditions that had been shown to have produced silicosis based on sampling with the impinger-count technique in the 1920's and 1930's.[42] To accomplish this, dust measurements were obtained by a wide variety of methods including horizontal elutriators operated at flow rates of 2.5, 10, and 50 liters/min, a $\frac{1}{2}$-inch steel cyclone sampling at 10 liters/min, 10-mm nylon cyclones sampling at 1.7 and 2.0 liters/min, a gross mass sampler, and a Greenburg–Smith impinger sampling 1 min out of 10 at 1 ft^3/min. By a contractual agreement, arrangements were made with a large monument manufacturer to simulate conditions, to the extent possible, that existed during operation of the facility in the 1920's.

The report contains much relevant sampling data pertaining to the correlations between various types of sampling units employed. Of particular significance is a series of regression equations that correlate each sampling method to the others. Briefly, the results of this study revealed concentrations of respirable dust of up to 49 mg/m^3 and concentrations of respirable free silica of up to 4.4 mg/m^3. On the average, the respirable dust concentrations ranged between 10 and 20 mg/m^3, of which 15% was free crystalline silica. Under the conditions of the study, it appeared that a concentration of granite dust of 10,000,000 particles/ft^3 of air, as determined by the impinger-count technique, was equivalent to approximately 0.2 mg/m^3 of "respirable" free silica. The report includes a discussion of the implications of the results of this study on a TLV developed specifically for silica as opposed to the formula approach currently being used in the industrial hygiene profession.

Combustion Products from Vinyl Chloride

O'Mara *et al.* have reported the results of an analytic study in which the combustion products of vinyl chloride monomer were determined.[43] The total combustion profile developed during the course of this study included an evaluation of flame temperatures, soot content, and analysis of combustion gases. Depending upon the amount of vinyl chloride–air premixing that was permitted prior to combustion, the temperature of the vinyl chloride flame ranged between 950° and 1466°C. Similarly, the amount of soot, or unburned carbon, in the vinyl chloride flame ranged between 3 and 6%, on a weight basis. Analysis of the combustion gases from the vinyl chloride revealed the following average composition: hydrogen chloride, 2700 ppm; carbon dioxide, 58,100 ppm; carbon monoxide, 9500 ppm; phosgene, 40 ppm; and only a trace of the vinyl chloride monomer. The authors concluded that, from the standpoint of potential health hazard, the gross quantities of hydrogen chloride present the most significant hazard associated with combustion of vinyl chloride monomer. Although it was recognized that, in the vicinity of the vinyl chloride fire, dangerous amounts of phosgene may be present, it was apparent that at those locations the atmosphere would already have been rendered intolerable by the high concentrations of hydrogen chloride. In addition, in peripheral areas, the pungent odor of hydrogen chloride would act as a warning mechanism to clear the area or to obtain necessary breathing apparatus for those required to fight the fire.

Correlation of Clinical and Environmental Measurements for Workers Exposed to Vinyl Chloride

Kramer and Mutchler have presented the results of a study in which a method was described for statistical consolidation and correlation of environmental measurements and clinical findings using, as an example, a group of healthy male workers exposed routinely to vinyl chloride for periods of up to 25 years.[44] The environmental aspects of this study were compiled on the basis of industrial hygiene surveys conducted in one or both of two manufacturing facilities using vinyl chloride in polymerization processes. The environmental sampling reported focused on exposure levels of men working in eight critical job classifications. Sampling for one or more of these classification was performed, with the exception of 2 years, for a period of over 20 years. Continuous monitoring of the work environment was accomplished during the most recent half of the total period of surveillance.

Of the 21 clinical parameters screened for correlation with environmental exposures, six were shown to indicate significant correlations with the exposure variables, cumulative time-weighted average exposure, and cumulative dose. These six clinical parameters were systolic and diastolic blood pressure, bromsulfalein (BSP), Icteris index, hemoglobin, and β-protein. The results of the environmental monitoring program, which was reviewed previously, indicated that, for most individuals in the study, the highest exposures occurred in the early phases of their careers and their later exposures were much lower. In the final analysis, much weight was placed on the readings observed for those employees who experienced high exposure levels especially during the early half of the surveillance period. For example, the average time-weighted exposures for all job classifications in 1950, the first year of the study, was 155 ppm, whereas the average exposure level 15 years later was approximately 30 ppm.

The authors concluded that the results of their study suggested that repeated exposures of workers to vinyl chloride at time-weighted average levels of 300 ppm or greater for a working lifetime would likely result in observable changes in physiologic and clinical laboratory parameters. Results of the study indicate the possibility of some impairment in liver function as a result of exposure to vinyl chloride even though no overt clinical disease was evident in any of the individuals studied.

CONTROLS OF SPECIFIC HAZARDS

As indicated earlier, specific environmental control problems that arise in the work place are normally not so unique that they do not lend themselves to application of fundamental control concepts. However, such occasions do occur from time to time in particular industrial operations. The information presented below, therefore, is representative of recently reported engineering approaches to particular industrial hygiene problems encountered in specific industries. It should be of interest to the practicing industrial hygienist, not because it is innovative in nature, but rather because it reveals a variety of engineering concepts and procedures that have been proven to be successful in controlling particular stresses.

Beryllium Decontamination of a Plant Shell

Gronka *et al.* have reported in detail the procedural considerations and accomplishments that were undertaken in order to effectively decontaminate a large vacated building that had formerly housed beryllium machining operations and a beryllium ceramics laboratory.[45] Personnel from the Pennsylvania Division of Occupational Health had conducted comprehensive wipe surveys throughout the building and found significant beryllium contamination. The initial study indicated that beryllium contamination amounted to approximately $8 \mu g/100 \text{ cm}^2$ of surface area in the machine shop, $5 \mu g/100 \text{ cm}^2$ in the furnace room, and in excess of $100 \mu g/100 \text{ cm}^2$ in the dust collectors in the beryllium oxide laboratory. Although limits for surface contamination by beryllium and its compounds had not been established at the time of the study, available information did suggest that floor and wall contamination should be less than $2 \mu g/100 \text{ cm}^2$ and that contamination of equipment should be less than $1 \mu g/100 \text{ cm}^2$. A commitment was made to adequately decontaminate the entire building using a combination of sand blasting, manual scraping, hydrobrushing, and manual scrubbing. Personnel involved in the decontamination operation were provided with mandatory medical surveillance and personal protective equipment including coveralls, boots, plastic boot covers, plastic gloves with liners, airline respirators, and respirators recommended by the manufacturer for protection against radioactive dusts. Clothing was washed daily in automatic washers installed on site. This comprehensive project, results of which were monitored throughout the operation by wipe sampling, was effective in reducing the surface contamination to less than 1 μg of beryllium per 100 cm² of surface area in all strategic areas of the building. Thus, because of close interagency cooperation, and the uncovering, identification, and resolution of this beryllium contamination problem, potentially significant exposures to beryllium oxide were averted.

Vacuum Metallizing Operation with Cadmium

A study was reported by Vigil in which the industrial hygiene control problem associated with use of new equipment for the plating of metal parts with cadmium was discussed.[46] Basically, the vacuum cadmium metallizing machine consisted of a cylindrical tank approximately 9 ft in length and 6 ft in diameter, equipped with an internally mounted jig assembly upon which parts to be plated could be mounted. Electric heating strips, which were equipped with retaining boats to hold cadmium pellets, were located along the base of the jig. After loading the machine with parts, cadmium pellets were placed in the boats and the large cylindrical tank was sealed. Air was then pumped out of the tank, the cadmium pellets were heated to the boiling point, and the resulting fumes condensed on the parts and other surfaces inside the tank. The machine operated on a cycle of 32 min and significant exposures of operators to cadmium fumes occurred during opening of the chamber and the unloading, cleaning, and reloading steps of the cycle. Before adequate controls were implemented, concentrations of cadmium ranged between 4.1 and 37.9 mg/m³ of air in areas where the fumes were introduced into breathing zones of workmen. As a result of the initial recognition of a problem, highlighted by the diagnosis of symptoms of overexposure to cadmium in three employees from the plating shop, a program of institution of additional control measures, in conjunction with a program of air sampling to determine the effectiveness of the modifications, was implemented. The engineering control modifications consisted primarily of increasing the time that the tank remained closed after heating, thus permitting more complete removal of cadmium fumes by the exhaust system and also allowing more time for the settling of dust and condensed fumes within the chamber prior to its being opened. In addition, the ventilation system was modified so that after the cylinder was brought back to ambient conditions, the chamber was opened no more than 1 inch with the exhaust system in full operation, thus providing a high-volume, high-velocity rush of air through the chamber, diluting the fumes within the tank. After institution of the engineering controls, concentrations of cadmium in areas occupied by workers were maintained below 0.1 mg/m³ with the exception of some periods during loading and unloading steps in the cycle, at which times the use of personal respiratory protective equipment was mandatory. The article points out that, although the process of vacuum metallizing presented potentially serious overexposure of personnel to cadmium, the operation was run safely by vigorous application of control procedures and proper monitoring of environmental conditions.

Control of Coal Dust by Water Spray

Tomb *et al.* have reported the results of a laboratory investigation conducted to study the effectiveness of doped and undoped spray water for control of respirable coal dust.[47] The basic objectives of the study were to evaluate the effects of droplet size, concentration, and velocity on the efficiency of water spray in suppressing levels of dust in the 0.6–10 μm diameter range, to determine the optimum combination of the parameters for obtaining maximum suppression efficiency, and to discover whether a nozzle's suppression efficiency could be increased by adding surface-active agents to the water. Four spray nozzles, operating over a range of flow rates and pressures typical of those found in underground coal mines, were used in the study. The most important factor resulting from the investigation was the development of the "nozzle parameter," P, which related the quantity of water discharged, the droplet velocity, and the mean volume diameter of the droplets to the suppression of the respirable coal dust. This parameter is defined as follows:

$$P = KQV/\bar{D}$$

where
    K = conversion constant (μm sec min/gal cm)
    Q = volume of water discharged (gal/min)
    V = droplet velocity (cm/sec)
    $\bar{D}$ = mean volume diameter of the droplets (μm)

This parameter provided a method for selecting a spray nozzle that would provide an optimum suppression efficiency for the quantity of water and line pressures available. The study also indicated that the suppression efficiency of the nozzle could be significantly increased for values of P less than about 15 by adding a surface-active agent to the water, due primarily to the reduction in droplet size caused by the decrease in liquid surface tension.

The authors point out that, although these relationships demonstrate that relatively high efficiencies can be obtained for capturing coal particles in the respirable range, these experiments were conducted in a coal tunnel where no attempt was made to determine the effect of tunnel-spray interaction on collection efficiency. However, they thought that the results could be used, on a relative basis, for selecting those operating characteristics of a nozzle which should provide optimum suppression efficiency.

Control of Airborne Dust Produced by Pneumatic Jackpicks

Scharf, in a continuing series of reports, has discussed the dust suppression capabilities of various water attachments for pneumatic jackpicks.[48,49] A newly designed coil-shaped attachment was demonstrated to have significantly better performance characteristics than a previously used cone-shaped device. In field tests, the coil attachment was more effective in reducing hazardous dust concentrations than the cone-shaped attachment and required significantly less water. Available information indicated that the percentage of dust reduction increased with an increasing percentage of water reaching the impact point of the steel to a certain optimum value. The optimum flow rate for water use with the coil attachment was 25 imperial gallons per hour. A practical method for approximating the percentage of water reaching the impact point of the jackpick steel from different water attachments was developed and is applicable for calibration use in the field.

Control of Contaminants in Hospital Clean Rooms

Graves reported on tests conducted to evaluate, qualitatively and quantitatively, the nature of airborne particulate present in a laminar airflow recovery room that was installed for kidney and heart transplant patients at the University of Michigan Medical Center.[50] Air sampling, primarily by means of an electrostatic precipitator, was conducted in the laminar airflow room, a control room, the outside make-up air supplying the laminar air room, and a baffle plate in the air conditioning system supplying the control room. Results of the testing program indicated that air filtration in the laminar airflow room was effective in reducing the quantity of dust to 20% of that present in the prefiltered air and to 24% of the amount present in a normal recovery room. Analysis of collected air samples showed the presence of eight metals in the dust collected within the recovery room, whereas dust collected in the prefiltered air and in normal recovery rooms showed 10 and 13%, respectively. Sodium chloride was the only crystalline material identified in the laminar airflow room air whereas silica and calcium sulfate were present in all other samples analyzed. No viruses or microorganisms of any type were isolated from samples of dust collected in the laminar airflow recovery room.

An evaluation of the effectiveness of control of gaseous contaminants and odors was conducted in a hard-wall, dust-free hospital room in a clinical research center by Wohlers et al.[51] The study was part of a long-range goal to improve the postoperative and burn patient care techniques by providing a known and controlled environment. Air supplied to the room being evaluated passed successively through a prefilter, a high-voltage and high-frequency unit (Cosa/ Tron), a high-efficiency particulate filter, and then into the room. The air-cleaning units studied were commercially available and were advertised as being effective in removing both gaseous and particulate matter from room air. Evaluation tests were conducted by introducing a "slug" of test gas into the return air duct of the room and monitoring the concentration of the gas, over a period of time, at fixed sampling stations within the room. Various test gases including nitrous oxide, carbon monoxide, sulfur dioxide, hydrogen sulfide, formaldehyde, and others were used for brief odor tests. The investigation demonstrated that, although the air-purifying system was effective for removing dust and particulate bacteria, there was essentially no effect of this system components, including the filters and charged electrodes, on removal of sulfur dioxide, hydrogen sulfide, formaldehyde, carbon monoxide, or nitrous oxide. Neither did there appear to be any effect of the system on subjective odor intensities of hydrogen sulfide, octanoic acid, caproic acid, or butyraldehyde. The decrease in contaminant concentrations within the room appeared to be a direct function of the dilution make-up air from the air conditioning system and the loss of air at the test room door and other places in the system.

An elaboration upon the study reported above was reported by Segall et al.[52] The same prototype hospital clean room evaluated by Wohlers et al. was used for this study. Tests were conducted over a 10-day period using three different concentration levels of sulfide generated by evaporation of dilute ammonium sulfide solution. Results of the study indicated that the charged electrode was not able to eliminate the odor of sulfide introduced into the system in the hospital clean room. In fact, the only case in which the difference in panel judgment (subjective odor response) corresponding to an "electrode on– electrode off" variation was found statistically significant indicated that the "electrode on" condition enhanced the odor rather than the expected reverse effect. The authors interpreted this as indicating that the use of the electrode did not inhibit, lessen, or eliminate the sulfide odor. The final conclusion from the study was that the odor-treatment unit installed in the air-cleaning facilities for the hospital room was not able to demonstrate reduction or elimination of odor of sulfide in air at concentrations ranging from 13 to 65 ppb in the hospital clean room studied.

Mercury Hazard during Fluorescent-Tube-Breaking Operations

A comprehensive survey at a steam-electric generating plant revealed a potential hazard posed by operations involving the breaking of fluorescent light tubes prior to disposal.[53] These tubes, each containing between 50 and 100 mg of elemental mercury, were crushed by processing them through commercially available tube breakers operated at the various steam plants. Concentrations of airborne mercury measured in the breathing zone of the breaker operators ranged from "negligible" to over 1 mg/m^3. Although the actual exposures of the operators were generally within acceptable limits, the potential for excessive concentrations was demonstrated. On the basis of an extended industrial hygiene survey, it was recommended that a local exhaust system be installed on, and incorporated with, the tube-breaking unit, replacing a dust collector bag that was standard on the units. Care had to be taken that the exhaust was vented from locations where recirculation into adjacent work areas was unlikely. In some situations local exhaust systems were not feasible and it was recommended that the tube-breaking operation be relocated to an outdoor location, away from occupied areas. In such cases, only the operator was to be permitted in the vicinity of the unit during operation and then he was required to wear personal respiratory protective equipment.

Reduction of Dust Exposures in the Slate Industry

Sacharov *et al.*[54] reported the results of surveys conducted in 1969 to determine the effectiveness of improvements that were to have been made in accordance with recommendations that followed previous surveys of dust conditions in the slate industry in Pennsylvania. These early surveys had indicated that excessive levels of dust were present in most of the industry. Recommendations were made to reduce the concentrations of dust to which workers were exposed. Basically, these recommendations specified that local exhaust ventilation systems be installed at strategic operations, adequate housekeeping programs be established, wet dust suppression systems be installed and/or improved, programs for periodic chest x-ray examinations be established, and a program of mandatory personal protective equipment usage be implemented until adequate engineering controls had been achieved. Basically, the results of the "follow-up" survey showed that, with the exception of the jackhammer and pin-setting operations, conditions within the slate industry were now characterized by exposures of workers to airborne dust being within acceptable limits.

Controlling Exposures to Toluene Diisocyanate

Linaweaver reported on a case of overexposure to high concentrations of toluene diisocyanate resulting from application of foaming chemicals into compartments of a U.S. Navy ship in attempts to salvage it after it had run aground.[55] The operation called for a diver to apply foam into several compartments below the main deck in attempts to displace water that had partially flooded the compartments, thus decreasing the weight, increasing the strength and stability of the ship, and preventing additional flooding. During the operation, the compressor that was being used to supply breathing air to the man failed and, as a result, he and another man attempting to rescue him were overcome by extremely high concentrations (unmeasured) of toluene diisocyanate.

As a result of this accident, a review of procedures and techniques utilized by the U.S. Navy was made and certain modifications of procedures were developed. These amounted to requiring careful physical examinations of personnel who would be assigned to such tasks, the use of protective clothing by all persons coming into contact with the foaming chemical, stringent requirements on the location of mixing operations, and requirements that adequate ventilation be provided during mixing and application of the foaming chemicals. As a direct consequence of the accident reported, it was made mandatory that standby self-contained breathing apparatus be available immediately in the event of failure of the primary source of air. In addition, provisions were implemented for the monitoring of TDI concentrations in and around mixing and foaming areas.

Dyson and Hermann have reported on an investigation of the gaseous state reaction between toluene diisocyanate and water.[56] Of particular interest was the possibility that humidified air could be used, in conjuction with local exhaust ventilation, as a mechanism for control of TDI. The effect of water vapor on the atmospheric TDI concentrations was determined quantitatively by means of a system for dynamically producing known concentrations of TDI in air in the presence of variable amounts of water vapor. The test results indicated that at $24°C$ and atmospheric pressure a maximum reduction of 50% was obtained for initial concentrations of TDI of 0.4 and 0.034 ppm, the percentage reduction apparently depending solely on the water vapor concentration. These data suggest that increased humidity would be only marginally useful and not quantitatively significant enough to justify the expense of using increased humidity as a control measure. The authors, as a result of questions raised during their studies, did suggest that it would be useful to know whether increased humidity with the concomitant production of TDI urea mitigates or aggravates the toxicologic effects of TDI alone.

General Applications of Ventilation Techniques

Siebert and Fraser reported on studies conducted in attempts to correlate experimental findings with empirically derived values for minimum exhaust flow rates for canopy-type hoods situated above hot processes.[57] The empirical equations used were modifications of Hemeon's basic equations for design of low- and high-canopy hoods for control of contaminants generated by hot sources. The report includes a treatment of the mathematical development of the applicable formulae. Basically, the experimental data, including measurement of hood temperature changes and smoke studies, indicated that there is a minimum exhaust flow rate for a low-canopy hood situated above a hot process. This exhaust rate varies with the temperature and surface area of the hot process—the higher the temperature and the larger the process, the greater the minimum exhaust requirements. The observed experimental minimum exhaust values were approximately one-third of those predicted by use of the modified empirical equations. However, when considering actual industrial applications, the authors agreed that the exhaust flow rates predicted from Hemeon's equations were indeed appropriate approximations of exhaust requirements.

Drivas et al.[58] have reported the results of attempts to experimentally characterize the ventilation systems in buildings. Tracer experiments using sulfur hexafluoride were used to obtain quantitative data regarding the actual residence time distributions in rooms and hallways of the building, as well as contamination caused by reentry into the building of exhaust fumes from laboratory hoods. The application of a mixing factor, ranging in values between 0.3 and 0.7 in small rooms without fans, was found to be of use. Of particular interest were the results of one experiment made to characterize the ventilation in an area serviced by a roof exhaust with air intakes both on an adjoining roof and at ground level of the test building. In this experiment, more of the exhausted air reentered the ground level intake of the same building than the roof intake of the adjoining building. In another series of experiments it was found that as much as 20% of the fumes exhausted from laboratory hoods was shown to reenter the ventilation system at various points in the building.

Control of Zinc during Welding Operations

Gregory et al.[59] have reported on the development of a method for control of fumes generated during welding operations on steels coated by hot-dip galvanizing, by zinc metallizing, or with zinc-rich paints. A control system has been developed for use in conjunction with gas-shielded metal arc (MIG) welding processes. This "fume extractor" was designed to completely surround the welding gun so that fumes are captured as close as possible to their point of origin. The article elaborates upon the demonstrated effectiveness of this system in controlling zinc fumes generated by the welding operations.

NIOSH Criteria Documents

As closing commentary to this chapter, mention is made of the criteria documents being prepared by the National Institute for Occupational Safety and Health under provisions of the Occupational Safety and Health Act of 1970. NIOSH is responsible for the development of criteria for recommended standards for environmental stresses encountered in American industrial operations. The specific mechanism required to accomplish this task requires a comprehensive and exhaustive review of the literature pertaining to the occupational health considerations for specific chemical and physical stresses. The resulting product of the in-depth interpretation of all available, relevant information is a document entitled "Criteria for a Recommended Standard . . . Occupational Exposure to (Specific Stress)." This publication is submitted to the U.S. Department of Labor as a statement of the National Institute for Occupational Safety and Health. The Department of Labor then reviews the document and, after necessary input has been obtained and modifications made, promulgates a legal standard under authority of the Occupational Safety and Health Act.

As of this time 15 "criteria documents" have been submitted to the Department of Labor by NIOSH. None of them, as yet, has been implemented into the occupational safety and health regulations by the Department of Labor. The federal standard for occupational exposure to asbestos was promulgated as an emergency standard although it is in basic agreement with the recommended standard outlined in the criteria document for asbestos. The criteria documents prepared to date by NIOSH include the following: inorganic arsenic, asbestos, beryllium, carbon monoxide, coke oven emissions, chromic acid, hot environments, inorganic lead, inorganic mercury, noise, sulfur dioxide, toluene, toluene diisocyanate, trichloroethylene, and ultraviolet radiation. With the exception of the coke oven emissions document, all publications include a recommended environmental level of the specific stress indicated. The coke oven emissions document is more appropriately termed criteria for a "work practices" standard.

In all criteria documents there are detailed rationale for, and methodology of, evaluating and controlling the specific stresses in the work environment. It is neither the intent, nor within the scope, of this chapter to present, or even summarize, these recommendations. Rather, the reader is encouraged to study these recommended practices and potential legal standards in light of his own interests. Theoretically, the concept of development of such documents will lead to a standardization of evaluation and control techniques throughout industrial operations that have associated with them potential exposures to specific contaminants covered by these documents. In that respect, it behooves all persons actively engaged in the profession of occupational health to become as actively involved as possible in activities that have an effect on the collection, interpretation, and review of information that will eventually become incorporated into legal environmental health standards.

REFERENCES

1. Lundgren, D. A., and McFarland, A. R., Application of a light-scattering aerosol counter and a four-stage impactor to industrial hygiene air sampling. *Amer. Ind. Hyg. Ass., J. 32,* 35–42 (1971).
2. Olin, J. G., Sem, G. J., and Christenson, D. L., Piezoelectric-electrostatic aerosol mass concentration monitor. *Amer. Ind. Hyg. Ass., J. 32,* 209–220 (1971).
3. Lilienfeld, P., and Dulchinos, J., Portable instantaneous mass monitor for coal mine dust. *Amer. Ind. Hyg. Ass., J. 33,* 136–145 (1972).
4. Carpenter, T. E., and Brenchley, D. L., A piezoelectric cascade impactor for aerosol monitoring. *Amer. Ind. Hyg. Ass., J. 33,* 503–510 (1972).
5. Palmes, E. D., and Gunnison, A. F., Personal monitoring device for gaseous contaminants. *Amer. Ind. Hyg. Ass., J. 34,* 78–81 (1973).
6. Nelson, G. O., and Shapiro, E. G., A field instrument for detecting airborne halogen compounds. *Amer. Ind. Hyg. Ass., J. 32,* 757–765 (1971).
7. McFee, D. R., and Bechtold, R. R., Pyrolyzer-microcoulomb detector system for measurement of toxicants. *Amer. Ind. Hyg. Ass., J. 32,* 766–774 (1971).
8. Morse, K. M., Bumsted, H. E., and Janes, W. C., The validity of gravimetric measurements of respirable coal mine dust. *Amer. Ind. Hyg. Ass., J. 32,* 104–114 (1971).
9. Seltzer, D. F., Bernaski, W. J., and Lynch, J. R., Evaluation of size-selective presamplers. II. Efficiency of the 10-mm nylon cyclone. *Amer. Ind. Hyg. Ass., J. 32,* 441–446 (1971).
10. Lamonica, J. A., and Treaftis, H. N., Investigation of pulsation dampers for personal respirable dust samplers. *U.S., Bur. Mines, Rep. Invest. RI-7545* (1972).
11. LaViolette, P. A., and Reist, P. C., Improved pulsation dampener for respirable dust mass sampling devices. *Amer. Ind. Hyg. Ass., J. 33,* 279–282 (1972).
12. Ash, R. M., and Lynch, J. R., The evaluation of gas detector tube systems: Benzene. *Amer. Ind. Hyg. Ass., J. 32,* 410–411 (1971).
13. Ash, R. M., and Lynch, J. R., The evaluation of gas detector tube systems: Carbon tetrachloride. *Amer. Ind. Hyg. Ass., J. 32,* 552–553 (1971).
14. Johnson, B. A., and Roper, C. P., The evaluation of detector tube systems: Chlorine. *Amer. Ind. Hyg. Ass., J. 33,* 533–534 (1972).
15. Johnson, B. A., The evaluation of gas detector tube systems: Hydrogen sulfide. *Amer. Ind. Hyg. Ass., J. 33,* 811–812 (1972).

16. Ash, R. M., and Lynch, J. R., The evaluation of gas detector tube systems: Sulfur dioxide. *Amer. Ind. Hyg. Ass., J. 32*, 490–491 (1971).

17. Roper, C. P., An evaluation of perchloroethylene detector tubes. *Amer. Ind. Hyg. Ass., J. 32*, 847–849 (1971).

18. Cralley, L. J., Identification and control of asbestos exposures. *Amer. Ind. Hyg. Ass., J. 32*, 82–85 (1971).

19. Subcommittee on Asbestos of the Permanent Commission and International Association on Occupational Health, Evaluation of asbestos exposure in the working environment. *J. Occup. Med. 14*, 560–562 (1972).

20. National Institute for Occupational Safety and Health, "Criteria for a Recommended Standard . . . Occupational Exposure to Asbestos." HSM 72–10267. NIOSH, Rockville, Maryland, 1972.

21. Reitze, W. B., Nicholson, W. J., Holaday, D. A., and Selikoff, I. J., Application of sprayed inorganic fiber containing asbestos: Occupational health hazards. *Amer. Ind. Hyg. Ass., J. 33*, 178–191 (1972).

22. Hill, T. A., Siedle, A. R., and Perry, R., Chemical hazards of a fire-fighting training environment. *Amer. Ind. Hyg. Ass., J. 33*, 423–430 (1972).

23. Linch, A. L., and Pfaff, H. V., Carbon monoxide—evaluation of exposure potential by personnel monitor surveys. *Amer. Ind. Hyg. Ass., J. 32*, 745–752 (1971).

24. Sidor, R., Peterson, N. H., and Burgess, W. A., A carbon monoxide-oxygen sampler for evaluation of fire fighter exposures. *Amer. Ind. Hyg. Ass., J. 34*, 264–274 (1973).

25. Anderson, D. E., Problems created for ice arenas by engine exhaust. *Amer. Ind. Hyg. Ass., J., 32*, 790–801 (1971).

26. Howlett, L., and Shephard, R. J., Carbon monoxide as a hazard in aviation. *J. Occup. Med. 15*, 874–877 (1973).

27. Noweir, M. H., and Pfitzer, E. A., Chemical analysis of decomposition products from carbon tetrachloride in air. *Amer. Ind. Hyg. Ass., J. 33*, 669–677 (1972).

28. Noweir, M. H., Pfitzer, E. A., and Hatch, T. F., Thermal decomposition of carbon tetrachloride vapors at its industrial threshold limit concentration. *Amer. Ind. Hyg. Ass., J. 34*, 25–37 (1973).

29. Rinzema, L. C., and Silverstein, L. G., Hazards from chlorinated hydrocarbon decomposition during welding. *Amer. Ind. Hyg. Ass., J. 33*, 35–40 (1972).

30. Noweir, M. H., Pfitzer, E. A., and Hatch, T. F., Decomposition of chlorinated hydrocarbons: A review. *Amer. Ind. Hyg. Ass., J. 33*, 454–460 (1972).

31. Anonymous, Bis-chloromethyl ether. *Amer. Ind. Hyg. Ass., J. 33*, 381 (1972).

32. Anonymous, Concentrates: Science. *Chem. & Eng. News 51*, 13 (1973).

33. Kallos, G. J., and Solomon, R. A., Investigations of the formation of bis-chloromethyl ether in simulated hydrogen chloride-formaldehyde atmospheric environments. *Amer. Ind. Hyg. Ass., J. 34*, 469–473 (1973).

34. Fannick, N., Gonshor, L. T., and Shockley, J., Exposure to coal tar pitch volatiles at coke ovens. *Amer. Ind. Hyg. Ass., J. 33*, 461–468 (1972).

35. National Institute for Occupational Safety and Health, "Criteria for a Recommended Standard . . . Occupational Exposure to Coke Oven Emissions," HSM 73–11016. NIOSH, Rockville, Maryland, 1973.

36. Hammad, Y. Y., and Corn, M., Hygienic assessment of airborne cotton dust in a textile manufacturing facility. *Amer. Ind. Hyg. Ass., J. 32*, 662–667 (1971).

37. Cheng, L., Formation of airborne respirable dust at belt conveyor transfer points. *Amer. Ind. Hyg. Ass., J. 34*, 540–546 (1973).

38. Fulwiler, R. D., Detergent enzymes—an industrial hygiene challenge. *Amer. Ind. Hyg. Ass., J. 32*, 73–81 (1971).

39. Fulwiler, R. D., Abbott, J. C., and Darcy, F. J., An evaluation of detergent enzymes in air. *Amer. Ind. Hyg. Ass., J. 33,* 231–236 (1972).
40. Fowler, D. P., Balzer, J. L., and Cooper, W. C., Exposure of insulation workers to airborne fibrous glass. *Amer. Ind. Hyg. Ass., J. 32,* 86–91 (1971).
41. Balzer, J. L., Cooper, W. C., and Fowler, D. P., Fibrous glass-lined air transmission systems: An assessment of their environmental effects. *Amer. Ind. Hyg. Ass., J. 32,* 512–518 (1971).
42. Ayer, H. E., Demment, J. M., Busch, K. A., Ashe, H. B., Levadie, B. T., Burgess, W. A., and DiBerardinis, L., A monumental study—reconstruction of a 1920 granite shed. *Amer. Ind. Hyg. Ass., J. 34,* 206–211 (1973).
43. O'Mara, M. M., Crider, L. B., and Daniel, R. L., Combustion products from vinyl chloride monomer. *Amer. Ind. Hyg. Ass., J. 32,* 153–156 (1971).
44. Kramer, C. G., and Mutchler, J. E., The correlation of clinical and environmental measurements for workers exposed to vinyl chloride. *Amer. Ind. Hyg. Ass., J. 33,* 19–30 (1972).
45. Gronka, P. A., Tomchick, G. J., Bobkoskie, R. L., and Suroviec, H. J., Beryllium decontamination of a plant shell. *Amer. Ind. Hyg. Ass., J. 32,* 199–202 (1971).
46. Vigil, T. S., Industrial hygiene aspects of a vacuum metalizing operation with cadmium. *Amer. Ind. Hyg. Ass., J. 32,* 203–208 (1971).
47. Tomb, T. F., Emmerling, J. E., and Kellner, R. H., Collection of airborne coal dust by water spray in a horizontal duct. *Amer. Ind. Hyg. Ass., J. 33,* 715–721 (1972).
48. Scharf, A., Control of airborne dust produced by pneumatic jackpicks with water attachments. Report III. *Amer. Ind. Hyg. Ass., J. 34,* 48–53 (1973).
49. Scharf, A., Control of airborne dust produced by pneumatic jackpicks. Report IV. Calibration of water attachments. *Amer. Ind. Hyg. Ass., J. 34,* 171–175 (1973).
50. Graves, I. L., Air-borne particles in a laminar air flow recovery room for kidney and heart transplant patients. *Amer. Ind. Hyg. Ass., J. 32,* 47–51 (1971).
51. Wohlers, H. C., Suffet, I. H., Blakemore, W. S., Kenepp, D., Coriell, L. L., and McGarrity, G. J., Gaseous pollutant evaluation of hospital clean rooms. *Amer. Ind. Hyg. Ass., J. 32,* 831–839 (1971).
52. Segall, S., Suffet, I. H., Wohlers, H. C., Blakemore, W. S., Coriell, L. L., and McGarrity, G. J., Gaseous odorant evaluation of a hospital clean room. *Amer. Ind. Hyg. Ass., J. 34,* 367–370 (1973).
53. Freeman, T. W., and Oppold, J. A., Mercury hazard and its control during operation of fluorescent tube breakers. *Amer. Ind. Hyg. Ass., J. 33,* 419–422 (1972).
54. Sacharov, K. M., Knauss, K. G., and Kubala, P. J., Reduction of dust exposures in the slate industry. *Amer. Ind. Hyg. Ass., J. 32,* 119–122 (1971).
55. Linaweaver, P. G., Prevention of accidents resulting from exposure to high concentrations of foaming chemicals. *J. Occup. Med. 14,* 24–30 (1972).
56. Dyson, W. L., and Hermann, E. R., Reduction of atmospheric toluene diisocyanate by water vapor. *Amer. Ind. Hyg. Ass., J. 32,* 741–744 (1971).
57. Siebert, G. W., and Fraser, D. A., Exhaust ventilation for hot processes. *Amer. Ind. Hyg. Ass., J. 34,* 481–486 (1973).
58. Drivas, P. J., Simmonds, P. G., and Shair, F. H., Experimental characterization of ventilation systems in buildings. *Environ. Sci. Technol. 6,* 609–617 (1972).
59. Gregory, E. N., Herrschaft, D. C., and Cole, J. F., Fume extraction when welding zinc-coated steels. *Amer. Ind. Hyg. Ass., J. 32,* 170–173 (1971).

Personal Protective Devices

WILLIAM A. BURGESS AND BRUCE J. HELD

INTRODUCTION

Personal protective devices have continued to receive attention during the review period under the impetus of the Occupational Safety and Health Act of 1970. The National Institute for Occupational Safety and Health (NIOSH) took over the testing of respiratory protective devices from the Bureau of Mines. The Bureau of Mines respiratory test schedules were updated and published in the *Federal Register* as Title 30 Code of Federal Regulations, Part II (30 CFR, Part 11).[1] Federally funded research to improve the test procedures in 30 CFR Part 11, to develop special-purpose protective devices, and to study respirator effectiveness in industry, emphasized national concern about protecting the worker. Industry continued to reevaluate its programs and update them. A better informed worker population questioned past practices and demanded the best possible protection. Just as World War I set the stage and direction of personal protection development during the early 1900's, so federal legislation in the early 1970's appears to be the basis of improved personal protective devices for many years to come.

RESPIRATORY PROTECTION

Application Information

The adequacy of available cartridges and canisters for protection against gases and vapors, particularly organic vapors, is a major concern of personnel responsible for respirator programs. The NIOSH test schedule in 30 CFR Part 11 for organic vapor cartridges has a single test against carbon tetrachloride.[1] The Respirator Manual,[2] prepared by the Joint Respirator Committee of the AIHA–ACGIH in 1963, showed that organic vapor cartridges with activated charcoal were not as effective against some solvents as they were against carbon tetrachloride. Recently, Freedman[3] and Nelson[4] defined the problem by classifying the breakthrough times of various organic compounds and families of compounds. Vapor pressure, molecular weight, chemical structure, and polarity were among the factors found to affect breakthrough patterns. Procedures for testing respirator sorbents are well described by these authors[3,5] and also by Ruch[6] and Reist[7]; the latter uses detector tubes for a qualitative indicator of breakthrough.

A discussion of the application of respirators for protection against toxic agricultural chemicals[8] emphasizes through omission that little research is going on in the area of pesticides and respiratory protection. A study by Blair[9] on abrasive blasting protective practices illustrates the lack of proper respiratory protection in this common manufacturing procedure. Many firms doing abrasive blasting use nuisance type respirators or no respiratory protection at all. Respondents to a survey questionnaire were, in general, not acquainted with the need for respirators. Attention to quality control in respirator programs is evident in the nuclear industry. As an example, Dow Chemical Company's Nuclear Division at Golden, Colorado is using a Q 127 penetrometer to test all new and cleaned respirators for leakage.[10] High-efficiency filters are also tested before issue.

Respirator selection has always been confusing for some air contaminants, especially under certain application conditions. Preparation of the respiratory protection provisions of NIOSH criteria documents has identified the inconsistencies of industrial practice and emphasized the need to formalize a means of selecting respirators. Hyatt proposed protection factors for respirators at the 1973 American Industrial Hygiene Conference[11] and the AIHA–ACGIH Respirator Committee recommended a respirator selection guide for protection against airborne particulates.[12] The Respirator Committee intends to make recommendations for all air contaminants in the near future.

In the past, medical examinations for respirator users has not been routine practice. However, OSHA now requires that such an examination be given a worker required to wear a respirator to be sure he is physically able to perform the work.[13] However, no guidelines are given to the examining physician regarding what might be or might not be acceptable physical conditions when wearing different types of respiratory protective equipment.

Design specifications for self-rescuers used in mines for protection against carbon monoxide resulting from fires and explosions has been proposed, based upon physiologic requirements and the composition of mine air after the incident.[14] Physiologic considerations included the effects of carbon monoxide, resistance to breathing, and air temperature. The concentration of carbon monoxide and carbon dioxide noted in mine atmospheres after fires is also presented. A review of four self-rescuers provides insight into the operation and performance of present devices. The limitations on the existing equipment is based on the level of carbon monoxide which it can handle, and the carbon dioxide concentrations in the environment.

The application of respirators for caisson operations was reviewed, and it was found that the only safe apparatus was a modified mixed-gas breathing device.[15] The discussion of the design deficiencies of the equipment available for this application should be extremely valuable to supervisors of respirator programs. Conventional air-purifying devices were found unsuitable, since work was in an enclosed area with the possibility of oxygen deficiency. The high air density also would result in a dramatic increase in breathing resistance. Due to the toxicity of high partial pressures of oxygen, open-circuit breathing apparatus was found unsuitable. Although open circuit compressed air breathing apparatus did not present a hazard, the use time does decrease significantly with increased ambient pressure. A special mixed gas breathing device was finally chosen as the respirator of choice for work at 1.5 atm.

The following application data are used for selecting respirators for protection against asbestos in the United Kingdom.[16,17]

	Chrysotile or amosite	Crocidolite
Dust respirators	Up to 40 fibers/ml	Up to 4 fibers/ml
Positive pressure dust respirators	200	20
Ultra-efficiency dust respirators	800	80
Positive pressure airline respirators	800	80

Effective methods of cleaning and disinfecting respirator facepieces have concerned supervisors of industrial respirator programs for many years. Much can be learned from techniques used by anesthesiologists. In one contribution, the effectiveness of iodine for disinfection of resuscitation equipment contaminated with bacteria was evaluated and effective disinfection was found using the method of Mallet. This procedure uses successive exposures to carbon dioxide followed by iodine at a relative humidity of 50%.[18] Similar success was noted by French investigators.[19] A review of various decontamination procedures available for medical facilities and equipment is also of value in developing an effective respirator program.[20]

A guide to the selection, use, and maintenance of breathing apparatus used in the fire service has been published by the National Fire Protection Association.[21] A series of instructional articles on the operation of a respirator program was presented in the National Safety News and included administration of the program, hazard assessment, selection of respirators, training, inspection, maintenance, and medical surveillance.[22]

A general discussion of respiratory protection and a useful chart for respirator selection was published in the French literature.[23] A discussion of the operation of a mine rescue station in Germany provides an excellent review of a modern training facility for breathing apparatus used in mine rescue conditions.[24] This article should be helpful to anyone setting up a respirator program.

New Developments and Design Trends

Emergency escape respirators in the United States are normally equipped with a mouthpiece for quick donning. A new German device utilizes a fold-up half-mask with the air-purifying element.[25] The complete device is packaged in a can that can be placed in the pocket for easy access. Since the device is not equipped with valves, the exhalation resistance is represented by the cartridge. It is claimed that this flow pattern extends the useful life of the filter.

Several supplied air suits have been developed during the reporting period. Although NIOSH has no schedule for certifying these suits at the present time, field use has proven that some of them afford a high degree of protection against airborne contaminants. G. Phillabaum of Mound Laboratory reported that the "bubble suit" developed there has been used over an extensive period in a plutonium-238 facility with highly satisfactory results.[26] Union Carbide at Oak Ridge, Tennessee, has also developed a lightweight fully enclosed environmental suit,[27] with a self-contained air regulator sensitive to a pressure less than one-quarter inch water gage, and equipped with full-flow, self-sealing, quick-detachable air and vacuum connections, and wiring and plugs for two-way communications.

Jansson of the M.I.T. Charles Stark Draper Laboratory reported two schemes to lower the resistance to breathing of self-contained closed-circuit devices.[28] Battery-powered fans are used to move the air. One system includes simple passive valves, while the other uses electronically controlled active valves.

A powered air-purifying respirator for coke oven workers was designed by Burgess.[29] The unit operates with a battery-powered fan that keeps the facepiece under positive pressure; this reduces the fitting problems inherent in ordinary air-purifying devices, thereby improving performance and increasing acceptance.

Solid state sources of oxygen continue to attract investigators. A mix of KO_2 pellets and pellets treated with $3\ CuO \cdot CuCl_3 \cdot 3\ H_2O$ as a catalyst packed in a

450 gm canister provided an adequate oxygen supply for 3 hr of work underwater.[30] Studies of a $NaClO_3$ source of oxygen showed that a candle 35 mm in diameter and 185 mm long will supply oxygen at a rate of 4.5 liters/mm for 30 min.[31] Martin describes a 1-hr closed-circuit breathing apparatus designed for use in coal mines.[32] A chlorate candle was selected as the oxygen source and lithium hydroxide as the carbon dioxide absorbent. The device is inexpensive, provides good voice communications, and requires low maintenance.

In a NASA funded program an analytical method was developed which permits each respirator component to be represented by an electric analog.[33] The individual components are then combined mathematically to create the complete model. The effects of system modification can be evaluated without testing a prototype device. This method was verified by laboratory testing of a typical respirator.

Work continues on the development of air-supplied plastic suits for protection against tritium and tritiated water. One suit with a double envelope within which air circulates reduced leakage to 0.001%.[34] A second innovative design provides air supply and exhaust by an aspirator.[35] No performance data are given for this system.

Ergonomic Studies

Impairment of maximum working capacity due to the wearing of dust respirators was studied in East Germany.[36] The most significant criteria were pulse rate changes and oxygen consumption. Reduced performance was noted in those subjects wearing respirators at work levels of approximately 560 kcal/hr. In the United States, Craig found that physical fitness is a factor in a person's endurance while wearing a respirator; however, for inexperienced men, the ratio of endurance when masked to endurance when unmasked is not affected by fitness.[37] In the United Kingdom, Bentley concluded that excessive breathing resistance during inspiration is a major factor in determining subjective tolerance to respirators.[38]

The impact on the worker of wearing compressed air-breathing apparatus was evaluated by monitoring pulse rate and physical strain identified under exercise conditions.[39]

An additional work physiology study, which demonstrates the strain incurred when wearing a respirator, indicates that subjects wearing respirators under work conditions showed increased blood lactate concentrations with a lowering of blood pH.[40]

Measurements of heart rate, blood pressure, skin temperature, and energy expenditure were used to evaluate the impact of respirators on workers.[41] As a result of these studies conclusions were drawn on design changes in the respirator and the necessary work–rest patterns for different jobs.

Shoemaker has reported on tests to minimize stresses imposed by wearing respirators.[42] The stresses can be categorized as psychologic, physiologic, mechanical, and functional. Severe interactions between these categories may be more detrimental than the mere summation of the individual stresses.

Respirator fit in relation to facial size has been under study through NIOSH- and AEC-sponsored projects. Hack at Los Alamos, in conjunction with McConville of Webb Associates, has developed test panels that represent 95% of the civilian male population with respect to face lengths and face width for full-face respirators and face length and mouth width for half-face respirators.[43,44]

One European respirator manufacturer provides half-masks in three sizes to fit a large percentage of the population. A fitting technique using a single facial measurement was evaluated to determine if it was helpful in choosing the proper mask size.[45] It was found that a single physical measurement did not permit proper mask selection, but rather the best fit could be obtained by simply trying on various mask sizes.

Anthropometric and physiologic data have provided the basis for an East German proposal on respirators which concludes that three or four facepiece sizes are necessary in oral–nasal masks for proper fitting, a 15–20° peripheral field is adequate when there is limited moving machinery in the work area, inhalation resistance should not exceed 10 mm H_2O, and mask dead space should not be greater than 300 cm.[10,46]

Testing and Evaluation

During the respirator chemical cartridge studies at the Lawrence Livermore Laboratory, Nelson and Harder also compared the effects of steady-state and pulsating flow.[47] A mechanical breathing simulator was used to evaluate the pulsating flow rates. Work rates from 208 to 1107 kg m/min and their equivalent respective steady-state flow rates of 14.0–71.4 liters/min were investigated. No significant differences were found in breakthrough characteristics between the steady-state and pulsating flows, even at the highest work rate and humidity conditions. The effective service life of the cartridges appeared to be inversely proportional to the flow rate at a given concentration. At the Los Alamos Scientific Laboratory, similar tests were run using respirator filter cartridges rather than chemical cartridges.[48] Solid monodisperse polystyrene latex aerosols were used, as well as liquid monodisperse dioctyl phthalate (DOP). The experimenters concluded that steady-flow rates may provide an overestimate of filter efficiency.

Respirator performance testing continued throughout the report period with emphasis on leakage of devices worn by human subjects. The performance of high-efficiency dust respirators was measured at Los Alamos in a quantitative DOP aerosol man test chamber.[49] Fifteen-hundred tests were run on 150 subjects using half- and full-face respirators. With five makes of half-mask respirators, 97–100% of the subjects obtained an efficiency of 90% or greater. Wearing approved full-facepiece respirators, 76–97% of the subjects obtained an efficiency of 99% or greater. Several papers were presented at the American Industrial Hygiene Conferences in 1972 and 1973 on respirator performance and fitting tests. Hyatt discussed the degradation problem of resin-impregnated wool felt respirator filters.[50] High humidity, liquid aerosols and mists, and NaCl aerosol were found to progressively neutralize the electrostatic charge on most of these filters, causing substantial losses in their filtering efficiency. Stawitcke discussed machine-powered demand respirator systems for coal miners[51] while Harris presented the results of field tests in mines using single-use dust respirators.[52] In the latter paper, only one brand of the three makes of single-use respirators tested was found acceptable by miners. Crooks[53] and Yankovich[54] discussed the use of various powered air-purifying respirators in underground coal mines. Harris also discussed protection afforded coal miners from half-mask dust respirators and their effectiveness in bituminous coal-mining operations.[55,56] It was concluded that there is much to be done to provide more effective and convenient respirators.

The application of sodium chloride aerosols had increased considerably in the United States over the past few years. Ferber reported on filter testing using sodium chloride and with penetration measurements down to 0.0005% using a flame photometer.[57] Hyatt used this tracer aerosol for quantitative man tests to measure respirator performance; a wide variation in the initial filtering efficiency of dust respirators was found.[58] The efficiency of some dust respirators ranged from 70–90% with a clean filter, but increased to 99% with a heavy loading. A study by White and Merrett at Chalk River, Ontario, used sodium chloride to measure respirator leakage through small orifices of known sizes.[59] Calculations were made relating the total volume of air leakage through the orifices in the respirators to the total volume of air breathed by the human subjects wearing the respirator.

A number of lawsuits in recent years have contested regulations prohibiting wearers of face masks from having excessive facial hair in the form of beards, sideburns, and moustaches. The suits generally charged that shaving facial hair is a loss of personal freedom and that a facepiece seal can be maintained without shaving. Los Alamos ran tests to determine the effects of facepiece seals when the wearer had different types of moustaches, beards, sideburns, or varying degrees of facial stubble.[60] It was shown that excessive facial hair will interfere with the respirator seal and reduce the degree of protection afforded by the respirator. Furthermore, if an adequate seal was obtained one day, it could change within a few days because of growing or trimming of the facial hair.

The filter-loading characteristics of various particulates on respirator filters conducted at a flow rate 30 liters/min with mass loadings of 1800 mg showed that soot, titanium dioxide, and sodium chloride rapidly clogged the filters, while oil mist and sand resulted in minimal increases in resistance to flow.[61]

Breakthrough curves for granular and pellet forms of activated charcoal were determined for methyl alcohol, ethyl alcohol, and pyridine and found to agree with theory.[62] Beech and walnut shell charcoals were evaluated for adsorptive capacity.[63] The protection time increases for increased grain size for benzene; however, in the case of HCN and NH_3 protection is enhanced by reducing grain size. The absorptivity of activated carbon for hydrogen sulfide was increased by 70% by impregnating the charcoal with a solution of potassium iodide–iodine.[64] The effectiveness of an activated charcoal against carbon disulfide was evaluated and found to have a capacity of 502 mg CS_2/gm charcoal at 57 ± 11 mg CS_2 per liter of air.[65]

A simple method of conducting a nondestructive test of adsorbent respirator cartridges is described using a small pulse of an assault vapor and noting the effluent pulse with a sensitive detector.[66]

Both sodasorb and barylime are commonly used as carbon dioxide scrubbers in closed circuit, self-contained breathing apparatus and in underwear rigs. The U.S. Navy has evaluated the effect of temperature and pressure on the ability of these absorbents to remove carbon dioxide.[67] The efficiency of the absorbents decreased as the temperature decreased ($3°–31°$ C) and as the pressure increased ($2–4$ atm at $30°$ C).

A comparison of open-circuit demand apparatus and rebreathers demonstrates the superiority of the latter in terms of use time per unit weight. The weight of both types of devices can be reduced by increasing the cylinder pressure to 500 bars.[68] A study of hose type respirators revealed serious limitations of this equipment.[69] If the equipment is used without a blower the hose diameter should not be less than 25 mm and the maximum hose length should be 5–10 m when the equipment is used at high work rates.

The significance of dead space of the respirator facepiece has been identified again in an East German study, which proposes a maximum CO_2 concentration of 2% under conditions of high breathing resistance and work rate.[70]

A mathematical model of the respiratory system of man and the breathing apparatus has been used to identify the relationship between breathing resistance and respiratory performance.[71]

Standards

In the United States, respirator test schedules have been published as Title 30 Code of Federal Regulations, Part 11 (30 CFR, Part 11).[1] The publication of the first part of a German Republic standard for industrial respirators was announced.[72] All respirators are discussed except self-contained breathing apparatus. That information will be published at a later date.

A British standard has been issued on positive-pressure-powered dust hood and blowers and includes a description of the appropriate leakage test[73]; a standard has also been issued for closed-circuit breathing apparatus and airline respirators.[74]

PROTECTIVE CLOTHING

Special-purpose protective clothing design continues to dominate the research in the United States. Martin compares physical, biophysical, and physiologic methods of evaluating thermal stress when wearing protective clothing.[75] For protection against extremely cold temperatures, a protective garment heater was developed by Grega in which fluid heated by a radioactive source flows through a passageway in the garment.[76] Westinghouse designed a thermoelectric heating and ventilating system for use in military clothing which weighs 10 lb unfueled and requires 0.26 lb of fuel per hr of operation.[77] Makarov compared the characteristics of basic forms of clothing for polar expeditions and attempted to define the optimum material for lightness and maintenance of a large volume of air under the clothing.[78] A camel-hair garment was most adaptable to the test conditions. An emergency survival suit was described by Curtic at the Second Conference on Portable Life Support Systems.[79] The suit is a thermally insulative inflatable garment designed specifically as a lightweight low storage volume garment for survival in subzero weather. When inflated with Freon, a subject standing at rest can survive air temperatures of $-450°$ F. Cold weather face masks were investigated at the Army Natick Labs under simulated Arctic conditions.[80] Two new experimental masks offered far better protection than did the standard Army mask.

For protection against high temperatures, Shitzer developed a thermal protective suit using independent regional control of coolant temperatures.[81] A John F. Kennedy Space Center report concludes that Nomex is the best general purpose nonflammable material for protective clothing.[82] The U.S. Army developed a new class of heterocyclic polyamides with outstanding thermal properties to be used for protective clothing for air and tank crewmen.[83]

General Electric developed an environmentally controlled suit consisting of an airtight outer garment attached by a bellows to the wall of a sterile chamber.[84] An undergarment provides for circulation of air near the skin of the wearer. The workman, wearing the undergarment and circulation system, enters the outer garment through a tunnel in the chamber wall without danger of spreading bacteria. A microwave radiation protective suit has been reported by Klascius.[85]

The Navy Clothing and Textile Research Unit introduced an environmental control unit (ECU) for a shipboard life support system[86] that uses wet ice in finned canisters for cooling and a closed circuit forced ventilation system with a battery-powered fan. Lithium hydroxide and potassium superoxide remove carbon dioxide and replenish oxygen. An integral oxygen monitor and low oxygen warning system monitor the suit environment. The impermeable suit has boots, gloves, and a communications headset.[87]

English scientists continue to add to the basic design information for protective clothing. Crockford has contributed an instructive chapter on protective clothing and equipment to a text on occupational health.[88] The same author has chronicled the development of protective clothing for fishing crews.[89] This study defined the needs of the trawlermen, evaluated present garments, and proposed improvements of protective clothing for this application. A series of measurements were used to characterize both conventional and new garments. Of special interest is an innovative scheme used to measure the air turnover of the microclimate by a gas dilution technique. It is interesting to note that the physical tests used in the study were more sensitive to differences in garment design than physiologic tests. This work is a model for clothing design studies for special occupations.

A method was devised for evaluating the heat and water vapor transfer characteristics of protective clothing using a skin simulator whose temperature and sweat rate could be controlled.[90] A method of calculating the thermal resistance of textiles used in protective clothing has been verified by experiment.[91] A study of the air movement under heat protective clothing revealed critical locations that should be observed in clothing design.[92]

The effectiveness of cleaning protective clothing contaminated with benzedine and dianisidine is enhanced by the use of a 2.5% solution of sodium hypochloride which changes color depending on the type and quantity of the contaminating amino compound.[93] The effectiveness of a fungicidal impregnant consisting of tributyl tin oxide–dichlorodiphenyl acetate and phenoyx acetate was proposed for protective clothing.[94] Fabric used in protective clothing can offer shielding from ionizing radiation when acid groups are formed in the cellulose and then treated with radiation-absorbing materials such as lead or barium.[95]

The application of vest-cooling panels has been explored by the Japanese using dry ice. A cooling vest with six panels containing dry ice was evaluated from 20° to 40° C and found to reduce skin temperature, heart rate, and sweat rate.[96] The incorporation of conductive fibers in textiles used in work clothing was found effective in reducing electrostatic charge and spark discharge in an explosive atmosphere.[97]

A study of the dose to the skin from particles containing radioactive strontium, cesium, and cobalt on protective clothing reveal that 1 to 2 μCi of each of the three nuclides presents a dose rate of 1 rad/hr over 1 cm^2 of skin.[98] Specific studies on strontium titanate as the contaminant revealed washing of the protective clothing removed only 60% of the particle activity. A second study of the hazard due to airborne radioactive contamination when removing protective clothing was based on the ratio of activity deposited on 1 m^2 of clothing and the resuspension of the activity in 1 m^3 of air.[99] Permissible limits on the contamination of clothing were prepared based on the resulting MPC of the airborne contamination.

Attention is again drawn to the dust exposure that can occur from protective clothing containing asbestos.[100] Naval fire-fighting helmets utilizing asbestos in a cloth cover caused exposure levels of somewhat over 2 fibers/cm^2. When the helmet was aluminized, the asbestos exposure was negligible.

Data obtained in a review of the fire-resistant qualities of clothing materials used by racing drivers should be helpful in the design of clothing for industry and the fire services.[101] A revised specification for PVC and polyurethane-coated fabrics used in protective clothing includes performance requirements and recommendations for the use, care, and maintenance of the material.[102] The Canadian Department of Labor has issued a regulation on protective clothing and equipment which defines the responsibility of both the employer and the worker.[103]

HEAD, EYE, FACE, FOOT, AND HAND PROTECTION

NIOSH is developing criteria that may serve as the basis for recommended performance, testing, and user standards for industrial and firefighting protective helmets.[104] The tests will be carried out at the NIOSH Testing and Certification Laboratory at Morgantown, West Virginia.

Hand and body protection were described in an article in *Occupational Hazards* in March 1973,[105] and foot protection was covered in three articles later in the year.[106] Quale discussed NIOSH criteria development for industrial protective gloves at the Boston AIHA meeting.[107]

Lasers dominated United States research in eye protection during the reporting period. One group of researchers evaluated commerically available laser eye protectors.[108] The report covers not only the test results to determine if the devices conform to the manufacturers' specifications, but also proposes guidelines for the design, selection, and use of laser eye protectors. A similar study was done by Holst.[109] Woodcock reported the development of an ocular laser filter with an optical density of 3.5 for all laser wavelengths and a luminous transmission of 60%.[110] Plastic goggles made from propionate and methacrylate were produced having a minimum optical density of 3.[111] A 3 mm water sheet contained between Lucite panes was developed for eye protection against IR laser radiation.[112]

A comparative assessment of eye protective devices and a system for acceptance testing and grading was proposed by Wigglesworth.[113] American Optical has developed an advanced method for evaluating eye protection using a systems approach.[114]

The emission from various welding processes in the range of 0.4–2.0 μm was measured to estimate the protection required of welding filters.[115] The permeability of 100 safety gloves of French manufacture to trichloroethylene was studied and physical and chemical damage, permeability, and solvent penetration data are presented.[116]

A unique device to protect the eyes of military personnel using optical sighting devices from laser radiation is based on a mirror which is destroyed within 20 nsec when exposed to energies of greater than 10 J/cm^2.[117]

The Construction Safety Association of Ontario has published a valuable report that includes methods for testing protective shoes for resistance to fatigue and penetration.[118] A revision of British Standard 1870 covers the design construction and materials for safety shoes and boots.[119] A standard covering protective clothing for protection up to 5 min against radiant heat and flame licks and up to 2 min against flame immersion has also been revised.[120] A standard for foundry footwear has now been issued by the British Standards Institute.[121]

Specifications for industrial safety helmets for electrical workers have been published by the American National Standards Institute and include general requirements, physical requirements, and test procedures.[122] West German standards for plastic-coated knitted gloves used in mines have been promulgated and include properties of the coated plastic and manufacturing and testing data.[123] A series of standards published in France cover general and special-purpose eye protection devices.[124,126]

REFERENCES

1. Respiratory protective devices; tests for permissibility; fees. Title 30. Code of Federal Regulations. Part 11. *Fed. Regist. 37,* No. 59 (1972).
2. "Respiratory Protective Devices Manual," Amer. Conf. Gov. Ind. Hyg., Amer. Ind. Hyg. Ass., Detroit, Michigan, 1963.
3. Freedman, R. W., Ferber, B. I., and Hartstein, A. M., Service lives of respirator cartridges versus several classes of organic vapors. *Amer. Ind. Hyg. Ass., J. 34,* No. 2, 55 (1973).
4. Nelson, J. O., and Harder, C. A., "Effect of Concentration on Respirator Cartridge Efficiency," University of California Radiation Laboratory 50007–72–3, pp. 6–8, 1973.

5. Nelson, G. O., and Hodgkins, D. J., Respirator cartridge efficiency studies. II. Preparation of test atmospheres. *Amer. Ind. Hyg. Ass., J. 33,* No. 2 (1972).

6. Ruch, W. E., Nelson, G. O., Lindeken, C. L., Johnsen, R. G., and Hodgkins, D. J., Respirator cartridge efficiency studies. I. Experimental design. *Amer. Ind. Hyg. Ass., J. 33,* No. 2 (1972).

7. Reist, P. C., and Cole, H. M., A simple procedure for the routine testing of respirator sorbents. *Amer. Ind. Hyg. Ass., J. 33,* No. 8 (1972).

8. Law, S. E., Respirators and masks. *Agr. Eng. 53(11)* (1972).

9. Blair, A. W., Abrasive blasting protective practices study—preliminary survey results. *Amer. Ind. Hyg. Ass., J. 34,* No. 2 (1973).

10. Skaats, C. D., "Test Development for Full Face Mask Respiratory Equipment," RFP–1997. Rocky Flats Division, Dow Chemical, Golden, Colorado, 1973.

11. Hyatt, E. C., Respirator protection factors and selection guide. *AIH Conf. 1973,* No. 118 (1973).

12. Held, B. J., and Hyatt, E. C., Letter to C. Powell, Sc.D., NIOSH, from AIHA–ACGIH Respirator Committee (1973).

13. Occupational safety and health standards. Title 29, Code of Federal Regulations. Part 1910. *Fed. Regist. 37,* No. 202 (1972).

14. Griffin, O. G., and Atherton, E., The physiological requirements for self-rescuers related to the performance of existing apparatus. *Ann. Occup. Hyg. 15,* 361 (1972).

15. Warncke, E., Development of the mixed gas breathing apparatus model BG 174 C2.2 for breathing protection under over pressure. *Draeger Rev. 24,* 1 (1971).

16. Luxon, S. G., The use of dust respirators against asbestos dust hazards in the United Kingdom. *Amer. Ind. Hyg. Ass., J. 32,* No. 11, 723–725 (1971).

17. H.M. Factory Inspectorate, Dept. of Employment, London, "Asbestos Regulations 1969: Respiratory Protective Equipment," Tech. Data Note 24. HM Stationery Office, London, 1971.

18. Roujas, F., Saint-Laurent, P., and Cassou, J., Decontamination of artificial respirators by ethylene oxide (Dep. Anesth.-Reanim., Hop, Henry Mondor, Creteil, Fr.). *Ann. Anesthesiol. Fr. 13,* 367–372 (1972).

19. Roquefeuil, B., Gaucher, M. and Du Cailar, J., Sterilization by ethylene oxide and its applications to respirators (Dep. Anesth.-Reanim, Cent. Hosp. Univ., Montpelier, Fr.). *Ann. Anesthesiol. Fr. 13,* 357–366 (1972).

20. Centi, R., Bisiani, M., Salicone, A., and Zaffiri, O., Decontamination of anesthesiological and reanimation equipment (Serv. Anest. Rianimazione, Osp. Magg. Trieste, Trieste, Italy). *Minerva Anestesiol. 37,* 340–345 (1971).

21. "Fire Officers' Guide to Breathing Apparatus for the Fire Service." National Fire Protection Association, Boston, Massachusetts, 1971.

22. Establishing and maintaining an effective respiratory protection programme. *Nat. Saf. News 103,* No. 4, 72–74, No. 5, 92–95, No. 6, 56–59 (1971); *104,* No. 1, 91–95, No. 2, 60–69, No. 3, 77–81, No. 4, 78–89, No. 5, 84–87, No. 6, 94–99 (1971).

23. Lardeux, P., La protection respiratoire individuelle, *Travail et Securité* No. 1, pp. 6–10. Paris, 1972.

24. Niemann, E., Aspect of a modern mine rescue station. *Draeger Rev. 29,* 17 (1973).

25. Haas, H., and Knapp, F., Draeger escape filter respirator parat. *Draeger Rev. 25,* 12 (1971).

26. Phillabaum, G. L., and Adams, P. C., The development of the Mound Laboratory supplied-air bubble suit. *Amer. Ind. Hyg. Ass., J. 35,* No. 1 (1974).

27. "Environmental Suit and Accessories," CAPE–2202, TID–4100, Suppl. 70 (F.S.). Y–12 Plant, Union Carbide Corp., Oak Ridge, Tennessee.

28. Jansson, D. G., Lower breathing impedance of self-contained closed-circuit respirators. *Amer. Ind. Hyg. Ass., J. 33,* No. 7 (1972).

29. Burgess, W. A., Design of a powered air-purifying respirator for coke oven workers. *Amer. Ind. Hyg. Ass., J. 32,* No. 11 (1971).

30. Rio, M., Potassium peroxide pellets for respirators (Air liquide, société anon. pour l'etude et l'exploitation des procédés Georges Claude). German Patent 2,159,493 (Cl. A 62db) (1972).

31. Ducros, H., Value of chemical oxygen in air sanitary evacuations (Lab. Med. Aerosp., Cent. Essais Vol., Bretignysur-Orge, Fr.). *Rev. Med. Aeronaut. Spatiale 10,* 71–74 (1971).

32. Martin, F. E., Chlorate candle/lithium hydroxide personal breathing apparatus. *NASA Spec. Publ. NASA SP.- 302,* 81–88 (1972).

33. Silver, L., Analytical modeling of respiratory protective devices. *Amer. Ind. Hyg. Ass., J. 32,* No. 12, 775–785 (1971).

34. Le Bourdonnec, Y., Colonna, P., and Renard, R., "Tests on Pressurized Clothing for Work in Environments Highly Contaminated with Tritium." Centre d'Etudes Nucléaires, Comissariat a l'Energie Atomique, Saclay, France, 1973.

35. Savornin, J., Protective equipment for personnel working in contaminated environments (to Commissariat a l'Energie Atomique). French Patent 2,112,034 (1972).

36. Selig, R., Mahrlein, W., and Schettler, R., The effect of dust respirators on the efficiency of miners. *Atemschutz* No. 2 (1973).

37. Craig, F. N., Blevins, W. V., and Froelich, H. L., Training to improve endurance in exhausting work of men wearing protective masks: A review of some preliminary experiments. Available National Technical Information Service CSCL 06/17 (1972).

38. Bentley, R. A., Griffin, O. G., Love, R. G., Muir, D. C. F., and Sweetland, K. F., Acceptable levels for breathing resistance of respiratory apparatus. *Arch. Environ. Health 27,* 273–280 (1973).

39. Gihl, M., Untersuchungen der Pulsfrequenz -eim Tragen von Atemschutzgeraten. *Draeger Heft* NR 292 (1973).

40. Stojiljkovic, Z., Brdaric, R., and Savic, S., Aerobic and anaerobic work capacity with an industrial protective mask. *Sigurnost Rud. 5,* 77–83 (1972).

41. Comte, T., Physical work capacity when wearing respiratory protective equipment. *Pr. Cent. Inst. Ochr. Pr. 21,* No. 77, 319–333 (1971).

42. Shoemaker, C. J., Stresses associated with protective mask wearing. AIHA Conf., 1972. No. 120 (1972).

43. Hack, A. L., Moore, T. O., Richards, C. P., Pritchard, J. A., and Held, B. J., Selection of a respirator test panel representative of U.S. face sizes. AIHA Conf., 1973. (1973).

44. McConville, J. T., Ethnic variability and respirator sizing. AIHA Conf., 1973. No. 128 (1973).

45. Sommer, H., Is it possible to determine half mask size in advance. *Draeger Rev. 27,* 27 (1972).

46. Herman, H., Studies of anatomical and physiological parameters for respirator facepiece design, Berlin (Eastern Sector). *Atemschutz Inform. 10,* No. 3, 56–61 (1971).

47. Nelson, G. O., and Harder, C. A., Respirator cartridge efficiency studies. IV. Effects of steady-state and pulsating flow. *Amer. Ind. Hyg. Ass., J. 33,* No. 12 (1972).

48. Stafford, R. G., Ettinger, H. J., and Rowland, T. J., Respirator cartridge filter efficiency under cyclic- and steady-flow conditions. *Amer. Ind. Hyg. Ass., J. 34,* No. 5 (1973).

49. Hyatt, E. C., Pritchard, J. A., and Richards, C. P., Respirator efficiency measurement using quantitative DOP man tests. *Amer. Ind. Hyg. Ass., J. 33,* No. 10 (1972).

50. Hyatt, E. C., Pritchard, J. A., Richards, C., Geoffrion, L., and Moore, T., Degradation of resin wool respirator filters. *AIHA Conf., 1973.* No. 27 (1973).

51. Stawitcke, F. A., and Crooks, T. P., Machine powered demand respirator systems for underground coal miners. *AIHA Conf., 1973.* (1973).

52. Harris, H. E., and DeSieghardt, W. C., Field testing of throwaway half-mask dust respirators. *AIHA Conf., 1973.* No. 31 (1973).

53. Crooks, T. P., and Gerken, G., Performance and acceptance of various powered respirators in underground coal mines. *AIHA Conf., 1973.* No. 114 (1973).

54. Yankovich, D., Powered air-purifying respirators for coal miners. *AIHA Conf., 1973.* No. 61 (1973).

55. Harris, H. E., and DeSieghardt, W. C., Factors affecting protection obtained by underground coal miners from half-mask dust respirators. *AIHA Conf., 1973.* No. 117 (1973).

56. Harris, H. E., Reist, P. C., Burgess, W. A., and DeSieghardt, W. C., Respirator useage and effectiveness in bituminous coal mining operations. *AIHA Conf., 1972.* No. 116 (1972).

57. Ferber, B. I., Brenenberg, F. J., and Rhode, A., Penetration of sodium chloride aerosol through respirator filters. *AIHA Conf., 1972.* No. 132 (1972).

58. Hyatt, E. C., Pritchard, J. A., Geoffrion, L. A., and Richards, C. P., Respirator performance using quantitative sodium chloride aerosol man tests. *AIHA Conf., 1972.* No. 113 (1972).

59. White, J. M., and Merrett, K. W., Measurement of leakage of a respirator using a NaCl aerosol when size of opening causing leakage is known. *AIHA Conf., 1972.* No. 134 (1972).

60. Hyatt, E. C., Pritchard, J. A., Richards, C. P., and Geoffrion, L. A., Effect of facial hair on respirator performance. *Amer. Ind. Hyg. Ass., J. 34,* No. 4 (1973).

61. Van der Smissen, C. E., Absorptive power of aerosol filters for respirators (Draegerwerke A-G., Luebeck, Ger.). *Staub 31*(9) (1971).

62. Bergstrom, G., Ekedahl, E., and Sillen, L. G. (Res. Inst. Nat. Def., Stockholm, Swed.)., Leaking curves for activated carbons with physically sorbed gases at low leaking concentrations. *FOA (Foersvarets Forstningsanst.) Rep. 5,* 1–9 (1971).

63. Smigelschi, T., Influence of some factors on the protection capacity of sorbents intended for the equipment of respiratory devices, Stan, Gh. (Rom.). *Rev. Chim. 23,* 304–307 (1972).

64. Draegerwerk, A.-G., Respirator filters for hydrogen sulfide. German Patent 2,114,197 (Cl. A 62d) (1972).

65. Petrovic, D., and Duric, D., Problems in protecting the respiratory system from carbon disulfide. *Hem. Vlakna 11,* 12–15 (1971).

66. Maggs, F. A. P., Nondestructive test of vapor filters. *Ann. Occup. Hyg. 15,* 351–359 (1972).

67. Cook, R. B., Temperature and pressure effects on sodasorb and baralyme. *U.S. Nat. Tech. Inform. Serv., AD Rep. AD–749708,* 1–30 (Eng.) (1972).

68. Warncke, E., Recent progress in self-contained respiratory protective equipment, Cologne, Germany (Fed. Rep.). *Arbeitsschutz* No. 6, pp. 240–242 (1972).

69. Reber, E., Limitations of hose-type respirators without blowers, Solothurn, Switzerland. *Schweiz, Arch. 37,* No. 10, 333–341 (1971).

70. Leers, R., Effects of carbon dioxide in the use of respiratory protective equipment, Berlin (Eastern Sector). *Atemschutz-Inform. 11,* No. 3, 49–54 (1972).

71. Heusinger, P., Breathing resistance and ventilatory flow—theory and methods of measurement for testing breathing apparatuses, Leipzig, Germany (Dem. Rep.). *Atemschutz-Inform. 10,* No. 1, 17–18 (1971).

72. Fahrbach, J., Respirator pamphlet (Part 1) of the German Respirator Committee—standard for the use of suitable respirators. *Staub 33,* 321 (1973).
73. "Specification for Positive Pressure, Powered Dust Hoods and Blouses," BS 4771. British Standards Institution, London, 1971.
74. "Specification for Breathing Apparatus," Part 1, BS 4667. British Standards Institution, London, 1971.
75. Martin, H. de V., Comparison of physical, biophysical, and physiological methods of evaluating the thermal stress associated with wearing protective clothing. *Ergonomics 15,* (1972).
76. Grega, M. G., Shivers, R. W., and Beckman, E. L., Suit heater. Australian Patent 415,410 (to the U.S. Atomic Energy Comm.) (1971).
77. Bernard, A. M., Thermoelectric heating and ventilating system. National Technical Information Service CSCL 06/17 (1971).
78. Makarov, N. I., Comparative characteristics of basic forms of climatic clothing of Polar expedition members of Vostok Station. National Technical Information Service HC (1972).
79. Curtis, D. L., "An Emergency Survival Suit," Second Conference on Portable Life Support Systems, National Technical Information Service, CSCL 06K. NASA-Ames Research Center, 1972.
80. Bensel, C. K., Johnson, R. F. Q., and Nichols, T. L., A human factors evaluation of cold weather face masks. National Technical Information Service CSCL 05/5 (1972).
81. Shitzer, A., Thermal protective garment using independent regional control of coolant temperatures. *Aerosp. Med. 44,* 49–54 (1973).
82. Reynolds, J. R., Fire and safety materials utilization at the John F. Kennedy Space Center. National Technical Information Service SOD CSCL 11D (1971).
83. Stapler, J. T., and Bornstein, J., High temperature polyamides from new herahydro-benzodipyrrole monomers. National Technical Information Service CSCL 11/9 (1972).
84. Carl, G. R., Air conditioned suit. National Technical Information Service C SCL 06K [U.S. Patent Application SN 84290 (1970)].
85. Klascius, A. F., Microwave radiation protective suit. *Amer. Ind. Hyg. Ass., J. 32,* No. 11 (1971).
86. Orner, G. M., and Audet, N. F., Environmental control unit for damage control suit system. Available National Technical Information Service CSCL 13/1 (AD–749025: TR–101; Report–2–71) (1972).
87. Audet, N. F., Reins, D. A., and Chadwick, A. H., Damage control suit system. Available National Technical Information Service CSCL 06/11 (AD–762428: TR–107) (1973).
88. Schilling, R. S. F., ed., "Occupational Health Practice." Butterworth, London, 1973.
89. Crockford, G. W., Protective clothing for fishing crews. *Text. Inst. Ind.* 121 (1970).
90. Votta, F., and Spano, L. A., "Flow of Heat and Water Vapor Through Protective Clothing," Tech. Rep. 71–5–CE. Clothing and Personal Life Support Equipment Laboratory, U.S. Army, Natick, Massachusetts, 1970.
91. Yankeievich, V. I., Calculation of the thermal resistance of the air layers in air-permeable clothing. *Tecknol. Tekst. Pro.* No. 2 (1971).
92. Kosceev, V. S., and Romanenko, M. Ja., The hygienic significance of air movement between clothing and skin. *Gig. Sanit.* 49–53, No. 3 (1973).
93. Genin, V. A., Decontamination of protective clothing contaminated with benzidine and dianisidine. *Bezop. Tr. Prom. 23,* No. 2 (1973).

94. Pawlowska, Z., and Liwkowicz, J., Use of a new organotin fungicidal impregnation for cellulosic fabrics. *Pr. Cent. Inst. Ochr. Pr. 21,* No. 17 (1971).

95. Ermolenko, I. N., and Lyubliner, I. P., Improvements in or relating to fibrous material for use in forming radiation-shielding fabric. British Patent 1,296,845 (1972).

96. Miura, T., Effect of a local-cooling vest with CO_2-ice as a cooling material on the physiological functions of man in hot environment. *J. Sci. Labor 47,* No. 7 (1971).

97. Tabata, Y., "Preventing the Build-Up of Static Electrical Charges in Work Clothing by the Use of Conductive Fibres," Tech. Note RIIS-TN-71-1. Research Institute of Industrial Safety, Ministry of Labour, Tokyo, 1971.

98. Stevens, D. C., Stephenson, J., and Bruce, G. S., The estimation of the dose to skin from radioactive particulate contamination of clothing. *Ann. Occup. Hyg. 14,* 1 (1971).

99. Scheidhauer, J., and Matevet, C., Transfer factor in air encountered when removing radioprotective clothing. *Radioprotection 7,* No. 2 (1972).

100. Lumley, K. P. S., Asbestos dust levels inside fire fighting helmets with chrysolite asbestos covers. *Ann. Occup. Hyg. 14,* 285 (1972).

101. "Fire-Resistant Clothing Report." Jim Clark Foundation, Edinburgh, 1971.

102. "Specification for Coated Fabrics for Protective Clothing." British Standards Institution, London, 1970.

103. Department of Labor, Regulations respecting the provision and use of protective clothing and equipment in federal works, undertakings, and businesses (Canada Protective Clothing and Equipment Regulations), SOR/72-108. *Can. Gaz. Part II 106,* No. 8 (1972).

104. Kamin, J. I., NIOSH research activities in protective helmets. *AIHA Conf., 1973.* No. 218 (1973).

105. Master blueprint for hand and body protection. *Occup. Hazards 35,* 00-00 (1973).

106. "Occupational Hazards," Vol. 36. Cleveland, Ohio, 1973.

107. Quale, T., and Kamin, J. I., Development of criteria for industrial protective gloves. *AIHA Conf., 1973.* No. 219 (1973).

108. Marston, D. R., Landieri, P. C., and Walker, P. D., Evaluation of laser eye protectors commercially available. National Technical Information Service CSCL 06/17 (1971).

109. Holst, G. C., Proper selection and testing of laser protective materials. *Amer. J. Optom. 50* (1973).

110. Woodcock, R. F., and Hovey, R. J., Research and development of an ocular laser protective filter. National Technical Information Service CSCL 06/17 (1971).

111. Sherr, A. E., Cordes, W. F., and Tucker, R. J., Plastic materials for eye protection from lasers. National Technical Information Service CSCL 0/17.

112. Specer, D. J., and Bixler, H. A., IR laser radiation eye protector. National Technical Information Service CSCL 06/17 (1971).

113. Wigglesworth, E. C., A comparative assessment of eye protective devices and a proposed system of acceptance testing and grading. *Amer. J. Optom. 49,* (1972).

114. La Marre, D. A., and Zdrok, J. Z., Developments in eye protection. *AIHA Conf., 1973.* No. 217 (1973).

115. Huebner, H.-J., Sutter, E., and Wicke, K., "Measurements of Radiant Power at Welding Processes and Consequences for Eye Protection Against IR Radiation" (translated by J. R. Kohr). National Research Council of Canada, Ottawa, 1972 [from *Optik 31,* No. 5, 462-476 (1970)].

116. "Resistance of Safety Gloves to Industrial Solvents" (La resistance des gants de protection aux solvants industriels), n° 491. Supplement to "Travail et securité, Editions INRS, Paris, 1972; No. 10 (1972).

117. Sztankay, Z. G., and Holland, R. J., A study of laser eye protection by direct initiation of thin explosive wafers. Available from National Technical Information Service CSCL 20/6 (1971).

118. "Foot Protection." Res. Publ. No. 2. Construction Safety Association of Ontario, Applied Research Dept., Toronto, Ontario, Canada, 1968.

119. "Specification for Safety Footwear," Part 1, BS 1870. British Standards Institution, London, 1970.

120. "Specification for Clothing for Protection Against Intense Heat for Short Periods," BS 3791: British Standards Institution, London, 1970.

121. "Specification for Gaiters and Footwear for Protection Against Burns and Impact Risks in Foundries," BS 4676. British Standards Institution, London, 1971.

122. "Safety Requirements for Industrial Protective Helmets for Electrical Workers," Class B, ANSI Z89.2-. American National Standards Institute, New York, 1971.

123. "Safety Gloves in Plastics-Coated Knitted Fabric (Schutzhandschuhe aus Kunststoff-beschichitetem Gewirk)," DIN 23 317, 318, and 324. German Standards Committee (Deutscher Normenausschuss), Berlin (Western Sectors), 1969.

124. "Prevention, Protection, and Safety—Eye Protection—Specifications for Eye Protection Equipment." Norme française homologuee NF S 77–101. Association française de normalisation, Tour Europe, Cedex 7, 92080 Paris La Defense, 1972.

125. "Prevention, Protection, and Safety—Eye Protection—Non Optical Test Methods for Eye Protection Equipment," Norme française homologuee NF S 77–103. Association française de normalisation, Tour Europe, Cedex 7, 92080 Paris La Defense, 1972.

126. "Prevention, Protection, and Safety—Eye Protection—Optical Testing Methods for Eye Protection Equipment," Norme française homologuee NF S 77-102. Association française de normalisation, Tour Europe, Cedex 7, 92080 Paris La Defense, 1972.

The Off-Job Environmental Health Stress as Related to the Workplace

LESTER V. CRALLEY AND LEWIS J. CRALLEY

INTRODUCTION

While the major focus of "Industrial Environmental Health," 2nd ed. has remained the same as that of the first edition and "Industrial Hygiene Highlights," i.e., the environmental health hazards of the workplace, it is recognized that the environmental stress of the worker must be considered in terms of its totality. Accordingly, those environmental stresses off the job must be placed in perspective as they relate in an additive manner to the on-job stresses. Only in this way can the individual increments be properly assessed.

HEALTH STATISTICS

The trend in death rates from 1900 to 1966 has been recently examined by Morison.[1] The greatest decrease is associated with the age group under 1 year and to a lesser extent with the age groups 1–4 and over 55. This has been brought about largely through the control of infectious diseases. Today, the great majority will live to be over 70. The death rate for both sexes, all ages, over the past two decades has not changed. The rate for 1950 was 964 while that for 1969 was 952 with excursions both above and below these values in the interim period.[2] However, when a comparison is made on a 5-year average basis over this period by 10-year age brackets and sex, a pattern of interest is developed (Table I). For females, the pattern is somewhat constant through the 54 age bracket with an accelerated decrease afterwards. In contrast, the pattern for

TABLE I

	Age grou					
	25–34		35–44		45–54	
Year	Male	Female	Male	Female	Male	Female
1965–1969	207	104	398	235	972	518
1960–1964	190	106	375	229	973	522
1955–1959	191	110	374	232	975	536
1950–1954	211	129	411	270	1,042	612

TABLE II

	Age grou					
	25–34		35–44		45–54	
Year	Male	Female	Male	Female	Male	Female
1965–1969	0.6	0.8	2.7	2.1	14.3	6.1
1960–1964	0.5	0.8	2.5	2.1	13.3	5.0
1955–1959	0.5	0.7	2.1	1.6	10.0	3.4
1950–1954	0.5	0.9	1.7	1.6	7.0	3.4

males is constant until the 64 age bracket with an increase for the bracket 65–74 and a decrease afterwards.

While the factors of smoking and alcohol doubtlessly play a major part in the pattern observed, the cause for this anomaly in the 65–74 age bracket warrants a greater examination, especially as it might be related to pre- and postretirement environmental health stresses. This is further emphasized in Table II, which compares the death rates on a similar basis for bronchitis, emphysema, and asthma.[2] The pattern for females has not changed substantially over the last 20 years. In contrast, the rate of increase in males in the 55 and over age brackets during this time period has been sharp.

Additional information on acute respiratory conditions is provided through the Health Interview Survey, which covers acute illnesses having their onset in

Five-Year Average Death Rate per 100,000 All Causes

by years							
55-64		65-74		75-84		Over 84	
Male	Female	Male	Female	Male	Female	Male	Female
2,324	1,120	5,081	2,760	9,786	6,823	20,508	19,170
2,286	1,165	4,955	2,829	9,921	7,326	21,501	19,383
2,293	1,217	4,811	2,946	10,054	7,722	20,347	18,831+
2,360	1,335	4,814	3,166	10,216	8,094	20,103	18,644

Five-Year Average Death Rate per 100,000
Bronchitis, Emphysema, and Asthma– White Male and Female

by years							
55-64		65-74		75-84		Over 84	
Male	Female	Male	Female	Male	Female	Male	Female
67.4	14.1	180.9	24.4	260.3	38.7	276.4	74.2
54.2	9.4	128.7	17.0	164.3	32.0	180.8	57.9
37.9	6.6	78.7	13.4	100.0	28.4	110.5	53.4
22.9	6.5	43.1	14.2	60.4	29.0	83.3	56.2

the 2-week period prior to the interview for which the individual either sought medical attention or experienced 1 or more days' restricted activity (Table III). As expected, the incidence decreased with age, but also the female rate exceeded that for males.[3]

There is but little doubt that environmental improvements, i.e., water treatment, sewage disposal, and food sanitation have placed an important part in the increase in life expectancy. Likewise, as longivity increases, the chronic degenerative diseases assume an even greater importance.[4] Of particular concern to this discussion is whether, conversely, the environmental health hazards of today will also contribute significantly to disability and causes of death. Statistical data are too meager to provide an answer. It is important, though, that this potential be kept under surveillance.

TABLE III

Incidence of Acute Conditions per 100 Persons by Sex and Age Groups (1971)

Condition group	All ages		Both sexes			
	Male	Female	Under 6 years	6-17	17-44	45 and over
All acute conditions	207.8	228.5	372.7	295.8	206.2	122.5
Respiratory conditions	111.1	121.6	213.3	163.5	103.7	63.7
Upper respiratory conditions	67.8	71.2	147.9	104.1	55.7	33.6
Common cold	51.3	53.2	–	–	–	–
Other upper respiratory conditions	16.5	18.0	–	–	–	–
Influenza	37.6	44.8	48.1	54.5	44.1	25.9
Influenza with digestive manifestations	5.2	6.3	–	–	–	–
Other influenza	32.4	38.6	–	–	–	–
Other respiratory conditions	5.7	5.5	17.2	4.9	3.8	4.3
Pneumonia	0.9	0.8	–	–	–	–
Bronchitis	2.7	3.0	–	–	–	–
Other respiratory conditions	2.2	1.7	–	–	–	–

COMMUNITY

Air, Water, and Food

During the last two decades an ever-increasing concern has been exhibited over the environmental health hazards associated with air pollution, water pollution, and food contamination. There is ample past evidence that, under unique circumstances, significant responses have resulted. Regulations have been established by the Environmental Protection Agency, the Food and Drug Administration, and state agencies to provide control. This is discussed in more detail in the chapter, "Impact of Governmental Environmental Regulations upon Industrial Processes," which follows. The complexity and magnitude of this problem have been well illustrated in publications associated with a symposium conducted by the National Academy of Sciences–National Research Council,[5] a workshop sponsored by the John E. Fogarty International Center and the National Institute of Environmental Sciences,[6] and a United Nations Conference on the Human Environment held in Stockholm in 1972.[7] All placed major emphasis on the need for additional information concerning the long-term health effect of environmental stresses, singly and in combination, and a more adequate program for monitoring the environment. Attention was also called to the large voids that exist in our present information which make an appraisal most difficult, if not impossible.

Similarly, the draft report of the Presidential Panel on Chemicals and Health under the President's Science Advisory Committee (now abolished and the responsibilities transferred to the National Science Foundation) expresses concern for the potentially deleterious effects on health from long-term exposures to chemicals in the environment.[8]

The sustained scientific interest in this area is attested by a forthcoming International Symposium entitled, "Recent Advances in the Assessment of the Health Effects of Environmental Pollutants" to be held in Paris in June 1974. This symposium, under the co-sponsorship of the Commission of the European Communities, the U.S. Environmental Protection Agency, and the World Health Organization, will cover the following aspects:

1. Assessment of exposure of general and selected population groups.
2. Metabolic aspects of exposure to environmental pollutants and measurement of pollutants and their metabolites in human tissues, fluids, and excreta.
3. Evaluation of suspected or observed health effects from exposure to environmental pollutants.

Even though it is recognized that under certain circumstances the environmental health stress from this source may be significantly additive to the on-job stress, it is beyond the scope of this section to do other than recognize the potential.

Noise

Noise is now accepted as one of the leaders in community pollution. In some instances, it goes beyond the category of annoyance to constitute an important increment in the potential to produce loss of hearing.[9-15] However, community annoyance is the major complaint. Noise levels, at 50 feet, exceed 70 decibels measured with an A-frequency weighting (dBA) for passenger cars and 80–90 dBA for motorcycles and trucks.[9] Garbage compactors and overhead jets may exceed 100 dBA.

The emergence of community noise as a major environmental problem is recognized in the Noise Control Act of 1972, which establishes statutory deadlines for initial noise control regulations. EPA is concentrating its initial major attention to noise control for trucks and planes, but is also actually working on rail, construction, industrial plant, office building, and residential noise control programs. As a part of the Noise Control Act of 1972, EPA has published a document entitled "Public Health and Welfare Criteria for Noise," July 27, 1973. This document does not suggest specific recommended levels of control. However, Cohen et al.,[9] in relating off-job noise stress to that on the

TABLE IV

'A' Weighted Sound Levels of Some Noises found in Different Environments[a]

Sound level, dBA	Industrial (and military)	Community (or outdoor)	Home (or indoor)
130			
120 Uncomfortably loud	Armored personnel carrier (123 dB) Oxygen torch (121 dB) Scraper-loader (117 dB) Compactor (116 dB)		
110	Riveting machine (110 dB) Textile loom (106 dB)		Rock-n-roll band (108-114 dB)
100 Very loud	Electric furnace area (100 dB) Farm tractor (98 dB) Newspaper press (97 dB)	Jet flyover @ 1000 ft. (103 dB) Power mower (96 dB) Compressor @ 20 ft. (94 dB) Rock drill @ 100 ft. (92 dB)	Inside subway car – 35 mph (95 dB)
90	Cockpit-prop aircraft (88 dB) Milling machine (85 dB) Cotton spinning (83 dB)	Motorcycles @ 25 ft. (90 dB) Propeller aircraft flyover @ 1000 ft. (88 dBA)	Cockpit-light aircraft (90 dB)
80 Moderately loud	Lathe (81 dB) Tabulating (80 dB)	Diesel truck, 40 mph @ 50 ft. (84 dB)	Food blender (88 dB) Garbage disposal (80 dB) Clothes washer (78 dB)

70	Diesel train, 40-50 mph @ 100 ft. (83 dB)	Living room music (76 dB)
60	Passenger car, 65 mph @ 25 ft. (77 dB)	Dishwasher (75 dB)
50 Quiet	Near freeway-auto traffic @ (64 dB)	TV-audio (70 dB)
40	Air conditioning unit @ 20 ft. (60 dB)	Vacuum (70 dB)
	Large transformer @ 200 ft. (53 dB)	Conversation (60 dB)
30 Very quiet	Light traffic @ 100 ft. (50 dB)	
20		
10 Just audible		
0 Threshold of hearing (1000–4000 Hz)		

^{a} Unless otherwise specified, listed sound levels are measured at typical operator-listener distances from source. Noise readings taken from general acoustical literature and observations by PHS.

job, used a reference limit 15 dB below that in the Walsh–Healey Act for assessing outdoor exposure durations of 8 hr per day or less. The authors cautioned that the above levels should not be construed as a suggested standard since more supporting data would be needed than were available at that time (1970). Goldsmith and Jonsson[11] and Koczkur et al.[16] have suggested that lower levels may be required to prevent undue annoyance.

HOME

Household Chemicals

The health hazard potential of household chemicals has become a subject of intense interest within the last decade. Poisoning in children has been and continues to be of top priority. Consequently, first attention was directed to educational programs to prevent children having access to these chemicals. It became evident, however, that rapidly developing technology, in which an ever-increasing number of chemicals were being made available both in conventional and aerosol packaging, would require a more vigorous program. The present-day concern extends to nonprescription drugs, cleansers and polishers, solvents, paints and lacquers, solders, glues, cements, pesticides, cosmetics, deodorants, etc. The concern also goes beyond child poisoning to the potential for chronic effects from long-term exposures at low levels. Sunshine lists about 25 fungicides, 80 herbicides, and 85 insecticides in use today.[17] Many are packaged for household use. Of the 40-odd herbicides, insecticides, and fungicides for which threshold limit values of exposure have been adopted or proposed for the workroom air, about one-half are recognized as being hazardous from skin contact with the concentrate.[18]

Poison Control Center Statistics

The National Clearinghouse for Poison Control Centers' tabulations for 1972 based on 160,824 individual reports submitted to the Clearinghouse showed that 72% of the reports occurred in persons under 14 years of age, 21% in persons over 15 years of age, and 7% in persons of unknown age.[19]

Medicines accounted for 52% of the cases reported. Sixty-two percent of the reports were of persons under 14 years of age, 32% for persons over 15 years of age, and 6% for persons of unknown age. Cleaning and polishing agents were of the second highest group, accounting for 13% of the reports. The remaining 35% of the reports related to petroleum products, cosmetics, pesticides, gases and vapors, plants, turpentine, paints, etc.

Of the 160,824 cases reported to the Clearinghouse, 40% were treated cases, 75% were from accidental ingestion, 2% from kicks trips, 2% from inhalation, 14% from self-poisoning, and 7% from other or unknown cause.

The report stressed that the above cases were only those reported to the Clearinghouse and were not to be construed as the total number occurring annually, as many cases are treated by physicians or hospitals not associated with Poison Control Centers and are not reported to the Clearinghouse.

These data attest that accidental poisoning from chemicals found in or around the home are an important source of health injury.

The American Association of Poison Control Centers has announced the inauguration of a bimonthly newsletter that will include information of observations on poisons, programs, and personnel of Poison Control Centers, and other information of general interest.[20]

Congress, acknowledging the need to develop a specific program in this regard, passed the Federal Hazardous Substances Labeling Act of 1960 and amended it in 1966 to require the proper labeling of the hazardous contents of household packages, the statement of necessary precautions for safe use, and the banning of substances so hazardous as to be dangerous in the household regardless of labeling. Regulations for labeling were developed by the Food and Drug Administration charged with the administration of this Act.

In 1970, the National Commission on Product Safety completed a 2-year investigation. It concluded that a critical need existed for hard data on actual injuries and developed a National Electronic Injury Surveillance System (NEISS) in cooperation with 14 hospital emergency rooms. This has now been expanded to include 119 emergency rooms.[21] Information was developed by product, percent by age of victim and sex, and rate per 100,000 population. In addition, a mean severity value was assigned in order to set priorities to allocate internal resources for further study.

On October 27, 1972, the President signed Public Law 92–573 establishing an independent Consumer Product Safety Commission. The Commission was assigned the responsibility of protecting the public against unreasonable risks of injury associated with consumer products and the specific tasks of evaluating the comparative safety of consumer products, developing uniform safety standards for consumer products where necessary, and promulgating research and investigation into the causes and prevention of product-related deaths, illnesses, and injuries.[22] The authority and responsibility established under the Federal Hazardous Substances Labeling Act were transferred to this Commission. The Food and Drug Administration is still responsible for food, drugs, and cosmetics.

NEISS data for the year 1973 for specific products of interest are presented in Table V.

The highest incidence in home and family maintenance products, as expected, falls in the 0–4 age bracket with the next highest in the 25–64 age bracket. The latter is of particular interest from its potential of being additive to the on-job environmental health stress. A high mean severity value has been assigned this classification of consumer products. The Bureau of Biomedical Science, Consumer Product Safety Commission, is now formulating plans whereby useful

TABLE V

Injuries Associated with Selected Consumer Products as Reported in Hospitals in the National Electronic Injury Surveillance System 1973

Description	Number of cases	Percent by age					Rate per 100,000 population
		0-4	5-14	15-24	25-64	65+	
Adhesives and related compounds	157	64.3	17.2	10.8	7.6	—	1.41
Antifreeze	55	36.4	1.8	27.3	34.5	—	0.53
Bleaches and dyes	586	70.6	7.3	4.8	16.0	1.2	4.96
Cleaners, caustic, solvents, etc.	1,095	61.5	6.4	10.1	20.7	1.3	10.24
Gasoline, kerosene, paint removers, etc.	1,039	45.8	18.1	16.0	19.2	0.9	12.41
Lubricants	103	57.3	9.7	15.5	16.5	1.0	0.93
Paint, varnish, shellac, etc.	264	57.2	15.5	9.8	17.0	0.4	2.14
Polishes and waxes	202	86.6	3.5	3.0	4.5	2.5	2.08
Cosmetics	594	56.2	5.4	13.0	23.4	2.0	5.45
Drugs	5,444	77.1	10.0	6.8	5.5	0.6	52.84
Pesticides	499	83.2	8.0	3.0	5.6	0.2	4.74

data from NEISS can be made available upon request. This is a much needed service.

Household Allergens

Although allergens found in the home environment in foods, fabrics, etc., constitute an important source of stress, the subject is too extensive in scope to discuss here except where the same allergens are found also in some industrial environments.

Two investigations, one by Rudner et al.,[23] the other by Badmann et al.,[24] show the importance of allergens, found both in the home environment and in industry, as a source of allergic contact dermatitis. Rudner et al. tested 1200 subjects suspected of having some type of contact sensitivity with 16 allergens. The percentages of the subjects with positive reactions to specific allergens tested were: nickel sulfate, 11%; potassium dichromate, 8%; p-phenylene-diomene, 8%; thimerool (merthiolate), 8%; ethylenediamine, 7%; neomycin sulfate, 6%; turpentine oil, 6%; formalin, 4%. Badmann et al. tested 4000 patients for sensitivity to a series of 20 allergens. Approximately 13% of the group tested reacted positively to each of potassium dichromate, nickel sulfate, and cobalt chloride; 20% to wood tars, 12% to turpentine; and 7% to formaldehyde.

There is not sufficient information at present to arrive at an opinion as to whether this source of exposure can be significantly additive to on-the-job environmental health stress. However, it is a potential that must be kept in mind especially when an occupational situation exists which cannot be satisfactorily explained by the job exposure per se. Not only is the opportunity readily afforded to "take a chance" with household chemicals, but also the consumer can arrive at various shades of meaning in the interpretation of the precautionary measures printed on the package.

Noise

Noise in the home, as in the community, is coming under greater scrutiny. Decibel levels may vary from the low 70's for radio, vacuum cleaners, etc., to 100 or more for loud music. That for lawn mowers, saws, food blenders, electric razors, etc., can be expected to range from 80 to 90 or higher. In as much as these sources present a limited exposure, they generally can be expected to contribute to the annoyance classification rather than loss of hearing. However, as control technology and application develops in the industrial and community sources, similar improvement can be expected in home products. Except for unique situations, home noise sources should not constitute an important increment to loss of hearing.

Hobbies

Home recreational activities have been growing at a phenomenal rate. The estimated 1972 hobby industry retail volume shown below is projected to exceed one billion dollars with a doubling within 10 years or less.[25]

Hobby	Estimated 1972 hobby industry retail volume ($)
Crafts: Packaged and bulk crafts of all types, includes paint-by-number, special tools and finishing materials, hardware and accessories. Art supplies and materials sold through traditional industry channels included.	306 million
Plastic Kits: Of all types, domestic or foreign sold in the U.S.A. Category includes adhesives, paints, display cases, tools, and finishing materials for this hobby.	202 million
Model Railroads: All scales, kit and ready-to-run; includes layouts, buildings, scenery, power, track, and accessories, domestic and imported.	112 million
Model Aeronautics and Radio Control: Includes balsa kits, rubber and engine powered; gas engines; ready-to-fly models; radio control systems for planes, ships, cars; fuel, batteries, accessories.	108 million
Model Car Racing: Home and commercial racing sets; all gauges, track and accessories, cars built-up and kit, controllers, power, parts, buildings, scenery, custom building equipment, etc.	101 million
Scale Model Miniatures: Includes assembled metal, plastic or wood collectors' items including vehicles, planes, ships, military miniatures, etc.	78 million
Stamps, Coins, and other Collectors' Items: (Volume estimates refer only to those moving through traditional "Hobby" channels of distribution.)	48 million
Science: Kits, set and accessories for chemistry, biology, electricity and electronics, physics, microscopes, geology, etc. Includes model rockets and accessories.	46 million
Hobby Toys/Games	44 million
Tools: Adhesives, finishing materials, balsa, architectural model materials and accessories not identified with a specific category.	36 million
Wooden Model Kits: Includes ships, vehicles, planes, etc.	10 million
TOTAL	$1,091,000,000

While some of the kits may contain potentially hazardous chemicals, these products come within the jurisdiction of the U.S. Consumer Product Safety Commission. With proper use of these kits, diversionary interest is provided the adult worker that can be a valuable means of allowing off-job recovery from job stress requiring high energy expenditure, close detail, etc. On the other hand, some hobbies such as woodworking, antique furniture restoration, gardening, etc., may entail significant exposures unless proper precautionary measures are observed.

Recreation

The phenomenal expansion of leisure activity during the last 10–20 years is an outgrowth of mounting free time and affluence. The growth during the past 10 years, as developed by the Chase Manhattan Bank, is given in Fig. 1.[26]

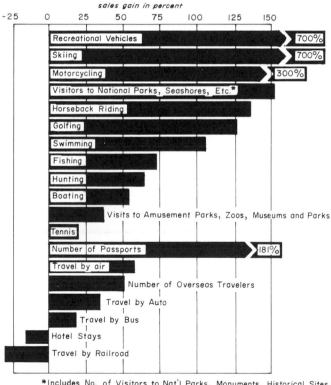

*Includes No. of Visitors to Nat'l Parks, Monuments, Historical Sites, Military Areas, Parkways, Seashores, Recreational Areas

Data: CMB

Fig. 1. Growth of leisure activities (1960–1971).

It is interesting to note the extraordinary increase in recreational vehicles, motorcycling, hunting, and boating. Noise can be an important environmental stress in these areas as well as in sports shooting.

Annoyance

Workers, both on and off the job, are exposed to two types of environmentally interrelated stresses. One includes the exposure to measurable doses of chemical or physical agents and the energy requirement to do the job. The other is an entity difficult to measure and evaluate. It is annoyance that may be reflected in task performance as well as biochemical changes, physiologic response, and nervous system reactions. Illustrative of the increasing interest in this area are recent publications by Buckley,[27] Chase,[28] and McQuade[29] which discuss the potential role of environmental stresses, resulting in tension and anger as a causation of chronic disease. A symposium was held on August 30, 1971 under the sponsorship of the Department of Environmental Hygiene of the Kårolinska Institute, Stockholm, in collaboration with the Swedish Environmental Protection Board and the U.S. Environmental Protection Agency to discuss methods for measurement of annoyance due to environmental factors.[30]

The following quotations from the proceedings illustrate the importance attached to this subject.

> The modern world is now paying increased attention not only to proved health hazards produced by such factors as food contamination, air pollution, or noise, but also to reactions only potentially related to disease states or of uncertain health significance. These apparent nondisease effects may include physiological responses, central nervous system reactions, biochemical changes, and annoyance in connection with sensory perception of pollutants, or even from such nonspecific factors as disorderliness or distasteful architecture. Such effects are much more widespread than overt toxic responses to environmental pollution. Because of the importance of defining and measuring such effects as annoyance, this symposium was convened.
>
> From the medical point of view the term "annoyance" implies an effect which may not be demonstrable pathogenic but which involves a negative factor for the individual's comfort and well-being. However, the demarcation between pathogenic processes and annoyance is not distinct since the line between health and disease is partly established by current attitudes in the community. A similar viewpoint is implied in the World Health Organization's definition of health: "A state of complete physical, mental and social well-being and not merely the absence of disease or infirmity." In many countries the logical consequence of this manner of considering the problem has been to regard even annoyance as a medico-hygienic problem and to attach great importance to subjective nuisances in the environment.
>
> The members of the symposium adopted as a definition that "Annoyance is a feeling of displeasure associated with any agent or condition believed to affect adversely an individual or group." In some human populations, annoyance arising from environmental conditions may be present in a majority of the people. In

terms of the numbers affected, annoyance is probably much more widespread than overt toxic effects arising from chemical or physical agents, and avoidance of toxicologic effects alone is not an adequate criterion of a suitable environment. For this reason, the need is urgent to have good methods to study annoyance.

Spontaneous complaints, such as letters to newspapers or health authorities may indicate the existence of annoyance but this crude measure should be replaced by better techniques. Methods applied to date have emphasized population survey techniques in determining annoyance, and the possibility of errors in application of survey methods has been strongly emphasized by members of the symposium. When these survey techniques have been properly and expertly developed and applied they have yielded valid and significant results related to annoyance, and these techniques have proved the data that are the basis of current knowledge of this subject in quantitative terms. Modern psychological and sociological research offers the possibility of application of many new and potentially more quantitative methods pertinent to research in annoyance. Their practical applicability and usefulness under field conditions has to be proved, however.

Several physiological parameters have been found in laboratory experiments to be related to reactions of annoyance, for example, epinephrine release into blood or urine. If a significant relationship between such physiological indicators and annoyance can be established in field studies, they may be useful indices and may supplement verbal reporting of annoyance.

Methods for indirectly measuring annoyance in groups, which include the study of population redistribution, economic costs of pollution or organizational response and governmental actions have generally not been established as valid indicators of annoyance. If they can be validated they may prove to be useful because of the ease of their application to large populations.

Research should emphasize methods capable of determining multiple factors contributing to annoyance, both in terms of conditions predisposing to development of annoyance, as well as synergistic or antagonistic relationships between several annoyance sources or other environmental conditions.

It is not possible presently to equate the role of annoyance as an additive stress to that rising from exposure to the on-job chemical and physical agents. There is a growing belief, though, that this factor must be considered in evaluating the stress-response pattern.

PERSONAL HABITS

Smoking

A comprehensive review of the health effects from smoking is presented in a report from the Surgeon General entitled, "The Health Consequences of Smoking (1972)."[31] It leaves no doubt but that smoking continues to be a major health problem and cites that smokers have higher death rates from cerebrovascular disease and from nonsyphilitic aorta aneurysm than nonsmokers. It is the most important cause of chronic obstructive bronchopulmonary disease and a major cause of lung cancer in men as well as a significant one in women. It exerts a retarding influence on fetal growth, is associated with an increased prevalence of peptic ulcer, and may produce exacerbation of allergic symptoms in nonsmokers who are suffering from allergies of diverse cause.[27]

Smoking is associated with an additive or synergistic effect when combined with respiratory exposure to asbestos, cement, chlorine, coal, coal gas, cotton, grain, iron oxide, mouldy hay, silica, uranium, and wood ("Industrial Environmental Health, the Worker and the Community", 1st and 2nd eds.).

Drugs

The synergistic effect of drugs on exposures to agents encountered in industry is well recognized by industrial physicians and toxicologists. Examples include the potentiating effect of alcohol on the toxicity of carbon tetra-chloride[32] and the synergistic action of phenobarbital on chloroform and carbon tetrachloride.[33]

Knowledge of the extent that workers occasionally or routinely use drugs becomes important, especially if these workers are also exposed to chemical agents in the working environment. A recent survey by Redfield[34] covering 303 employment applicants for a company in Oregon provides some information of this nature; however, it is not known how applicable the data from this study are to industry as a whole in the United States. Of the 303 applicants, 136 part-time students and 167 nonstudents, 86% consumed alcohol occasionally or regularly; 28% smoked marijuana occasionally or regularly; 6% used psychedelics occasionally; 1% used sedatives occasionally; 9% used speed drugs occasionally or routinely; and 0.3% used opiates occasionally; 66% of the nonstudents smoked compared to 29% for the students. No information was presented on the extent the applicants occasionally or regularly used more than one of the above drugs. From the percentages given, however, it is obvious that many of the same applicants used tobacco, marijuana, and alcohol.

Additional information on the seriousness of alcoholism in workers is presented in a special report to the U.S. Congress.

It is not within the scope of this discussion to more than emphasize the potential of drugs in combination with certain environmental chemical stresses. Educational programs directed toward this area can provide an important means of communication with the worker in specific relevant chemical job stresses.

SUMMARY

Information on the magnitude and complexity of the exposure of workers to environmental health stress in the community and home preclude conclusions based upon hard facts. Scientific concern, however, has been voiced through publications, workshops, symposia, and conferences. This awareness has resulted in the formulation of governmental programs directed to this issue. One area of relevance, though, needs additional attention. That is, whether community and home conditions are such as to permit adequate recovery from job stresses to avoid a day-to-day buildup. This applies to such specific factors as annoyance, lack of sleep, proper nutrition, diversionary recreational activities, home humidity and temperature, hobbies, smoking, and the use of drugs.

REFERENCES

1. Morison, R. S., Dying. *Sci. Amer. 229,* 55–61 (1973).
2. Personal Communication. National Center for Health Statistics, Public Health Service, U.S. Department of Health, Education and Welfare, Rockville, Maryland, 1973.
3. "Current Estimates from the Health Interview Survey, U.S.," Ser. 10, No. 79. National Center for Health Statistics, Public Health Service, U.S. Department of Health Education and Welfare, Rockville, Maryland, 1971.
4. Dingle, J. H., The ills of man. *Sci. Amer. 229,* 77–84 (1973).
5. Lee, D. H. K., and Minard, D., eds., "Physiology, Environment and Man." Academic Press, New York, 1970.
6. Lee D. H. K., ed., "Environmental Factors in Respiratory Disease." Academic Press, New York, 1972.
7. "Health Hazards of the Human Environment." World Health Organ., Geneva, 1972.
8. Chemical threats to health examined. *Chem. Eng. News 17,* No. 38, 11 (1973).
9. Cohen, A., Anticaglia, J., and Janes, H. J., Sociocusis—hearing loss from non-occupational noise exposure. *Sound & Vibration 4,* 12 (1970).
10. Jonsson, E., Kajland, A., Paccagnella, B., and Sorensen, S. Annoyance reactions to traffic noise in Italy and Sweden. A comparative study. *Arch. Environ. Health 19,* 692–699 (1969).
11. Goldsmith, J. R., and Jonsson, E., Health effects of community noise. *Amer. J. Pub. Health 63,* 782–793 (1973).
12. Young, M. F., and Woods, D. L., Sources and measurement of highway noise. *J. ASSE (Amer. Soc. Saf. Eng.) 17,* 38–41 (1972).
13. Flugrath, J. M., Modern-day rock-and-roll music and damage-risk criteria. *J. Acoust. Soc. Amer. 45,* 704–711 (1969).
14. Outlook, noise pollution control are in the making in U.S. *Environ. Sci. Technol. 7,* 1098–1100 (1973).
15. Jensen, P., Control of environmental noise. *J. Air Pollut. Contr. Ass. 23,* 1028–1034 (1973).
16. Koczkur, E., Broger, E. D., Henderson, V. A., and Lightstrong, A. D., Noise monitoring and sociological survey in the city of Toronto. *J. Air Pollut. Contr. Ass. 23,* 105–109 (1973).
17. Sunshine, I., ed., "Handbook of Analytical Toxicology." Chem. Rubber Publ. Co., Cleveland, Ohio, 1969.
18. "Threshold Limit Values for Chemical Substances in Workroom Air." Amer. Conf. Govt. Ind. Hyg., Cincinnati, Ohio, 1973.
19. "Tabulations of 1972 Reports," National Clearinghouse for Poison Control Centers,

Bulletin May–June 1973. Food and Drug Administration, Bureau of Drugs, U.S. Department of Health, Education and Welfare, Bethesda, Maryland, 1973.

20. Poison control newsletter. *Amer. Ind. Hyg. Ass., J. 34,* 480 (1973).

21. "Product Safety NEISS News." Food and Drug Administration, U.S. Department of Health, Education and Welfare, Bethesda, Maryland, 1972.

22. "NEISS News," Vol. 1, No. 6. U.S. Consumer Product Safety Commission, Bethesda, Maryland, 1973.

23. Rudner, E. J., Clendenning, W. E., Epstein, E., Fisher, A. A., Jillson, O. F., Jordan, W. P., Kanof, N., Larsen, W., Mailbach, H., Mitchell, J. C., O'Quinn, S. E., Schorr, W. F., and Sulyberger, M. D., Epidemiology of contact dermatitis in North America: 1972. *Arch. Dermatol. 108,* 537–540 (1973).

24. Badmann, H. J., Calnan, C. D., Cronin, E., Fregert, S., Hjorth, V., Magnusson, B., Mailbach, H., Malten, J. E., Meneghini, C. L., Pirila, V., and Wilkinson, D. S., Dermatitis from applied medicaments. *Arch. Dermatol. 106,* 335–337 (1972).

25. Communication. Hobby Industry Association of America, Inc., New York, 1973.

26. Growth of Leisure Activities, 1960–1971, "Business in Brief," No. 109. Chase Manhattan Bank, New York, 1973.

27. Buckley, J. P., Sights–sounds–stress. *Communiqué 2,* 21–22 (1973).

28. Chase, D. J., Worth the stress? *Chem. Eng. (New York) 79,* 78–82 (1972).

29. McQuade, W., What stress can do to you. *Fortune 85,* 102–108 and 139–141 (1972).

30. Lindvall, T., and Radford, E. P., eds., Measurement of annoyance due to exposure to environmental factors. *Environ. Res. 6,* 1–36 (1973).

31. "The Health Consequences of Smoking. A Report of the Surgeon General: 1972," DHEW Publ. No. (HMS) 72–7516. Public Health Service, Health Services and Mental Health Administration, U.S. Dept. of Health, Education and Welfare, Washington, D.C., 1972.

32. Patty, F. A., ed., "Industrial Hygiene and Toxicology," Vol. II. Wiley (Interscience), New York, 1965.

33. Cornish, H. H., Ling, B. D., and Borth, M. L., Phenobarbitol and organic solvent toxicity. *Amer. Ind. Hyg. Ass., J. 34,* 487–492 (1973).

34. Redfield, J. T., Drugs in the workplace–substituting sense for sensationalism. *Amer. J. Pub. Health 63,* 1064–1070 (1973).

Impact of Governmental Environmental Regulations upon Industrial Activities

PATRICK R. ATKINS

During the last decade several major pieces of environmental legislation have been produced which are having profound effects on the public and the business community. The legislation covers a broad spectrum of environmental problems and touches on every aspect of industrial activity. The Occupational Safety and Health Act,[1] the Clean Air Act of 1970,[2] the National Environmental Policy Act,[3] the Federal Water Pollution Control Act Amendments of 1972,[4] and pending legislation concerning comprehensive land use planning are separate laws that act in concert to require that industry and, in some cases, the general public take numerous and at times difficult steps to ensure that the environment is protected.

Many of the concepts in these acts are new. The wording of the legislation is often imprecise. The requirements of some portions of the laws have been shown to be impossible to meet on the mandated schedules. The requirements of the nation and our knowledge of the resources and capital available to us are constantly being refined. For these and other reasons, the environmental legislation picture is not static. Legislation that has been law for four or more years is still "growing" as the result of almost continuous examination and interpretation by the courts, by industry, and by the responsible enforcement agencies. The intent of the Congress in each portion of the legislation is under examination, and each new interpretation can result in new requirements. Thus, as the laws mature, their impact on the nation can change.

The environmental legislation of import today is designed to involve as many people as possible. Public hearings, public disclosures, public comments, notifications, the right of challenge, citizen suits, etc., are the norm. It is obvious that one major intent of the legislation was to ensure that all interested and affected parties could participate in the regulatory process. However, this ability to participate was provided without placing commensurate responsibilities on the individuals involved. As a result, it appears that without a complete understanding of the issues involved, a policy is developing which places a great deal of responsibility on American industry to meet rather stringent environmental control guidelines and to fulfill a growing number of obligations to the employees, to the individuals directly affected by a company's actions, and to the general public. The purpose of this chapter is to discuss briefly several major regulations, to outline the actions that these law prescribe for industry, and to show how policy decisions based on an incomplete understanding of the situation can produce disconcerting results. A secondary purpose is to encourage full participation by industry at all levels of the regulatory process to hasten the time when reasonable and equitable legislation is developed in all areas of environmental protection.

OCCUPATIONAL SAFETY AND HEALTH ACT OF 1970

The Williams–Steiger Occupational Safety and Health Act was enacted on a relatively low-keyed basis with little fanfare. The purpose of the Act is "to assure so far as possible every working man and woman in the nation safe and healthful working conditions...." The Act created two agencies: (1) the Occupational Safety and Health Administration (OSHA) in the Department of Labor to administer and enforce the requirements of the legislation and the National Institute for Occupational Safety and Health (NIOSH) in the Department of Health, Education, and Welfare to conduct the necessary primary research and manpower development. In addition, the Act created the Occupational Safety and Health Review Commission to act as an appeals board for parties aggrieved by OSHA actions.

Requirements of the Act

The Act requires that:
1. Occupational safety and health standards be developed and promulgated initially using national consensus standards and established federal standards; then adding emergency standards and standards developed through a prescribed procedure outlined in Section 6(b) of the Act.
2. Federal action be taken to enforce the standards at least for the initial period of the Act, until and if states can develop acceptable (to OSHA) programs of their own.
3. A training and education program be established to develop expertise in the field and produce a corps of safety and industrial health manpower.

4. The necessary research be conducted to provide the information needed to set and enforce proper standards.
5. The states be encouraged to develop the capabilities to administer and enforce their own occupational safety and health programs after approval by the federal agency.

The Standards

Under the Act, an industrial establishment is required to provide a working environment that meets the stipulations of several hundred safety and health standards, maintain detailed records on a variety of subjects, conduct periodic sampling and monitoring programs in several areas, and live up to the General Duty requirements of the Act, which specify that a place of employment be provided free of recognized hazards that may cause death or serious physical harm. In addition, industry is encouraged to participate in research activities, training programs, and the critique of proposed standards.

The original standards included in the Act were several hundred consensus standards or established federal standards. A national consensus standard is any safety and health standard that has been adopted and promulgated by a nationality recognized standards-producing organization, if the development was subject to review and comment by a cross-section of groups. An established federal standard was defined as any operative occupational safety and health standard established by any agency of the United States and in force on the date of enactment of the Act. From the period April 28, 1971, until April 28, 1973, these types of standards, referred to as "interim standards," were the backbone of the Act.

As of April 28, 1973, additional standards, referred to as "permanent standards," can be incorporated into the regulation by the Secretary of Labor, if certain criteria are met. The permanent standards are to be based on research, demonstrations, and experiments, taking into consideration the latest scientific information, feasibility, and experience. Standards can be proposed by the Secretary of Labor or an advisory committee appointed by the Secretary. Outside parties such as employers or employees may request that a standard be developed, modified, or revoked. In addition, NIOSH may make recommendations for new standards. Public participation in permanent standard development is required, but the Secretary of Labor has wide latitude in determining the manner in which this participation is accomplished. The entire standard-setting process can require a considerable amount of time—a minimum of 18 months, if all the time schedules are met. Since the probability of delay is great, many new standards will require considerably more time than this.

The third type of standard utilized by the Act is the emergency standard. The

Secretary of Labor can at any time issue an emergency standard by publishing it in the *Federal Register* if he determines that is necessary to protect workers from immediate danger. A permanent standard must be promulgated within 6 months after the publication of the emergency standard.

Recently, a new approach to standard setting was initiated by the Occupational Safety and Health Administration. A series of 415 mini-standards will be developed and promulgated within two years. These mini-standards will utilize the expertise of three consulting agencies to develop medical surveillance procedures, engineering methodology for control and monitoring techniques. Published data and "accepted" TLV levels will be used to set the mini-standard levels. In this way, OSHA plans to produce standards on a much shorter time base than is required for the lengthy process outlined initially.

Industry Activity

An industrial establishment is required to meet the requirements of the OSHA Standards. Unlike several other environmental acts, the Occupational Safety and Health Act regulations do not require prior approval before a practice or process can be utilized. No permit system is specified by the Act. However, the employees have the opportunity to submit a complaint to OSHA if a violation is suspected and an inspection by an OSHA representative will follow. If a violation is found, a citation may be given and corrective action will be required. In addition, unsolicited visitations by OSHA inspectors are utilized to ensure compliance with the standards.

If an employer suspects a violation he has the opportunity to request a variance. To receive a variance, he must show that compliance cannot be reached within the specified time frame because of manpower, training, equipment, or materials delays or that equivalent safety and health protection will be achieved by an alternate method. If an employer is aggrieved by a standard, he has the opportunity to challenge its validity by filing a petition in the U.S. Court of Appeals within 60 days from the promulgation of the standard.

In addition, employers can participate in the standard development procedure by requesting that the Secretary develop, modify, or revoke certain standards, by submitting written comments on various proposed standards, by participating in public hearings, and by serving on advisory committees. These approaches are often frustrating and are always time consuming, but participation at these levels can be effective.

CLEAN AIR ACT OF 1970

The Clean Air Act of 1970 superseded the 1967 legislation on this subject and reversed the trend toward nonuniform emission standards around the nation. The new legislation encourages the use of uniform standards to ensure that all sources are controlled to the highest degree possible without regard to the location of the source. The new legislation set up the mechanism for the development and enforcement of uniform new source performance standards to be applied to all facilities constructed after the effective date of the Act. In addition, the regulations contain requirements that each state develop implementation plans to achieve uniform national air quality goals by utilizing methods acceptable to the Federal Environmental Protection Agency. The deadlines established by the Act are unrealistic and, in their efforts to comply with the timetable, the various agencies have sometimes rushed into areas without the proper amount of study. Some of the timetables are now being altered by court action and, perhaps, this trend will be reinforced by legislative action in the near future.

The Environmental Protection Agency promulgated primary (human health related) and secondary (welfare related) air quality goals in 1971 and developed model implementation plans for the states to utilize as examples of programs that would result in the attainment of the air quality goals. All state plans were received in 1972, reviewed, and approved, at least in part, in May of that year. The deadline for attainment of the national primary air quality goals was set as July 1975, three years after implementation plan approval.

In areas where stationary control alone was not capable of producing air quality equivalent to the National Air Quality Goals, transportation control measures were also required as part of the implementation plan. These transportation control plans have caused some delay in the acceptance of state implementation plans and several issues in this area are yet to be resolved.

Several recent court decisions have seemingly extended the Congressional intent of the Clean Air Act and markedly reduced the flexibility for implementing the requirements of the Act. Several of these decisions have played a role in making the social and economic implications of the legislation more apparent. These decisions include the following.

1. The imposition of the Supreme Court's nondegradation ruling, which requires that the state implementation plans contain regulations to maintain the present air quality in those areas where the air is already cleaner than that required to meet the national air quality goals.
2. The upholding of the court-imposed regulation on air quality approval for complex sources.
3. The yet unresolved question of the Environmental Protection Agency's transportation control program for new large urban areas.
4. The recent interpretation in the First Circuit Court of Appeals (Federal) which prevents any state from granting variances that extend beyond the federally imposed air quality achievement date of mid-1975 (post-attainment of air quality goals).

5. The decision in the Fifth Circuit Court of Appeals (Federal) which seemingly declares that it is improper for any state to grant variances which are effective until mid-1975 (the preattainment period).

Regulations

In 1971 the Federal Environmental Protection Agency promulgated national air quality goals for five "criteria" pollutants. These pollutants were: particulate matter, sulfur dioxide, carbon monoxide, nitrogen oxides, and total oxidants. Criteria documents showing the need for control and the feasibility of control of these pollutants were developed before the national air quality goals were promulgated. The states were then required to develop implementation plans to achieve the air quality goals by controlling existing sources. New sources were placed under the auspices of the federal government for regulation development. Enforcement of these regulations, however, was left a state responsibility.

The states, constrained by the requirements of the Act, pressured by unrealistic deadlines, and influenced by the model plans developed by the Federal EPA, produced implementation plans with many similarities. For example, allowable emission levels are determined in the majority of states by sliding scale process weight or fuel input tables, which require higher levels of control as the size of the process increases. Several states do utilize more simplified methods such as a uniform allowable pollutant concentration in the process exhaust stream, regardless of the size of the source, but these types of regulations are used mainly in the less industrialized states.

The states were free to choose the dates when their implementation plans would become effective. Some specified immediate compliance, others chose compliance dates 1–2 years from the date of the plan promulgation, and most chose the federally-mandated deadline of mid-1975 for compliance. Many states included provisions for variances up to, and in some cases beyond, the mid-1975 primary air goal achievement deadline. Public hearings are required before these variances can be granted. Recent court interpretations have indicated that these variance procedures, even though approved by the EPA, may be illegal. Complete resolution of this question will require additional time. The interim period will be one of some confusion and uncertainty on the part of the agencies and industry.

As a result of the tight energy situation and the questions concerning the availability of reliable sulfur dioxide control technology, several states have recently modified the regulations and timetables for sulfur dioxide emission control to allow for the use of intermittent control strategies (curtailment during periods of limited dispersion) and tall stacks. However, the courts have not yet accepted these methods for achieving the national air quality goals, and the issue is also unresolved at present.

The states have developed permit programs in conjunction with the emission regulations. These programs require that operating permits be obtained in a specified time frame for all existing sources. In addition, the permit system requires that construction permits be obtained *prior* to the commencement of construction of any *new* potential air contaminant source. This construction permit in no way obligates the control agency to issue an operating permit after the unit is completed. The operator must then apply for and receive an operating permit based on actual emission testing after the unit is on-line and available for sampling. Public hearings may or may not be required, based on the judgment of the agency.

All states were required to include in their plan statements that all information on emissions would become information available to interested citizens upon request. Provisions were included to handle proprietary information, but the case-by-case approval of the administrator of EPA is required. Other regulations—including emergency episode plans, start-up, shut-down, and malfunction procedures, emission inventory requirements, and ambient or source monitoring—differ from state to state, but are present in some form in many of the plans.

One particularly interesting part of the Act is a provision that requires the states to promulgate regulations on existing sources if the Federal EPA establishes New Source Performance Standards that limit the emissions of any pollutant other than the five criteria pollutants. This section III(d), is still under review and further interpretation will probably be required before the intent is completely clear. However, present interpretation of this provision appears to give the federal agency broad powers to require that additional state regulations be developed on short time schedules.

One of the interesting dichotomies that has developed as a result of the interpretation process that is continuing to modify the Act is that even though a source is located in an area where the primary, and perhaps the secondary, national air quality goals are being met, that source must comply with the state's emission limitation on the prescribed timetable. Thus, even though the goal of the Act is being met, i.e., desirable air quality is being maintained, more control must be accomplished if the emission regulations require it.

A second and much more insidious dichotomy is developing in the Clean Air Act. The nondegradation requirements specified by the Supreme Court (yet to be promulgated by the EPA) require that the state plans must in some way be modified to limit industrial development in clean areas where the air quality is much better than the goals established by the Act. Simultaneously, the complex source regulation suggests that the states will have to include in their plans statements that will prohibit the further development of fringe areas where the air quality could be affected by large complexes that could generate heavy automobile traffic and secondary pollutants. Finally, the air quality goals themselves limit development in already established urban areas. Therefore, these three segments of the Act, if applied rigorously, will make it increasingly difficult, if not impossible, to pursue further development in almost any area of the nation.

Industry Activity

One of the more salient points of the Clean Air Act is that it requires "prior approval" for new activities. In the case of industry expansion, the permit system requires that a permit to construct be obtained long before actual construction begins and that a permit to operate be obtained very soon after a unit begins operation. Therefore, detailed planning and submission of these plans for review is now required before a decision can be made to begin construction on a new project. This will force many industries to modify their construction procedures. No longer will it be possible to begin a project with the idea of completing the design and engineering as the program progresses.

Industry is required to obtain the necessary information to assure the control agencies that the emission points under construction or in operation are in compliance with the regulations. This requires that the industry develop the expertise and capability to perform source and ambient sampling or obtain outside help. The states may check these emissions by having agency sampling teams perform emission testing or by requiring that the industry obtain additional outside assistance from firms with recognized expertize in emission testing. In most cases, the agencies seem willing to rely on the industry data if the industry has demonstrated competence in the sampling area. Hopefully, this will continue to be the case especially as more and more firms become proficient in sampling. Industry is required to maintain emission data and in many cases maintain ambient air quality data for periodic submission to the proper agencies. These regulations vary from state to state, but the trend toward more required data seems well established.

Activity in the area of nondegradation planning, stationary emission control for sulfur dioxide and NO_x, and the question of variances are yet to be resolved. The resolution of these and other questions can markedly affect the impact of the Clean Air Act on American industry and can have a significant effect on the degree of activity that will be required of the industry to meet the requirements of this legislation. Ample opportunity is provided for industry representatives to be involved in the regulatory process. Early participation at the development stage through advisory committees, direct contacts with the agency technical staff and contractors as they search for data, and publication of industry data in the technical literature are helpful tactics. In addition, participation in public hearings and participation by commenting directly to the EPA on proposed standards can be influential. In most cases, the agencies seem willing to receive and evaluate all the input from responsible sources, especially if care is taken to fully document all the information. Finally, after a regulation is promulgated, it may be challenged in the courts if the requirements are unrealistic.

FEDERAL WATER POLLUTION CONTROL ACT AMENDMENTS OF 1972

The Federal Water Pollution Control Act Amendments of 1972 were developed to "restore and maintain the chemical, physical and biological integrity of the Nation's waters." By July of 1983, wherever possible, water quality is to be suitable for contact recreation and for protection and propagation of fish and wildlife. The program is to be administered by the states, if the states can develop plans for enforcement which meet the criteria of the EPA. If, however, the state plan does not receive federal approval, the water quality program, specifically entitled the National Pollutant Discharge Elimination System (NPDES), will be administered by the Federal Environmental Protection Agency. If the state chooses, it can also operate a separate water quality program and compound the burdens on the discharger. A planning system is to be instituted to conduct areawide, statewide, and basinwide planning using the results of the different limitation programs as a guide for determining whether additional measures will be needed. To date, the court-related activity on the Act has been minimal. However, a number of suits have been filed as the result of the publication of several sets of effluent limitation guidelines and some judicial interpretations of the Act may be forthcoming.

The Requirements of the Act

The Act requires that the Federal Environmental Protection Agency set industry-by-industry effluent limitation guidelines for the discharge of any pollutant that may be released from a point source into any body of water, and utilize these guidelines to develop permits that will maintain the best level of water quality attainable. Three levels of guidelines are required. The Level I guidelines, Best Practicable Technology, are to represent the best performance being achieved by well-operated plants within each industrial category. The Level II guidelines, Best Available Technology, are to be based on the application of the best control and treatment measures that can or could be economically achieved. The Level III guidelines, New Source Performance Standards, will apply to plants that are constructed after the guidelines are published (in proposed form) and will require stringent control measures that might not be feasible on existing facilities.

The Act also requires that NPDES permits be issued for all discharges to ensure that all sources achieve Level I guidelines by 1977 and Level II guidelines by 1983. The Act sets as a goal, but not a legally binding requirement, that zero discharge of pollutants be achieved by 1985. The Act requires that water quality control standards be reviewed and revised where necessary and used as guides to test the effectiveness of the limitation guidelines program. In addition, the Act also contains a requirement that bodies of water which are "clean" cannot be degraded by wastewater discharges that differ greatly from the existing water quality. Finally, the Act requires that toxic substances be identified and that Toxic Effluent Limitation Standards be developed for these substances without regard to source. These standards must contain an "ample margin of safety" for "toxic" substances and they need not be based either on economic feasibility or the availability of treatment technologies.

As in the Clean Air Act, the timetables specified in the amendments are unrealistic and require that many steps be taken without the proper study or input. Portions of the regulatory programs and the compliance programs will require more time than the Act allows. Just how this additional time will be obtained has not yet been determined.

The Regulations

As required by the Act, the Environmental Protection Agency is developing Effluent Limitation Guidelines, New Source Performance Standards, and Pretreatment Standards for industrial dischargers. These guidelines and standards are to be used by the states that have approved programs to administer the NPDES programs and by the Federal Environmental Protection Agency to develop discharge permits for all sources. A limited number of these permits have been issued and the goal of December 31, 1974, has been set as the target date for issuance of all major permits. In some cases, it appears that the discharge permits will be issued before the effluent guidelines are established.

The permit system requires best practicable technology to be utilized by 1977 and best available technology to be utilized by 1983. The states and regional offices of EPA may require more stringent limits than the guidelines state, and several have chosen this course. The permits are issued for a time period not to exceed 5 years, and the time frame is at the option of the state or regional EPA agency. The permits require a certain amount of continuous monitoring, usually for flow, temperature, and pH, and periodic sampling for effluent characterization. Periodic reports to the control agency are required.

The Toxic Effluent Standards have been proposed for nine materials and public hearings are now underway to receive comments concerning these proposed standards. When promulgated, these standards will apply to the permitted discharges, even though the permits may not have placed limitations on the materials designated as toxic.

Industrial Activity

The Federal Water Pollution Control Act Amendments of 1972 require that all existing and future dischargers obtain National Pollution Discharge Elimination System permits from the state (if appropriate) or the regional EPA office. Existing sources should have applied in 1971 under the Corps of Engineers Refuse Act Program and all new sources must apply at least 180 days before the discharge is to begin. These permits require detailed information on incoming water quality, treatment system effectiveness, sludge disposal methods, and outlet water quality. Trace contaminants as well as major pollutants are of importance. All discharge permits require that public notice be given so that comments can be received. Public hearings may be required. The industry should be represented at the hearing and prepared to respond to comment.

Recently, the guidelines that have been published have contained a statement describing how a party faced with circumstances not considered in the guidelines development process can apply to the Administrator of the agency for relief from the guidelines. The statement places the burden of proof on the discharger and requires that he document his case well.

The permits issued will specify the limitation on pollutant discharges. The permits may be written on a "gross emission" basis with no credit allowed for pollutants present in the intake waters; but in some cases, net emissions may be used if it can be shown that the influence of substances in the inlet water has a significant impact on discharge water quality. If the industry uses pretreatment schemes to make the inlet water more suitable for plant use, all constituents removed from the water must be disposed of on land. The permit will also specify the monitoring and reporting requirements placed on the discharger. The industry is obligated to meet the guidelines and provide the necessary data to show compliance.

Industry can participate in the regulation development activities in several ways. The publication of technical data on wastewater generation, treatment, and discharge is of benefit. Cooperation with EPA contractors preparing development documents will usually prove fruitful. Participation at advisory committee meetings, testimony at public hearings, and direct comments on proposed regulations are also of use. Finally, the effluent guidelines can be challenged in court within 90 days after they are promulgated, and permits can be challenged at the public hearings or, failing that, in the courts. It is best to become involved in the regulation development as early as possible in order to obtain regulations that are reasonable.

NATIONAL ENVIRONMENTAL POLICY ACT

The National Environment Policy Act was passed in 1970. Its purposes are: "To declare a national policy which will encourage productive and enjoyable harmony between man and his environment, to promote efforts which will prevent or eliminate damage to the environment and biosphere, and stimulate the health and welfare of man; to enrich the understanding of the ecological system and natural resources important to the Nation; and to establish a Council on Environmental Quality."

The Act requires that all agencies of the Federal Government work with the Council on Environmental Quality and utilize a systematic interdisciplinary approach to determine the best course of action for any decision-making that may have an impact on man's environment. The Act requires that all decisions that might significantly affect the quality of the human environment be made only after a detailed statement is prepared describing the environmental impact of the proposed action, any adverse environmental effect that will result, alternatives to the proposed action, the relationship between short-term use of the environment and long-term productivity, and any irreversible and irretrievable commitments of resources. The statement must be reviewed and approved by all federal agencies that have expertise or jurisdiction in the area.

The Council on Environmental Quality is a three-man executive council that assists the President in the preparation of the annual Environmental Quality Report, monitors conditions and trends in environmental quality, reviews and monitors the environmental impact statement program, conducts studies related to ecological systems and environmental quality, and advises the President on environmental quality matters.

The Regulations

The National Environmental Policy Act requires that all Federal agencies prepare a comprehensive and detailed environmental impact statement before taking any "significant" action. The actions that are covered include legislative recommendations, project funding, project licensing, *permit issuance,* rule making, etc. Thus, any industrial activity requiring a federal permit, is subject to the environmental impact statement requirement.

The environmental impact statements prepared by the agencies must fulfill the purposes of the Act (as specified earlier). Guidelines for federal agencies were issued by the Council on Environmental Quality on August 1, 1973. Section 1500.8 of those guidelines contains an eight-part listing of the major items which must be included in an impact statement. If an industry is involved in the action, the primary agency involved will normally require that the industry prepare and submit an environmental document that will be used as the basis for preparation of the Draft Environmental Impact Statement. This document must be reviewed by all appropriate agencies, and, if the primary agency judges it to be necessary, a public hearing will be held to receive comments on the draft statement. The agency must allow a minimum of 90 days for review and comment, develop a final impact statement incorporating the proper comments, file the completed document, and wait an additional 30 days before taking any action. In some cases, the 90-day review period can be shortened by filing the final version with comments before the 90 days are up. Then the 30-day waiting period and the remainder of the 90-day review period can run concurrently.

Industrial Activity

If an industry is involved in an activity that will require federal action, it is normal to expect that the agency that must take the action will require the industry to prepare a detailed document describing the proposed project and its environmental impact. Since this process can require a great deal of time, the industry must initiate the activity at an early date. For example, if a project is planned for a state that does not administer the NPDES permit system, a federal discharge permit will be required and an impact statement may be necessary. The industry should plan on a minimum time requirement of 18–24 months for the completion of the impact statement process. The EPA has recently suggested that a conference be scheduled by an industry interested in a project that will require federal permits. The conference should be held at least 24 months before the project is to begin to allow ample time for impact statement preparation, should one be necessary.

The goals, guidelines, and procedures of the impact statement process are reasonably well fixed. Some consideration is being given to a relaxation of the impact statement requirements for energy-related developments, but if this relaxation occurs, it will apply only until the energy situation becomes less chaotic. Industry input at this time will probably have little effect on the requirements of the Act. However, additional experience with the impact statement process may lead the agencies to the conclusion that the requirements of the Act can be met with more streamlined procedures and more concise impact statement documents.

LAND USE PLANNING

There is a strong effort throughout the country to begin comprehensive land use planning. In many areas, especially where states have adopted environmental policy type legislation similar to the National Environmental Policy Act, existing laws are being used as a means of implementing land use planning procedures. An air or water pollution control agency can and does deny permits to industries that meet all the requirements of the air and water pollution laws if in the view of the agency, the overall good of the area will not be served by the industrial development. Thus, the agency can take on the role of land use planner and can markedly affect the growth patterns in the area. The agencies involved in activities of this type are normally not adequately staffed to make comprehensive land use planning decisions. The physical environment, which should be factored into the land use decision-making process, becomes the major item for consideration.

Whether we like it or not, land use planning is being practiced in many parts of the nation today. Almost everyone agrees that something should be done to optimize our land use decisions. Thousands of governmental agencies make decisions that determine how land will be used. Yet much land is unplanned, or poorly planned, as evidenced by urban sprawl, developments around airports, and industrial developments that are incompatible with the area. Most will agree that some land use planning is needed, but performing this planning function poses a difficult problem. Industry needs relief from the layer upon layer of permits and delays which it faces in attempting to site new facilities. Planners need to know what developments will be allowed in the various areas of the country so that industrial facilities, public works, housing, etc., can be properly sited. Land use planning, by definition, restricts the use of private lands, and in that way significantly affects its value to the owner. In addition, land use planning can deny the use of certain resources to entrepreneurs. Therefore, land use planning regulations will be difficult to develop.

The U.S. Senate has passed Senate Bill 268 which is a land use planning bill. This bill urges the states to develop land use policies, provides funds to this end, provides funds for the inventory of land and natural resources, and requires the states to regulate "areas of critical environmental concern—areas as defined and designated by the state on non-federal lands where uncontrolled or incompatible development could result in damage to the environment, life or property or the long-term public interest which is of more than local significance, to include fragile or historic lands, natural hazard lands, renewable resource lands, and such additional areas as the state should designate." Key facilities such as large public facilities, energy-generating facilities, and large scale private developments that might produce an impact of more than local significance are also to be covered in the planning process.

A similar bill is in committee in the House of Representatives, but no date on a possible House vote is available at this time. Areas of concern, including prohibition of certain activities such as strip mining on certain lands, the question of how to deal with government owned land, coastal zone planning, wetlands area management, and control of the state programs to prevent misuse or overuse of the land use planning capability, have yet to be resolved.

It is apparent that some type of land use planning measure will become law within the next few years. This legislation will be very influential in setting the development patterns throughout the nation. Industry should be aware of these developments and should provide knowledgeable qualified individuals who can participate in the development phases of the Act and the regulations that will be generated to satisfy the goals outlined by the Act.

The nondegradation requirements of the Clean Air Act and the Water Pollution Control Act plus the National Environmental Policy Act and the equivalent state Environmental Policy Acts are reasonably effective land use planning mechanisms which place a great deal of emphasis on the physical environment issues. Hopefully, any true land use planning measure that comes from the Congress will look at the broad picture and include the many economic and social issues not properly viewed by today's legislation.

SUMMARY

A comprehensive web of environmental legislation surrounds our society. This legislation has an impact on all facets of industrial activity. It is impossible to make a product or perform a service without being involved with environmental regulations. Therefore, all industry should set about to equip itself with well-trained, competent individuals to work within the framework of the environmental legislation of today and influence the legislation that will be generated in the future. There are ample areas where individuals can become involved in the regulation development process, but a thorough understanding of the issues is required. The existing laws are available for review, and numerous environmental publications are published which will keep an individual informed of current developments. These are necessary steps if an industry is to be well informed in the environmental area and aware of the requirements facing industrial activity now and in the future.

REFERENCES

1. Occupational Safety and Health Act. 29–USC–651 *et seq.* P.L. 91–596, 91st Congress, S.2193, U.S. Department of Labor, Washington, D.C., 1973.

2. Clean Air Act. 42–USC–1857 *et seq.* P.L. 91–604, U.S. Environmental Protection Agency, Washington, D.C., 1970.
3. National Environmental Policy Act. 42–USC–4321 *et seq.* P.L. 91–190, U.S. Environmental Protection Agency, Washington, D.C., 1969.
4. Federal Water Pollution Control Act Amendments of 1972. 33–USC–4321 *et seq.* P.L. 92–500, 92nd Congress, S.2770, Council on Environmental Quality, Washington, D.C., 1972.
5. Mullins, D. L., and Werner, S. M., eds., "Guidelines for Federal Agencies Under the National Environmental Policy Act." 1973.
6. Mallino, D. L., and Werner, S. M., eds., "Occupational Safety and Health—A Policy Analysis." Government Research Corporation, Washington, D.C., 1973.
7. Denning, D., "Emerging Growth Policies—Total Environmental Considerations." U.S. Chamber of Commerce, Washington, D.C., 1973.
8. "Land Use Policy and Planning Bills—A Legislative Analysis." American Enterprise Institute, Washington, D.C., 1973.
9. Dorcey, A. H. J., and Fox, I. K., Critique of water pollution control act. *J. Environ. Eng. Div., Proc. Amer. Soc. Civil Eng. 100,* No. EE1, p. 141 (1974).

Index

345

ENVIRONMENTAL SCIENCES

An Interdisciplinary Monograph Series

EDITORS

DOUGLAS H. K. LEE

National Institute of
Environmental Health Sciences
Research Triangle Park
North Carolina

E. WENDELL HEWSON

Department of
Atmospheric Science
Oregon State University
Corvallis, Oregon

DANIEL OKUN

Department of Environmental
Sciences and Engineering
University of North Carolina
Chapel Hill, North Carolina

Merril Eisenbud, ENVIRONMENTAL RADIOACTIVITY, Second Edition, 1973

James G. Wilson, ENVIRONMENT AND BIRTH DEFECTS, 1973

Raymond C. Loehr, AGRICULTURAL WASTE MANAGEMENT: Problems, Processes, and Approaches, 1974

Lester V. Cralley, Patrick R. Atkins, Lewis J. Cralley, and George D. Clayton, editors, INDUSTRIAL ENVIRONMENTAL HEALTH: The Worker and the Community, Second Edition, 1975

A 5
B 6
C 7
D 8
E 9
F 0
G 1
H 2
I 3
J 4